Gerontology for the Health Care Professional

Third Edition

Edited by

REGULA H. ROBNETT, PhD, OTR/L
Professor
Department of Occupational Therapy
University of New England

WALTER C. CHOP, MS, RRT
Professor Emeritus
Respiratory Therapy Department
Southern Maine Community College

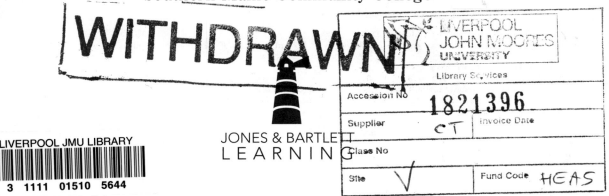

JONES & BARTLETT
L E A R N I N G

World Headquarters
Jones & Bartlett Learning
5 Wall Street
Burlington, MA 01803
978-443-5000
info@jblearning.com
www.jblearning.com

Jones & Bartlett Learning books and products are available through most bookstores and online booksellers. To contact Jones & Bartlett Learning directly, call 800-832-0034, fax 978-443-8000, or visit our website, www.jblearning.com.

Substantial discounts on bulk quantities of Jones & Bartlett Learning publications are available to corporations, professional associations, and other qualified organizations. For details and specific discount information, contact the special sales department at Jones & Bartlett Learning via the above contact information or send an email to specialsales@jblearning.com.

Production Credits
Executive Editor: Rhonda Dearborn
Editorial Assistant: Sean Fabery
Associate Director of Production: Julie C. Bolduc
Production Assistant: Brooke Appe
Marketing Manager: Grace Richards
VP, Manufacturing and Inventory Control: Therese Connell
Composition: Cenveo Publisher Services
Cover Design: Scott Moden
Photo Research and Permissions Coordinator: Amy Rathburn
Cover Images: (woman sitting with caregiver) © Alexander Raths/ShutterStock, Inc.; (group with laptop) © iStockphoto/Thinkstock; (older man smiling) © Diego Cervo/ShutterStock, Inc.; (couple with dog) © Stephen Coburn/ShutterStock, Inc.; (doctor with walking patient) © iStockphoto /Thinkstock; (woman with dumbbell) © Robert Kneschke/ShutterStock, Inc.
Printing and Binding: Edwards Brothers Malloy
Cover Printing: Edwards Brothers Malloy

To order this product, use ISBN: 978-1-284-03887-3

Library of Congress Cataloging-in-Publication Data
Gerontology for the health care professional / [edited] by Regula H. Robnett and Walter C. Chop. — Third edition.
    p. ; cm.
Includes bibliographical references and index.
ISBN 978-1-284-03052-5 — ISBN 1-284-03052-0
I. Robnett, Regula H., editor of compilation. II. Chop, Walter C., editor of compilation.
[DNLM: 1. Geriatrics. 2. Aged. 3. Aging—physiology. 4. Geriatric Assessment. WT 100]
RA564.8
618.97—dc23
                                    2013027708

6048
Printed in the United States of America
17 16 15 14   10 9 8 7 6 5 4 3 2

BRIEF CONTENTS

CONTENTS

v

INTRODUCTION

Thank you for choosing to open this textbook and read this page. *Gerontology for the Health Care Professional, Third Edition* is designed with you in mind. Our goal is to make this textbook as reader-friendly as possible, and to demonstrate that we are thoroughly committed to interprofessional healthcare practice.

As you read each chapter, we encourage you to consider the role of each of the healthcare professions listed below. While this is not an exclusive list and, most of the time, only a small portion of all the possible professions will actually be involved in working with any given client, we do want you to at least think about how this profession *could* be involved, and if a consultation or referral would be in order. You may need to investigate some of the following professions to understand exactly what they are. Further research is certainly encouraged.

The most prominent healthcare professionals involved in gerontological care are:

- Alternative Medicine Practitioners
- Art Therapists
- Athletic Trainers
- Audiologists
- Cardiovascular Technologists
- Case Managers
- Counselors
- Dental Practitioners
- Dieticians/Nutritionists
- Emergency Medical Practitioners
- Gerontologists
- Horticulture Therapists
- Imaging Technologists
- Massage Therapists
- Medical Laboratory Practitioners
- Medical Records Health Information Specialists
- Music Therapists
- Neuropsychologists
- Nursing Practitioners
- Occupational Therapy Practitioners
- Orientation and Mobility Specialists (low vision)
- Orthotists
- Physical Therapy Practitioners
- Physician Assistants
- Physicians
- Polysomnographers

- Prosthetists
- Psychiatrists
- Psychologists
- Radiological Technologists
- Recreation Therapists

- Rehabilitation Teachers (low vision)
- Respiratory Therapists
- Social Workers
- Speech and Language Pathologists
- Visual Care Specialists

We are fortunate to be living in this day and age, because information is now at our fingertips as it has never been before. Certainly not everything available online can be relied upon, and therefore we need to read what is out there in cyberspace with critical and questioning eyes. However, for those who want to learn, the floodgates have opened and the world of information is there for the learning.

The *Third Edition* begins with chapters on the different aspects of aging, including:

- Demographics (Chapter 1)
- Social (Chapter 2)
- Physiological (Chapter 3)
- Cognitive and psychological (Chapter 4)
- Sensory and functional (Chapter 5)

Later chapters explore various issues that, although not exclusive to older people, are of primary importance to the older population. These issues include:

- Pharmacology (Chapter 6)
- Nutrition (Chapter 7)
- Dental health (Chapter 8)
- Sexuality (Chapter 9)
- Housing and the continuum of care (Chapter 10)
- Policy and ethical issues (Chapter 11)
- Plain language (Chapter 12)
- Speculation on the future of our aging society (Chapter 13)

The *Third Edition* includes updates and new information, including:

- New chapter on dental issues
- New epilogue
- More case studies
- More on policy and legislative issues, patient advocacy, ethics, elder abuse, cultural issues, communication, and social theories of aging
- Latest information on obesity
- Updated information, statistics, and census data
- Expanded information on dementia, sleep disorders, and medication therapy management

Explore, enjoy the learning process, and thank you for your interest in learning about, and possibly working with, older people.

ACKNOWLEDGMENTS

It takes many individuals to create the final product that becomes a textbook. We would like to thank those who have contributed to the process that has made the *Third Edition* of *Gerontology for the Health Care Professional* possible. They are:

- All of the contributing authors whose hard work and dedication created the substance of this text: Nancy Brossoie, Charles Gregory, David Sandmire, Jessica Bolduc, Ann O'Sullivan, John Murray, Thomas Nolin, Christine Ruby, Sue Stableford, Marji Harmer-Beem, Kathryn Thompson, Nancy MacRae, Ellen Menard, Laney Anne Bruner-Canhoto, and Paul Ewald.
- All of the good people at Jones & Bartlett Learning, especially Katey Birtcher, who strongly encouraged us to proceed with a third edition. Also the following editorial and production staff for keeping us on task: Teresa Reilly, Julie Bolduc, Kristin Sladen, Toni Ackley, Amy Rathburn, and Bill Brottmiller.
- Our loving families, whose ongoing support and encouragement kept us going.

If we inadvertently left anyone out, we ask for your forgiveness.

CONTRIBUTORS

Jessica J. Bolduc, DrOT, MS, OTR/L
Portland, Maine

Nancy Brossoie, PhD
Center for Gerontology
Virginia Tech
Blacksburg, Virginia

Laney Anne Bruner-Canhoto, PhD, MSW, MPH
Director
Performance Improvement, Disability and
    Community Services
Assistant Professor
Family Medicine and Community Health
University of Massachusetts Medical School
Shrewsbury, Massachusetts

Paul D. Ewald, PhD
Provost
Notre Dame de Namur University
Belmont, California

Charles J. Gregory, PhD
Professor
Southern Maine Community College
South Portland, Maine

Marji J. Harmer-Beem, RDH, MS
Associate Professor
Dental Hygiene Program
University of New England
Portland, Maine

Nancy MacRae, MS, OTR/L, FAOTA
Associate Professor
Occupational Therapy Department
University of New England
Portland, Maine

Ellen Menard, MBA, BSN, RN
Patient Advocacy Expert
Ellen Menard, Inc.
Sarasota, Florida

John K. Murray, MPH, RRT, RPSGT
Department Chair
Cardiopulmonary, Sleep Technology and
    Exercise Science
Northern Essex Community College
Haverhill, Massachusetts

Thomas D. Nolin, PharmD, PhD
Assistant Professor
Department of Pharmacy and Therapeutics

University of Pittsburgh, School of
  Pharmacy
Pittsburgh, Pennsylvania

Ann O'Sullivan, OTR/L, LSW, FAOTA
Family Caregiver Support Program
  Coordinator
Southern Maine Agency on Aging
Scarborough, Maine

Christine M. Ruby, PharmD, BCPS
Assistant Professor
Department of Pharmacy and Therapeutics
University of Pittsburgh, School of
  Pharmacy
Pittsburgh, Pennsylvania

David A. Sandmire, MD
Professor
Biology Department
University of New England

Sue Stableford, MPH, MSB
Director
Health Literacy Institute
University of New England
Portland, Maine

Kathryn H. Thompson, PhD, RD
Professor
University of New England
Biddeford, Maine

REVIEWERS

Jodi Blair, PhD
Adjunct Professor
Allen Community College
Burlingame, Kansas

Erin Cattoor, MSN, RN
Clinical Assistant Professor of Nursing
Maryville University
St. Louis, Missouri

Bruce Elliott, PT, MS, DPT
Professor
University of Hartford
West Hartford, Connecticut

**Kathleen Evanina, RN, CRNP-BC,
APRN, PhD-c, DNP-c**
Professor
Marywood University
Olyphant, Pennsylvania

Dorcas C. Fitzgerald, PhD, RN, CNS
Faculty (Professor) Emeritus
Youngstown State University
Warren, Ohio

Vivienne Friday, EdD
Assistant Professor
Iowa Western Community College
Council Bluffs, Iowa

Steven D. Karnes, MHA
Assistant Professor
Ferris State University
Big Rapids, Michigan

Ralph Lucki, RRT, MEd
Professor, Program Director and
   Division Chair
West Virginia Northern Community
   College
Wheeling, West Virginia

DEMOGRAPHIC TRENDS OF AN AGING SOCIETY

WALTER C. CHOP, MS, RRT

I refuse to take seriously society's idea that at the arbitrary age of 65 I am suddenly a lamp going out.
—Eugene S. Mills, quoting an elder in *The Story of Elder Hostel*, 1993*

Chapter Outline

America: An Aging Society

Global Aging

Gender and Age

Race and Aging

Geographic Distribution: Where U.S. Older
   Adults Live

Marital Status

Economic Status

Health Care

Long-Term Care

Behavioral Objectives

Upon completion of this chapter, the reader will be able to:

1. Describe why the "graying of America" is occurring.
2. Identify the fastest growing segment of the population.
3. Discuss life expectancy in terms of gender.
4. Contrast aging by races in the United States.
5. Identify the states where the largest number of individuals 65 and older live.
6. Discuss older adults in the context of their lifestyles (married or living alone).
7. Contrast the economic status of those older than 65 years in terms of race and marital status.
8. List disease conditions older adults are most likely to experience.

*© University Press of New England, Lebanon, NH. Reprinted with permission.

9. Discuss healthcare expenditures for those older than 65 years and the demand placed on the healthcare system by them.
10. Describe pertinent issues related to the demographics of housing and long-term care of older adults.

Key Terms

Age cohort
Baby boom generation
Demographics of aging
Elderly, elders
Long-term care
Medicaid

Medicare
Old-old
Social Security
Third-agers
Young-old

AMERICA: AN AGING SOCIETY

The graying of America continues to accelerate as the first of the **baby boom generation** (those Americans born between 1946 and 1964) turned 65 years of age in 2011. From that time on, approximately one American will turn 65 years of age every 8 seconds for the next 18 years. This will have dramatic consequences on our entire society, especially our healthcare system.

In 1900, only 4% of Americans, or 1 in 25, were older than 65 years of age. The population of those older than 65 numbered 3.1 million in 1900. (See **Figure 1-1**.)

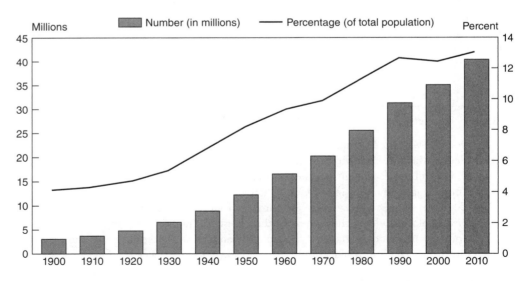

FIGURE 1-1   Population 65 years and older by size and percent of total populations: 1900 to 2010.
Source: Data from U.S. Census Bureau, decennial census of population, 1900 to 2000; 2010 Census Summary File 1.

As of April 1, 2010, this same **age cohort** numbered 40.3 million, representing 13% of the total population.[1] To put this in perspective, the population of those older than 65 years has increased by more than 2 million people (7% of the population) since 1990, whereas the younger-than-65 age group has increased by only 4%.

Projections for the year 2030 estimate that 22% of Americans, or 70.2 million, will be older than the age of 65. To get a true feel for the changing demography of the United States, note the baby boom bulge on the population chart in **Figure 1-2**. You can easily envision the top-heavy appearance of this same chart 25 years from today.

An even more dramatic aging trend exists among those older than 85 years of age, often referred to as the **old-old**. This age cohort is expected to increase from 5.5 million

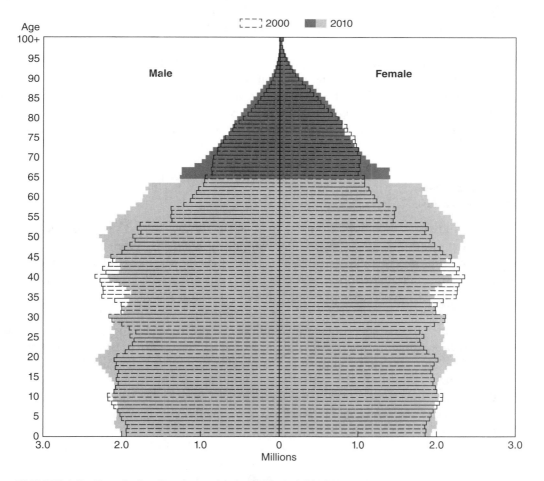

FIGURE 1-2   Population by age and sex: 2000 and 2010.
Source: Data from U.S. Census Bureau, Census 2000 Summary File 1 and 2010 Census Summary File 1.

in 2010 to 6.6 million in 2020, a 19% increase for that decade.[2] The number of those **elderly** exceeding 100 years of age reached 53,264 in 2010.[2]

Looking beyond the **demographics of aging**, let us now consider what the term *old age* implies. *Old age* is a difficult and complex concept to grasp because our idea of aging is constantly changing. What we thought of as old in the 19th century is considered middle age now. Policy makers have used the age of 65 as a marker in establishing policies affecting older adults. Some biologists, however, tell us that a person's biological age is more important than the person's chronological age when determining an individual's health status.[3] Bernice Neugarten was the first to coin the term **young-old**, which denotes relatively healthy and financially independent **elders** of any age, although usually those between 55 and 74 years of age.[3] The so-called old-old usually refers to those older than age 75 whose activities are often limited by functional disabilities. The French have a similar method of categorizing older adults. They use the terms **third-agers**, or *elder*, when referring to those persons 65 to 85 years of age. Their term *old-old* refers only to those individuals older than age 85.

Whatever classification of aging you choose to use is a matter of preference, as long as you realize the limitations and variations implied by the term *old age*. The salient point to note is that there is a great amount of variability among old-agers. Whereas many individuals moving into the third age and beyond are of sound mind and body as well as financially secure, others in this same age cohort are experiencing functional declines as well as healthcare or financial needs.

GLOBAL AGING

As of mid-year 2008, 506 million individuals worldwide were 65 years of age or older. This represents 7% of the world's population. By 2040 it is estimated that 1.3 billion persons will be 65 or older worldwide. This raises the percentage globally to 14%. For the first time in human history, people over 65 years of age will outnumber children under 5 years of age. This likely will occur between 2015 and 2020.[4]

As of 2008, approximately 62% of the world's population over 65 years old live in developing nations—an estimated 313 million people. By 2040, today's developing countries will be home to over 1 billion people over age 65. This represents 76% of all individuals worldwide over 65 years of age. A number of these less-developed nations are also experiencing a downturn in natural population increase (births minus deaths). A similar decline has already occurred in the industrialized nations. As this rate of downturn in natural population continues to accelerate, elders will make up an ever-greater proportion of each nation's total population.[4]

The world's oldest country is Japan, currently with 21.6% of its population over the age of 65 years, closely followed by Italy and Germany with 20%. The world's 25 oldest countries are all in Europe (see **Figure 1-3**), except for Japan.[4]

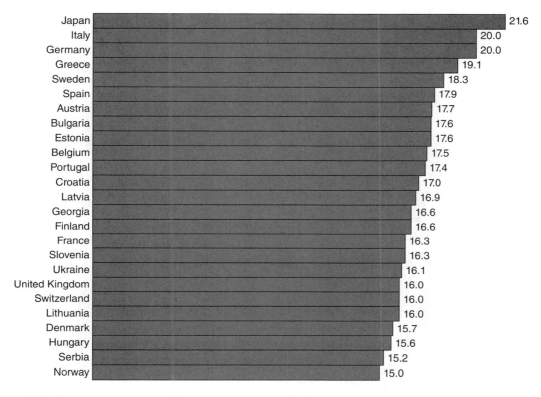

FIGURE 1-3 The world's 25 oldest countries: 2008.
Source: Data from U.S. Census Bureau, International Database.

GENDER AND AGE

Women make up the majority of elderly people in almost every country in the world. Today in the United States, and throughout most countries, women can expect to live, on average, 5 years longer than men. As of 2010, life expectancy was 81.1 years for women and 76.1 years for men.[1] Life expectancy projections for 2030 are 84.17 years for women and 78.32 years for men.[1] In fact, as of 2009, among those 85 years and older, there are only 32 men for every 100 women (**Figure 1-4**). This greater longevity in women is because heart attacks, cancer, and stroke—the major killer diseases—have been and still are more common in men, although men have closed the longevity gap somewhat due to the increase in cardiovascular disease among women. Other factors influencing female longevity may have to do with women's greater sensitivity to changes in their body condition, which make them more likely to seek out earlier medical intervention. Women may also handle stress better and have better social support systems than their male counterparts do.

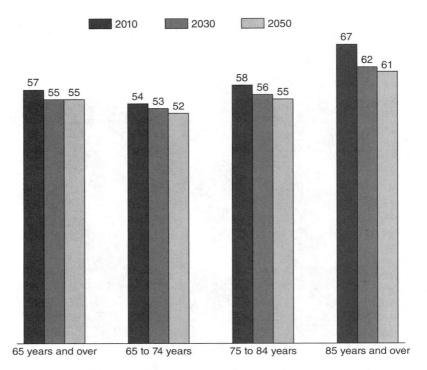

FIGURE 1-4   Percentage of females by age group: 2010, 2030, and 2050.
Source: Data from U.S. Census Bureau, 2008.

RACE AND AGING

In the United States, the aging baby boomer generation will contain a far greater racial and ethnic mix than did any generation preceding it. This results from both increasing immigration from primarily nonwhite countries and a lower fertility rate among the white population.[2] The U.S. Census Bureau predicts that nonwhite populations will account for nearly half (42%) of the U.S. population by 2050 (see **Figure 1-5**).[5]

Life expectancy for nonwhite Americans is less than it is for whites. African American men and women currently live on average 6 and 5 years less, respectively, than their white counterparts.[2] However, if a black person of either gender lives to age 65, his or her life expectancy is much closer to whites than it was at birth.[2] Other ethnic minorities in the United States, including Mexican Americans and Native Americans, have life expectancies lower than African Americans.[2] Even with their relatively low percentages, the population of minority older adults is growing at a faster rate than their white counterparts. The U.S. Census Bureau projects that minority populations will represent 42% of all the elderly people by 2050, up from 20% in 2010.[5] Of these groups, Native Americans have the shortest life expectancy of any minority group (45–50 years of age) and also the lowest standard of living.

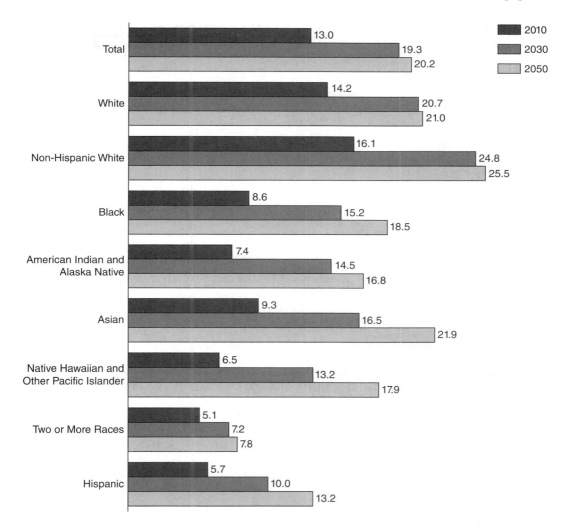

FIGURE 1-5 Percentage age 65 and over by race and Hispanic origin for the United States: 2010, 2030, and 2050.
Note: Unless otherwise specified, data refer to the population who reported a race alone. Populations for each race group include both Hispanics and non-Hispanics, unless otherwise specified. Hispanics may be of any race.
Source: Data from U.S. Census Bureau, 2008.

Therefore, besides an overall increase in the number of older Americans, there will also be a more heterogeneous mix of ethnic and cultural backgrounds. This will require healthcare providers to become even more culturally sensitive, acquiring new knowledge and skills to better recognize and respect cultural differences. Healthcare professionals will also need to understand the diseases, disorders, and concerns more common not only to specific age groups, but also to particular ethnic groups (**Table 1-1**).

TABLE 1-1 Leading Causes of Death Among U.S. Adults Aged 65 or Older in 2007

Cause of Death	Percentage of All Deaths
Heart Disease	28.2
Cancer	22.2
Stroke	6.6
Chronic Lower Respiratory Diseases	6.2
Alzheimer's Disease	4.2
Diabetes	2.9
Influenza and Pneumonia	2.6
Unintentional Injury	2.2
All Other Causes	24.9

Source: Data from CDC, National Center for Health Statistics, National Vital Statistics System, 2007.

In some elderly minority groups, social factors may play a role in reinforcing negative health patterns and behaviors. These factors may contribute to shorter life spans of certain minorities, as in the case of African Americans. Yet this same minority can expect to outlive their white counterparts if they live to age 80. At this point a racial mortality crossover phenomenon occurs in which life expectancy for blacks exceeds that for whites.

GEOGRAPHIC DISTRIBUTION: WHERE U.S. OLDER ADULTS LIVE

Persons 65 years and older constituted approximately 14% or more of the total population in 17 states in 2010: Florida (17.4%), West Virginia (16.1%), Maine (15.9%), Pennsylvania (15.5%), Iowa (14.9%), Montana (14.9%), Vermont (14.6%), Hawaii (14.5%), North Dakota (14.5%), Rhode Island (14.4%), Arkansas (14.4%), Delaware (14.4%), South Dakota (14.3%), Connecticut (14.2%), Ohio (14.1%), Missouri (14.0%), and Oregon (14.0%)[2] (**Figure 1-6**).

In 13 states, the 65-plus population increased by 25% or more between 2000 and 2010 (**Table 1-2**): Alaska (50.0%), Nevada (47.0%), Idaho (32.5%), Arizona (32.1%), Colorado (31.8%), Georgia (31.4%), Utah (31.0%), South Carolina (30.4%), New Mexico (28.5%), North Carolina (27.7%), Delaware (26.9%), Texas (26.1%), and Washington (25.3%). The 12 jurisdictions with poverty rates over 10% for elderly during 2010 were District of Columbia (13.1%), North Dakota (12.1%), New Mexico (12.0%), Mississippi (11.9%), Louisiana (11.5%), Kentucky (11.2%), South Dakota (11.1%), New York (10.9%), Alabama (10.7%), Georgia (10.7%), Texas (10.7%), and Arkansas (10.2%).[1]

This trend seems to indicate, for the most part, movement toward warmer states, with the exception of Alaska and the Rocky Mountain states of Utah, Wyoming, and Colorado. It is difficult to determine why older people migrated more often to the states that they did. Often warmer states seemed to be more appealing. Perhaps other reasons could

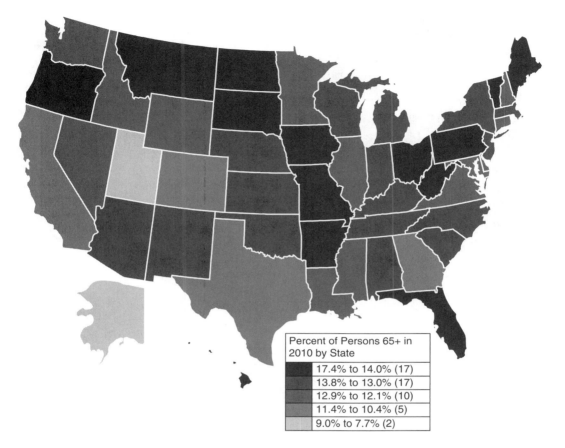

FIGURE 1-6 Percentage aged 65 and over of state population: 2010.

Source: Data from Administration on Aging, U.S. Department of Health and Human Services, 2010 Population Estimates from the U.S. Bureau of the Census.

involve lower cost of living, pleasant surroundings, or less dense populations. Older individuals moving to these states are generally affluent and well educated. They may also have existing ties to these new areas such as family, friends, or previously purchased retirement property. Many are also seeking escape from a metropolitan life to the relative safety and comfort of rural or small-town USA. The south had the largest number of individuals over age 65 whereas the northeast had the largest proportion of those over 65.[1]

In general, older Americans have a tendency to change residences less frequently than their younger counterparts do. This has led to an increased "graying" of certain communities. A number of counties have elderly populations exceeding 20% of the whole population. Many of these counties are located in the nation's predominantly agricultural heartland, where older persons have stayed while the youth have moved on.

TABLE 1-2 Population Aged 65 and Over and Percentage Change for Regions, Divisions, and States in 2010

State	Number of Persons 65 and Older	Percent of All Ages	Percent Increase from 2000 to 2010	Percent Below Poverty 2010
US Total (50 States + DC)	40,437,581	13.1%	15.3%	9.0%
Alabama	659,822	13.8%	13.7%	10.7%
Alaska	55,233	7.7%	50.0%	5.7%
Arizona	886,604	13.8%	32.1%	7.7%
Arkansas	421,476	14.4%	12.5%	10.2%
California	4,269,690	11.4%	18.3%	9.7%
Colorado	553,147	11.0%	31.8%	8.1%
Connecticut	507,837	14.2%	7.9%	6.6%
Delaware	129,586	14.4%	26.9%	7.7%
District of Columbia	69,061	11.4%	−0.9%	13.1%
Florida	3,273,940	17.4%	16.4%	9.9%
Georgia	1,037,287	10.7%	31.4%	10.7%
Hawaii	198,094	14.5%	22.5%	6.8%
Idaho	195,438	12.4%	32.5%	7.9%
Illinois	1,614,730	12.6%	7.5%	8.4%
Indiana	843,780	13.0%	11.7%	6.8%
Iowa	454,205	14.9%	4.0%	6.7%
Kansas	377,391	13.2%	5.8%	7.7%
Kentucky	580,394	13.4%	15.0%	11.2%
Louisiana	560,160	12.3%	8.5%	11.5%
Maine	211,336	15.9%	14.9%	9.5%
Maryland	710,761	12.3%	18.2%	7.7%
Massachusetts	905,896	13.8%	5.2%	8.7%
Michigan	1,364,431	13.8%	11.6%	8.0%
Minnesota	685,349	12.9%	14.8%	8.3%
Mississippi	381,372	12.8%	11.2%	11.9%
Missouri	841,075	14.0%	11.3%	9.1%
Montana	147,181	14.9%	21.4%	7.0%
Nebraska	247,518	13.5%	6.5%	7.5%
Nevada	325,935	12.1%	47.0%	7.6%
New Hampshire	178,625	13.6%	20.3%	6.1%
New Jersey	1,190,312	13.5%	6.9%	7.2%
New Mexico	273,572	13.2%	28.5%	12.0%
New York	2,627,101	13.5%	7.1%	10.9%

TABLE 1-2 Population Aged 65 and Over and Percentage Change for Regions, Divisions, and States in 2010 *(continued)*

State	Number of Persons 65 and Older	Percent of All Ages	Percent Increase from 2000 to 2010	Percent Below Poverty 2010
North Carolina	1,240,390	13.0%	27.7%	9.9%
North Dakota	97,863	14.5%	3.7%	12.1%
Ohio	1,626,201	14.1%	7.8%	7.7%
Oklahoma	509,065	13.5%	11.8%	9.3%
Oregon	535,754	14.0%	21.9%	7.9%
Pennsylvania	1,965,118	15.5%	2.5%	7.9%
Rhode Island	151,918	14.4%	−0.3%	8.2%
South Carolina	634,522	13.7%	30.4%	9.8%
South Dakota	117,070	14.3%	8.3%	11.1%
Tennessee	856,664	13.5%	21.6%	9.7%
Texas	2,619,733	10.4%	26.1%	10.7%
Utah	251,016	9.0%	31.0%	6.0%
Vermont	91,238	14.6%	17.1%	6.8%
Virginia	982,313	12.2%	23.7%	7.4%
Washington	832,650	12.3%	25.3%	6.9%
West Virginia	298,119	16.1%	7.8%	9.9%
Wisconsin	779,383	13.7%	10.6%	7.1%
Wyoming	70,225	12.4%	20.8%	6.8%
Puerto Rico	579,135	14.6%	35.3%	39.6%

Note: Data from Administration on Aging, U.S. Department of Health and Human Services. Population data is from U.S. Census Bureau 2010 Population Estimates. Puerto Rico population data is from the U.S. Census Bureau's international Data Base. State level poverty data is from the Census 2010 American Community Survey. National level poverty data is from the 2010 Current Population Survey/American Social and Economic Survey.

MARITAL STATUS

In the United States, in 2010, older men were more likely to be married than older women: 72% of men compared to 42% of women.[2] (See **Figure 1-7**.) What accounts for this, in large part, is the fact that women outlive men, thus increasing the ratio of widows to widowers. Internationally, as of 2008, 40% of women aged 65 and over were widowed as compared to 13% of men in this same age group.[1] Figures were similar to this in the United States in 2010.[2] Worldwide divorce rates of older persons is relatively low. In the United States, divorce in the over-65 population has remained relatively low (12.4% in 2010), but this is an increase from 5.3% in 1980.[1] To date, worldwide divorce rates of

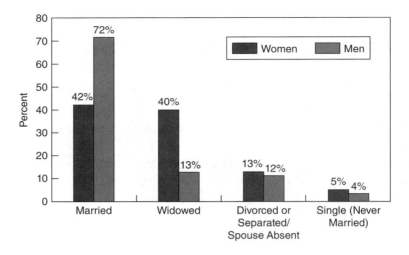

FIGURE 1-7   Marital status of persons 65+, 2010.
Source: Data from Administration on Aging, U.S. Department of Health and Human Services, 2010 Current Population Survey, Annual Social and Economic Supplement of the U.S. Census Bureau.

older people are relatively low because divorce is considered less socially acceptable by this older generation. However, in the United States and worldwide, the number and percentage of divorcing elders are likely to increase as younger generations, who tend to find divorce a more acceptable option, reach old age.

ECONOMIC STATUS

The economic status of elderly Americans is more varied than any other age group. Looking solely at income, on average, persons 65 years and older receive less income than those younger than 65. In 2010, the median income of males older than 65 was $25,704, as compared to $15,072 for females.[1] These figures may be somewhat misleading, however, because older adults have greater tax advantages, often have their home mortgages paid off, and are covered by **Medicare** insurance.[6]

Sources of income for those 65 years and older in 2009 were as follows: **Social Security** (38%), asset income (11%), public and private pensions (19%), earnings (29%), and all other sources (3%).[1]

As of 2010, poverty levels for older adults were 9%. In terms of race, poverty figures for those older than 65 years show 6.8% of whites at the poverty level, compared with 18% of African Americans and 18% of Hispanics. Older women had almost twice the poverty rate of older men (10.7% vs. 6.7%). Women age 65 and older have much higher poverty rates than men; this is true in every racial and economic group, especially among those who live alone.[7] The highest poverty rate among the elderly (40.8%) was experienced by Hispanic women who lived alone.[8]

HEALTH CARE

According to a 2000–2009 assessment of general health, 40% of noninstitutionalized persons age 65 years and older claimed their health was good to excellent. This compares with individuals 18–64 years of age, 65% of whom considered their health to be good to excellent.[2] There was not a significant difference between the genders; however, only 26% of older African Americans and 28% of older Hispanics rated their health as good to excellent.[8]

More than half of elderly persons have at least one chronic condition. In 2007–2009, the most frequently occurring conditions among older adults were uncontrolled hypertension (34%), diagnosed arthritis (50%), heart disease (32%), cancer of any type (23%), diabetes (19%), and sinusitis (14%).[8] Heart disease, cancer, and stroke account for 6 of every 10 deaths among those older than 65 years. Other diseases that rank high as causes of death in older adults include chronic obstructive pulmonary disease (COPD), pneumonia, influenza, and diabetes. According to the 2010 U.S. Census, 37% of noninstitutionalized elderly people have some kind of disability. Unfortunately the proportion of people with disabilities increases with age, leading to 56% of those over 80 reporting a severe disability.[8] Alzheimer's disease, confirmed on autopsy, is the leading cause of cognitive impairment in older adults.

Those 65 years and older visit a physician, on average, 6.8 times per year as compared with 3.8 visits per year in the younger-than-65 cohort. In 2007, approximately 1 person in 3 (12.9 million total) older than the age of 65 had a hospital stay. This is three times the comparable rate for persons of any age. Average length of stay in the hospital was 5.6 days for those over 65, as compared to 4.8 days for persons of all ages.[2] By 2030, with an estimated 71 million Americans older than the age of 65, healthcare spending is projected to increase by 25%.[9]

Healthcare expenditures are unbalanced. Most healthcare dollars are spent near the end of a person's life. Healthcare spending per person for those over age 65 was $14,797 in 2004, which was 5.6 times higher than spending per child ($2,650 in 2004) and 3.3 times higher than spending in those aged 16–64 years ($4,511 in 2004).[10] It has been estimated that by the year 2025, nearly two-thirds of the U.S. healthcare budget will be devoted to services for older adults.[10] This will place incredible demands on the healthcare system and its professionals. The question remains as to whether we will be ready to handle this staggering demand for healthcare services, to say nothing of affording the astronomical costs.

LONG-TERM CARE

As of 2012, approximately 9 million persons older than the age of 65 required some form of **long-term care**, whether in a nursing home, an assisted living center, or at home with some form of provider-based healthcare service.[11] It is estimated that by the year 2020 this number will increase to 12 million. Since 1966, when Medicare and **Medicaid** were introduced, the number of adults 65 and older requiring nursing home care has more than tripled from 2.5 million to 9 million. The average annual cost for a private room in a skilled nursing home is $73,000.[12,13]

In the population of those older than 85 years, one in four are eligible for placement in long-term care. Because this represents the fastest-growing segment of the population, the demand for nursing home beds will increase dramatically. Right now the number of nursing home beds is increasing by only half the rate at which this age cohort is increasing.

Elders who find themselves in long-term care facilities will, on average, use their life savings within 1 year.[11] At that point they may become eligible for public assistance or Medicaid. Considering the sharp increase in need, the question that begs asking is: Where will the funds come from to continue support of this program? This presents another problem for our ever-aging society, especially considering the ongoing debates to cut healthcare benefits such as Medicare.

As a result of the trend to get patients out of the hospital and back home as soon as possible, home health care has seen a dramatic increase. Expenditures for home health services were $70.2 billion in 2010. This is expected to grow at an annual rate of 8% for the years 2009–2019, partly due to shifting of long-term care services from institutional to home settings.[6] The advantage of home care is that it allows older persons to remain in the community, which can be more beneficial than living in a long-term care facility, from both a personal and a financial perspective. With an ever-increasing need for efficiency as a result of runaway costs, healthcare providers are being asked to become ever more productive and proficient in their delivery of elder services in alternative settings.

SUMMARY

Demographics clearly indicate that the United States, as a nation, is growing older. On January 1, 2011, one American began turning 65 years of age every 8 seconds. This aging baby boom generation will effect massive societal changes. These changes will occur in terms of gender, race, geography, marital status, economics, and health care. The number of women will continue to surpass the number of men, with aging African Americans, Hispanics, Native Americans, Asians, and Pacific Islanders increasing by a greater percentage than whites. Some states will be harder hit by an aging boom than others. Social Security and other government entitlement programs are likely to be stretched perhaps to the breaking point, or at least to the point where they need major revamping. The healthcare system, perhaps most of all, will experience demands never previously encountered.

Healthcare professionals will be at the forefront of this aging tidal wave as it washes over and through our healthcare systems. Although hospital admissions and lengths of stays have been on the decline since 1996, this may not be the case from 2011 to 2030 as baby boomers descend upon healthcare institutions. Even without dramatic increases in hospital admissions, long-term care and home care are expected to experience a dramatic rise in patient volume. It is not unrealistic to expect that two out of three healthcare professionals will be working in either long-term care or home care in the future. The majority of the patients in these settings will be older adults. Therefore, it benefits healthcare professionals to have an understanding of trends and projections as they relate to the "graying of America."

Review Questions

1. As of January 1, 2011, one American will turn 65 every _____ for the next 18 years.
   A. 8 minutes
   B. 8 seconds
   C. Hour
   D. Week

2. The fastest-growing segment of the population consists of individuals who are
   A. 1–18 years of age
   B. 24–40 years of age
   C. 30–50 years of age
   D. 50–65 years of age
   E. Older than 85 years of age

3. The young-old, according to Bernice Neugarten, refers to those who are
   A. 45–55 years of age
   B. 55–74 years of age
   C. 65–75 years of age
   D. 60–80 years of age

4. Women can expect to live, on average, _____ years longer than men.
   A. 2
   B. 5
   C. 7
   D. 10

5. Which ethnic group of those older than 65 is expected to increase at the least rapid rate between 1990 and 2030?
   A. African Americans
   B. Native Americans
   C. Whites
   D. Hispanics

Learning Activities

1. List what you believe will be some trends set by the baby boomer generation as it ages.
2. Design an elder community in a U.S. location. What factors would you consider in the design? Where would you place this community?
3. Which healthcare services and/or products are likely to be required by an aging population?
4. What will be possible roles and responsibilities of future healthcare professionals in long-term care facilities and home care?
5. Visualize yourself and your friends as older than 65 years of age. Where will you be living? What will you be doing? What will be your hobbies/roles? What will society be like?

REFERENCES

1. Wenner CA. *The Older Population: 2010. 2010 Census Briefs.* Washington, DC: U.S. Census Bureau, 2011.
2. U.S. Department of Health and Human Services, Administration on Aging. *A Profile of Older Americans: 2011.* Retrieved July 15, 2013 from http://www.aoa.gov/Aging_Statistics/Profile/2011/docs/2011profile.pdf
3. Neugarten B. The rise of the young-old. In R Gross et al. (Eds.), *The New Old: Struggling for a Decent Aging.* Garden City, NY: Doubleday Anchor, 1978.
4. Kinsella K, Wan H. *An Aging World: 2008.* Washington, DC: U.S. Census Bureau, U.S. Government Printing Office, 2009.
5. Vincent, GK, Velkoft, VA. The next four decades—The older population in the United States 2010–2050. Population estimates and projections. *Current Population Report*; May 2010. PS-25-1138 US Department of Commerce. Retrieved July 15, 2013 from http://www.census.gov/prod/2010pubs/p25-1138.pdf
6. Centers for Medicare and Medicaid Services. *National Health Expenditure Projections 2009–2019: Forecast Summary.* Retrieved July 15, 2013 from http://www.cms.gov/Research-Statistics-Data-and-Systems/Statistics-Trends-and-Reports/National-HealthExpendData/downloads/proj2009.pdf

7. Jacobson, LA, Kent, M, Lee, M, Mather, M. *America's Aging Population.* Population Reference Bureau, Feb 2011; 66(1). Retrieved July 15, 2013 from http://www.prb.org/pdf11/aging-in-america.pdf
8. National Center for Health Statistics. *National Vital Statistics Report.* 2012; 61(9).
9. Centers for Disease Control and Prevention, Merck Company Foundation. *The State of Aging Health in America 2007.* Whitehouse Station, NJ: Merck Company Foundation, 2007.
10. Hartman M, Catlin A, Lassman D, Cylus J, Heffler S. U.S. health spending by age, selected years through 2004. *Health Affairs*, November 6, 2007, pages W1–W12. Doi: 10.1377/hlthaff.27.1.w1.
11. U.S. Care, Inc. Likelihood of Needing Long-Term Care. Retrieved on February 10, 2009, from http://www.uscare.com/whyltc.html
12. Benz C. 40 Must Know Statistics About Long Term Care. *Morningstar.* Aug. 9, 2012. Retrieved June 10, 2013, from http://news.morningstar.com/articlenet/article.aspx?id=564139
13. Brandon E. Planning to Retire. Retrieved February 10, 2009, from http://usnews.com/blogs/planning-to-retire/2009/02/05/how-much-does-long-term-care-cost.html

SOCIAL GERONTOLOGY

NANCY BROSSOIE, PhD, and
WALTER C. CHOP, MS, RRT

Life is not a journey to the grave with the intention of arriving safely in a pretty and well-preserved body, but rather to skid in sideways, thoroughly used up, totally worn out, and loudly proclaiming, "Wow—what a ride!"

—Peter Sage

Chapter Outline

Behavioral Objectives

Upon completion of this chapter, the reader will be able to:

1. Define *gerontology* and how it differs from *geriatrics*.
2. Explain why taking a biopsychosocial perspective to understanding aging is important.
3. Define *ageism*.
4. Identify common myths about aging.
5. Discuss *infantilizing* and why it is harmful to the health and well-being of older adults.

6. Describe how older adults are portrayed in the media and how that influences social thinking about older adults.
7. Describe the diversity found in the lifestyles of older adults.
8. Describe some of the social roles adults might hold in later life.
9. Describe the challenges faced by grandparents raising grandchildren.
10. Identify major sources of income for older adults.
11. Describe how different ethnic groups treat older adults.
12. Identify strategies associated with a successful retirement.
13. Identify reasons why health promotion and disease prevention programs are beneficial to aging individuals.

Key Terms

AARP
Ageism
Biopsychosocial
Caregiver
Convoy of support
Discrimination
Fictive kin
Geriatrics
Gerontology
Gray Panthers
Healthy People 2020
Infantilizing
Long-distance caregiver

Long-term care insurance
Myths about aging
Older adult
Older Americans Act (OAA)
Polypharmacy
Retirement
Sandwich generation
Senior Service America (SSA)
Senior Volunteer Corps
Social roles
Social Security
Stereotypes

GERONTOLOGY

The aging process begins the moment we are born. As we age, our bodies and minds grow, develop, and mature. During childhood, the course of our development is influenced by many factors including our personal characteristics, our family background, how we are raised, where we grow up, and who raises us. Similarly, our development throughout adulthood continues to be influenced by our health, attitude, and behaviors and our interactions with family, friends, and the environment around us. Therefore, it is shortsighted to limit discussions about aging to matters of physical health and decline. Aging is a complex process influenced by many other personal and social factors.

Gerontology is the scientific study of aging that examines the biological, psychological, and sociological (**biopsychosocial**) factors associated with old age and aging. The factors that affect how we age are broad in scope and diverse: biological factors include genetic background and physical health; psychological influences include level of cognition, mental health status, and general well-being; and sociological factors range from personal relationships to the cultures, policies, and infrastructure that organize society.

Although sometimes confused with the term *gerontology*, **geriatrics** is a medical term for the study, diagnosis, and treatment of diseases and health problems specific to older adults. Geriatricians (medical doctors who specialize in geriatrics) increasingly recognize the importance of social and psychological influences when treating patients. In this chapter, key issues in gerontology are presented to facilitate your understanding about the lifestyles of older adults and how they may influence health status.

In the field of social sciences, the term **older adults** is used to describe people age 65 years and older, and is the preferred term when speaking about aged individuals. The term *patient* is medically oriented and can refer to a person of any age. The term *elderly* has the social connotation of being white haired and medically fragile. Because many people age 65 and older do not have gray hair and live vibrant healthy lifestyles, the term *older adult* has a more positive connotation and therefore is preferred and used in this chapter.

HISTORICAL PERSPECTIVES ON AGING

Throughout history, older adults have been generally valued for the experience, insight, and wisdom they can share with others. Leadership is frequently bestowed upon older adults because of a social belief that wisdom and experience are acquired over time; however, conferring respect and responsibilities to older adults has not always been consistent. It tends to occur more in preindustrial or agrarian societies where families are intergenerational and members are dependent on one another for survival and support. For example, in 2004, hours before a tsunami in the Indian Ocean reached the shore, villagers from small fishing communities followed the leadership of their village elders and fled to safety. The suggestions of the elders were followed because the elders held the respect of the others and possessed the ability to interpret environmental cues that signaled impending danger, cues that were passed down to them from village elders long ago.[1]

In industrial societies, older adults are generally less valued than they are in agrarian societies. During the 20th century, as industrialization in the United States expanded, family members became less dependent on each other for support, frequently leaving older adults to manage for themselves, many in poverty. In 1964, President Johnson launched the War on Poverty, which fought for the development of rights, opportunities, and social services for all poor Americans to help lift them out of poverty. From this initiative, the **Older Americans Act** (OAA) of 1965 was passed into legislation specifically to address the needs and rights of older adults. The OAA continues to be reauthorized and is expected to be reauthorized indefinitely. It is one piece of legislation that represents the United States' commitment to promoting the rights and welfare of older adults.

AGEISM

How we treat older adults is influenced by many social factors including our personal assumptions, expectations, and fears about growing older.[2] Fears about aging are generally based on a lack of understanding about the aging process. Unfortunately, many people believe that old age means being burdened with or suffering from physical disabilities, poor health, the inability to think clearly and quickly, and having a negative outlook on life. These inaccurate assumptions are examples of **ageism**, that is, systematic labeling and **discrimination** against people who are old.

Ageism is based on stereotypes, **myths about aging**, and language that conjure up negative images of older adults. Ageism is to old age as racism is to skin color and sexism is to gender. Ageist thinking is detrimental to society and can result in limited opportunities (e.g., employment and workplace discrimination) and reduced access to resources (e.g., healthcare discrimination) for older adults. In its worst form, ageism leads to elder abuse, mistreatment, and neglect.[3]

AGEIST STEREOTYPES

Ageist comments place older adults into set roles or categories, called **stereotypes**. For example, older adults are sometimes characterized as senile, grumpy, set in their ways and manners, and slow to accept new ideas and learn new skills. Similarly, older adults also may be portrayed as eccentric or overly happy about life, perceiving it as rosy and carefree. When members of a younger generation see ageist stereotypes portrayed in their own families and communities, they are likely to engage in ageist practices and thoughts, which may lead them to believe that older adults are different and perhaps less than worthy of respect and kindness.

Ageist attitudes permeate all facets of society, especially when money is involved. Negative connotations about older adults being "greedy geezers" first surfaced in a March 1988 issue of the magazine *The New Republic*. In that issue, older adults were described as wealthy with financial and social advantages, yet eager to siphon public money (i.e., **Social Security**) that should be dedicated to poor and needy children.[4] However, it must be realized that older adults paid into Social Security their entire working lifetime, and thus deserve remuneration.

Over the last 50 years there has been some gradual improvement in attitudes toward older adults in the United States, thanks to greater public education and awareness, the OAA, increased media attention, and the appearance of more positive role models in television and movie roles. This, however, has done little to reverse the deeper undercurrents that run below the surface of ageism, as some people continue to view older adults as drains on public resources.

MYTHS ABOUT AGING

Older adults are not a homogeneous group. They do not all look, think, or act alike. They are as unique as younger adults. Making blanket assumptions and generalizations about older adults simply perpetuates myths. The following statements are examples of myths that promote ageism. Although the statements may be accurate for some individuals, they are not true for older adults as a cohesive group:[3,5]

Myth 1: Older adults are either very rich or very poor.
Myth 2: Older adults are senile (have defective memory or are disoriented or demented).
Myth 3: Older adults are neither interested in nor have the capacity for sexual relations.
Myth 4: Older adults are miserable and unhappy with the state of their lives.
Myth 5: Older adults are very religious.
Myth 6: Older adults are unable to adapt to change.
Myth 7: Older adults are unable to learn new things.
Myth 8: Older adults generally want to live in nursing homes.
Myth 9: Older adults urinate on their clothing.
Myth 10: Older adults tend to be pretty much alike.

AGEIST LANGUAGE

Ageist language is insensitive to older adults because it is used without much thought or understanding of how ageist terms hurt and degrade an individual. Some ageist terms you may have heard before include the following:

Geezer	Old duffer	Biddy	Old buck
Hag	Dirty old man	Fossil	Old battleax
Q-tip	Old coot	Blue hair	Little old lady
Boroi (Japanese slang for old and worn)			

Ageist phrases in conversation also disparage older adults:

Over the hill	Out to pasture	Gone senile	One foot in the grave
Old school	Older than dirt	Set in their ways	Ol' man _____ (fill in name)

AGEIST ATTITUDES OF HEALTHCARE PROFESSIONALS

Unfortunately, healthcare professionals are not immune to promoting ageist attitudes when treating older patients.[6,7] Providers who view older adult patients sympathetically as "poor old dears" who can do little to care for themselves are actually placing little value on older adults' abilities. Calling an older patient "honey" or "dear" may be socially acceptable in some cultures, but generally carries a negative connotation. This **infantilizing** of older adults encourages dependency because it devalues the individual and does not foster independence. Although those are more subtle aspects of ageism, they are not person-centered and should be avoided.

Other ageist terms used by medical professionals in describing patients in conversation or in medical charts include the following:[8]

"The wheelchair (or the stroke, hop fracture, or other condition) in room number...."
MFP (measure for pine box)   Bed blocker   TMB (too many birthdays)
VAC (vultures are circling)   GOMER (get out of my emergency room)

Research has shown that healthcare professionals are significantly more negative in their attitudes toward older patients than they are toward younger patients.[7] Although not appropriate, their negative attitudes can be attributed to several reasons:

- A need to justify why the medical needs of the older adult were not addressed or met
- Feelings of frustration about not being able to manage the demands of the job
- Feelings of helplessness from not being able to save or cure patients' medical problems
- Increased awareness or reminder of one's own life and mortality

Awareness is the first step in overcoming an ageist attitude. To avoid making ageist comments and remarks as a healthcare professional, it is important to recognize and explore your personal feelings and attitudes about growing older. Stopping the spread of ageism is everyone's responsibility and starts at home.

THE MEDIA'S ATTITUDE TOWARD OLDER ADULTS

The media regularly perpetuate the stereotypes of older adults through inaccurate and sometimes demeaning portrayals of older adults in print, advertising, and entertainment. This is puzzling considering that older adults have the ability to purchase the products supporting the media, and thus should be able to facilitate change in the industry. Yet limited efforts have been made to alter how older adults are depicted. Perhaps as more members of the baby boom generation reach old age, positive changes will emerge.

The entertainment industry plays a major role in perpetuating age stereotypes. More often than not, older adults are portrayed as "more comical, stubborn, eccentric and foolish than other characters."[9] They are also often depicted as "narrow-minded, in poor health, floundering financially, sexually dissatisfied, and unable to make decisions."[9] Movie scripts tend to feature older adult characters only when they are reclusive (*Finding Forrester*), dying (*The Notebook*), or facing their own mortality (*The Bucket List*). It is uncommon to watch older adult characters on the big screen portraying everyday people (*Return to Me*) in a manner that does not romanticize their lives (*Cocoon*) or portray them as behaving comically (*Grumpy Old Men*).

Television show scripting is no different. Although we do see older adults on special programming, it is unusual to see a realistic portrayal of an older person on a television show. Again, this programming decision is puzzling considering that television shows are targeted for specific demographic audiences who are apt to buy the sponsors' products. Older adults watch television more than any other age group and generally have the discretionary income to buy the products advertised during commercials. Yet limited efforts have been made to accurately depict the lives of older adults on television, with the exception of selected actors such as Judi Dench, Betty White, and a few noteworthy others.[9]

Print and television advertisements tend to portray older adults at their worst—when they have some kind of physical ailment or have the desire to look and feel younger. We see older actors in commercials for laxatives, skin moisturizers, gas elimination medications, analgesics, and hair coloring products, just to name a few. This would not be as detrimental to the image of the older adult if we also saw older adults in other types of commercials advertising general-use products.

SOCIAL ROLES IN LATER LIFE

Social roles are useful in identifying, defining, and validating each member of society. A social role not only defines a position, but also includes social norms and expectations that dictate behaviors and attitudes within social groups such as families, workplaces, and communities. Some social roles remain with us throughout our lives (e.g., father, cousin, grandmother), whereas other roles change or transform as new levels of accomplishment or development are reached. For example, a person may transition from being a student to a teacher or from a worker to a retiree. In late life, social roles are more apt to remain constant (e.g., neighbor, club member, and community resident); however, the level of participation in those roles may fluctuate as changes in health, finances, and mobility occur. Nonetheless, older adults continue to participate in many of their social roles, even when faced with diminished capacities and capabilities.[10]

A new social role frequently faced by older adults is assumed at **retirement**. Adjusting to the changes in social status that result from leaving the workforce can be difficult for many people. By the time most older adults are ready to leave the workplace (regardless of position held) they have reached a higher status, which has earned them respect and support from their social networks of colleagues, friends, and acquaintances. Transitioning from a position of daily recognition and involvement to one with limited recognition and possible isolation from others can be psychologically difficult.[11] Although no single solution exists for everyone, adjusting to the loss of social roles accompanying retirement can be made easier with planning and preparation.

Becoming a **caregiver** for a family member or friend is a social role most of us do not think about until we find ourselves in the midst of providing care. Caregiving responsibilities often emerge slowly or begin suddenly after an illness or accident. Sometimes the need for assistance occurs so slowly that neither the caregiver nor the care recipient recognizes the full extent of decline over time.[12] For many older adults, providing care for a spouse is a subtle process that gradually increases and transitions into a full-time job before other family members are aware of the situation.

Many older adults are hesitant to take on the role of care recipient because they have a strong desire to remain independent and are unwilling to relinquish their roles and responsibilities to other people, even when they recognize they need help. Many are quite adamant about not accepting support until they reach a point where they cannot function without help. When that time comes, adult children are apt to intervene, although many are ill prepared to take on the caregiving role. Although each family is different, researchers have found a common pattern to family caregiving within the United States. Generally, older adults depend on the oldest daughter (or daughter-in-law) to provide assistance with activities of daily living and rely on the eldest son for support with financial and estate matters.[13] This does not mean that other family members will not be asked to help or will not offer to help. It simply means that, culturally, older adults expect specific assistance from these offspring.

In the past few years, more attention has been placed on the phenomenon of grandparents raising grandchildren. In 2010, the U.S. Census estimated that 2.5 million grandparents had full responsibility for providing for their grandchildren's basic needs. Approximately 1 million of those children did not have a parent actively involved in their lives.[14] The role of becoming a surrogate parent in late life can be demanding because it requires engaging in all aspects of the child's life including associating with teachers and other parents who are much younger. This new social role can be quite fulfilling and simultaneously challenging—especially when undertaken with a fixed retirement income and having to cope with the social stigma of the adult child's problem and inability to parent.

CULTURAL PERSPECTIVES ON CAREGIVING AND OLDER ADULTS

Most Western societies, including the United States and Western Europe, stress individualism (that is, the needs of the individual are addressed before the needs of the group). Other cultures, such as those in Asia and the Pacific Islands, are collectivist societies; that is, members place the needs of the family or collective group (which may be an intergenerational family) before the needs of the individual. Differences between individual and collective perspectives naturally inform how groups perceive older adults and place responsibility for providing care and support. Understanding how groups differ can assist in the planning and provision of effective healthcare services, no matter where the care is provided.

In an individualistic society, older adults are generally free to remain living independently and managing life as they see fit as long as they can afford it and they are not placing themselves or others in immediate danger. In a collectivist society, the resources of the older adults are pooled with other family resources. The activities of daily life are shared rather than lived separately. As a result, living expenses are reduced because the older adult lives with other family members. For example, in India, when an aging parent joins a younger household, he or she is welcomed as a member of the household. Even though the household may not have planned to include the older adult, family members willingly make accommodations for the aging family member.[15] In a Filipino household, the youngest daughter is expected to care for the older adult at home until she marries, and then moves the older adult with her to her husband's home.[16]

The social role of the older adult within the household varies by social expectations. Some ethnic groups revere elders as authority figures who reside in positions of power within the family and community. Other ethnic groups take an almost opposite view and see older adults in terms of added responsibility, if not burden, to family and society.

In the Vietnamese culture, a grandparent shares household authority with the father of the household. His or her place in the family is highly regarded.[17] In contrast, in the old Athabascan Indian culture in Alaska, older adults were seen as burdens—a drain on food and resources in the harsh and demanding climate. Older adults were expected to contribute as much as possible until the day came when the chief of the tribe would leave them to die in the wilderness in an effort to preserve resources for the healthy and strong members of the tribe.[18]

Family life and a respect for the knowledge and wisdom of the elder are central to Asian culture. This has, however, decreased somewhat in the Asian American population with modernization and assimilation into American society. However, Asian cultures remain strongly collectivistic and believe family life is central to their existence.[19,20]

Even though collectivism may appear to be an effective approach to managing family and social resources, sometimes it has not been perceived as beneficial to people with disabilities. People with disabilities often are viewed as an embarrassment to the family because they are not strong enough to contribute their fair share of family responsibilities. As a result, they are frequently disowned, abandoned, and left to beg on the street to get their needs met, further increasing the collectivist society's disdain for them. Because individuals with special needs (physical, cognitive, and behavioral) generally do not have strong support from within the collectivist society to lead a productive and successful life, they are challenged to determine their own life course.[15]

In the United States and in other individualistic societies, the strong belief in individualism has produced legislation that has protected the rights of people with disabilities (e.g., the Americans with Disabilities Act) and provides accommodation for people with physical and mental health needs in communities and the workplace. Coupled with legislation through the OAA, significant strides continue to be made to ensure that older adults are legally protected to lead full and productive lives.

A great deal of research has been conducted in the United States on family dynamics and the roles and responsibilities of family members. The United States has become a mobile and independent society where intergenerational households and the reliance on family for support are no longer assumed the norm. However, among some racial groups, such as African Americans, families still tend to maintain extensive kin networks that continue to provide help, especially to young family members and neighbors. Community institutions, including the church, are also viewed as very important sources of physical and emotional support.[12] Likewise, Hispanic Americans, who make up 10.3% of the U.S. population,[21] maintain close family relationships that promote family solidarity. They have more contact with their children than their non-Hispanic counterparts have with their own children.[22] As members of the baby boom generation surpass age 65, additional studies will need to be conducted to specifically address how different ethnic groups are coping and meeting the needs of their aging parents.

SOCIAL RELATIONSHIPS

Social relationships contribute to better physical health and provide individuals with great emotional and psychological benefits including better sense of belonging, increased self-worth, and feelings of security—all of which contribute to improved psychological well-being.[23] The importance of retaining relationships does not diminish over the lifespan. Older adults desire and engage in social relationships like younger adults, although their relationships are likely to reduce in number and type. Opportunities to socialize are also likely to be reduced as personal health declines or mobility becomes more difficult, resulting in fewer social engagements and relationships.

Research on personal relationships has also shown that as we age and our health declines, we intentionally distance ourselves from some of our relationships, retaining only the ones from which we can benefit and know we can maintain.[24] We do this because we recognize that relationships should be reciprocal. If we no longer have the ability, energy, or resources to exchange support, we let go of those relationships. The people we choose to retain in our social circle in late life tend to be people from whom we draw strength and value most, like family members. Kahn and Antonucci aptly described the evolution of the personal social network as a **convoy of support**, moving with the individual through life challenges and transitions.[25]

Relationships maintained in late life can serve a variety of purposes and take place within a variety of contexts. The following sections provide additional insights into some of the different types of relationships older adults enjoy.

Computers and Social Media   Computers play a large role in keeping older adults connected to family and friends, reconnecting old friends, and developing new relationships. Accessing the Internet is gaining popularity as friends encourage friends to "get connected" through social networking sites. Like their younger counterparts, older adults are keeping in touch through email and social media (e.g., Facebook) rather than relying on letters and telephone calls. Computers have enabled older adults to remain in touch and stay current with activities in the lives of children, grandchildren, and friends who have moved away. (See **Figure 2-1**.) Similarly, chat rooms and online dating services have also enabled older adults to establish new relationships for companionship and love.[26]

For older adults who have never used a computer, learning to operate one may be initially challenging. However, many community centers provide periodic classes on how

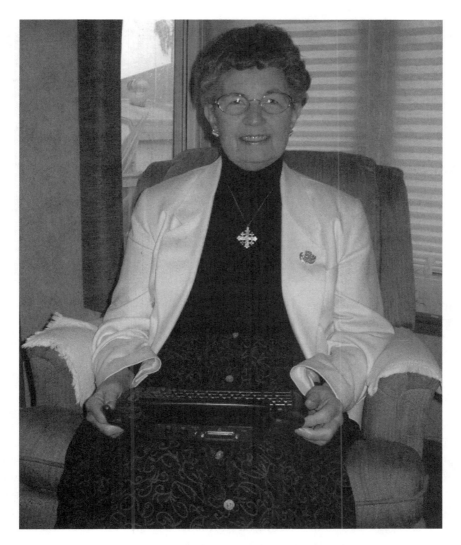

FIGURE 2-1   Email is an easy way for older adults to maintain communication with family and friends.
Source: Courtesy of C. Ernest Williams.

to send email, surf the web, access social media sites, play games, and use word-processing programs.

The Aging Couple   Like other adult couples, some older adults have been married or in a committed relationship for decades, whereas others have more recently become a couple later in life. (See **Figure 2-2**.) Older men who find themselves single generally have no problem finding female companionship because, statistically, women continue to outlive

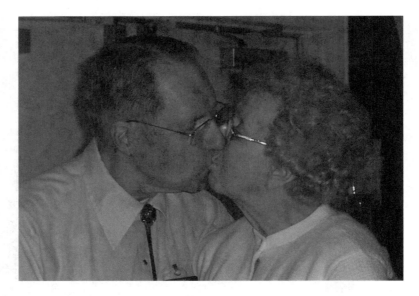

FIGURE 2-2 Expressions of love and affection.
Source: Courtesy of Theodore N. Brossoie.

men. The 2010 U.S. Census estimates that by age 85 there are 100 women for every 54 men.[27]

Couple relationships that have endured into old age have probably experienced and overcome many challenges and crises along the way. Health problems aside, one of the earliest challenges faced in later life occurs around the transition into retirement. For some, it is a time of deep soul searching, redefining social roles, and wondering what the future of the relationship will be like.[28] When children leave home and people transition out of jobs, their roles change and they are faced with establishing new roles for themselves and with their partner. If a couple successfully weathers these challenges, their feelings for each other can actually become enriched and strengthened. However, problems can arise when each person experiences this internal struggle at different times. For example, if one person is ready to retire while the other one is not, or one wants to sell the family home and move to a warmer climate and the other does not, problems in the relationship often arise. In response, some couples spend considerable time reflecting on the value, purpose, and usefulness of their relationship during this stage of life. For many, this is just another one of life's challenges that they will share and work through together. Others, however, will see it as a reason and opportunity to dissolve their relationship.

Many other couples choose not to grow old together. Maybe they have stayed together for the sake of the children, or perhaps they became absorbed in work or other activities over the years to avoid having to deal with relationship issues. These couples may share their lives but might not be emotionally engaged. They may be genuinely fond of each other but view their relationship as more of a business partnership than a marriage. Similar to a marriage of convenience, each partner does his or her own thing. Sometimes one or both partners in this type of relationship engage in extramarital affairs even into late life, which can bring about the final unraveling of the marriage.

Although some relationships worsen or dissolve with age, others actually get better and experience a renewal or rebirth. Communication often improves and affection and intimacy can become recharged. Late life can be the most satisfying years of a marriage for the couple who finds contentment in their relationship and has come to accept one another for who they are.[29]

In many ways, late life relationships among same-sex couples are no different than for heterosexual couples. Aside from sexual orientation, the main difference is public visibility. For some lesbian, gay, bisexual, and transgendered (LGBT) elders born more than 65 years ago, a lifetime of social marginalization, persecution, and denial of civil rights because of sexual orientation has forced them to keep their partnerships secret. Even though many LGBT couples have built lives that contradict negative social identities, many remain reluctant to reach out to the greater community for support services in late life.[30,31] The challenge for healthcare professionals in offering services to members of the LGBT community is gaining access and providing care that respects personal choice and right to self-determine care.

Aging Parent and Adult Child   Relationships between aging parents and adult children also tend to be as varied as spousal relationships.[32] Within most families, there is a fair degree of positive involvement between the generations. Many parents often continue to provide emotional, physical, and financial support to their adult children and grandchildren to help them manage their lives. Ideally support is provided without strings attached and out of good intentions. An underlying reason for helping out may in part be the hope or unspoken agreement that similar help will be reciprocated when needed in later years.[28]

However, strained relations can develop between a parent and child in adulthood. Verbal finger pointing—unfair fighting with "you never" or "you always" statements—can upset relationships, as can favoritism toward some family members over others. Sometimes parental disapproval of a lifestyle or friends generates family disharmony.

Feelings of disappointment coupled with shame may lead older parents to preserve their own public image instead of their son's or daughter's needs and feelings.[28] However, if affection and communication remain open between a parent and adult child, their psychological well-being will benefit and their relationship will grow stronger.[32]

One relatively recent challenge faced by many older adults has been the increased prevalence of substance abuse (alcohol and drug) and incarceration rates among their adult children. Subsequently, many older adults are forced to deal with the addictive behaviors of their adult child (or grandchild), a task many are ill prepared to undertake. Studies indicate that the problems of adult children are a significant cause of depression in older adults; the greater the child's problem, the greater the parent's depression. Older adults continue to want the best for their children, no matter what their age, and are often emotionally affected by the challenges and failures their offspring encounter.[33]

In many families, adult children are unaware of the daily routines, habits, and needs of their parents until a health problem arises and additional support in the home is needed. Like their children, most older adults want to live independently and do not want to live with other family members.[12] They also do not want to share their financial information or include their children in their decision-making processes. Older adults want to retain control over their lives.

When additional support or care is needed, approximately 83% of support received comes from family members.[12] One study estimated that 24% of caregivers of older adults lived with the person they were caring for, 42% lived within 20 minutes away, and 15% lived more than 1 hour away—referred to as **long-distance caregivers**. Nearly 7 million Americans are long-distance caregivers for an older relative.[12,34]

As family caregiving evolves and continues over time, it demands more of the adult child caregiver's time, often leaving less time for his or her own family. This can be especially challenging for caregivers simultaneously providing care to their own children. Adults found in this position are often referred to as the **sandwich generation** because they are caught between two caregiving roles—caring for a child and caring for a parent. In the United States, the average woman can expect to spend more time caring for an aging parent than she did caring for her children.[35]

Never-Married or Childless in Late Life   Approximately 4% of the population in the United States age 65 and older have never married.[36] Also notable is the increase of women in the United States who have never borne a child (nearly 20%)—a rate that has nearly doubled since the 1970s.[36]

The reasons for remaining single and for not bearing children are numerous and personal. Still, social roles and expectations of older adults are often centered around couplehood and families. This narrow perspective leads some people to wonder how never-marrieds and childless people receive support later in life and from whom.

Although some people may assume that never-marrieds and childless couples have been deprived of the emotional support of family in late life, research suggests otherwise. Happiness, life satisfaction, loneliness, and self-esteem appear to be unrelated to contact with adult children during late life.[37] Many never-marrieds and childless couples have adjusted by adapting their social network to include relationships generally thought to be held by partners and children. These **fictive kin** are treated as family and linked by close emotional bonds.[38] Sometimes a niece or a nephew takes on the social role of a child, or a sibling takes on some of the traditional roles of a spouse. Despite the social pressure to marry and bear children, those who do not conform to social pressure are not emotionally unstable in later life. Never marrying or remaining childless is not something to be pitied or viewed as a curiosity. It is simply another way of life.

Friendships   Friendships established early in life often continue into old age, especially if they begin during midlife. Unlike relationships with family members who are connected by blood ties and replete with social roles and expectations, friendships exist because the individuals involved share similar interests and want to maintain the relationship. Like younger adults, older adults tend to establish friendships with people similar to themselves: same gender, similar social and economic status, and from the same town or community. However, as friendships deteriorate as a result of increased distance, poor health, or death, new ones are formed if the older adult has the access and opportunity to build a new connection. The ability to form new relationships is essential because an important outcome of friendship is enhanced psychological well-being. Research indicates that friendships have an even stronger influence on well-being than do familial relationships, although the precise relationship remains unclear.[39]

Studies have also shown that women have more friends than men do because they view and engage in friendships differently.[40] Women perceive friendships to be sources of ongoing emotional and physical support and prefer to surround themselves with friends who can help them address the daily challenges they face. When a friendship ends, it is replaced with a new one. Thus, women are intentional about managing their friendships so that they maintain the desired complement of friends to help them process the events in their life. Men, however, prefer to rely on their spouse, partner, or close family members for help and emotional support rather than friends. Males' friendships are based on specific activities such as a sport or a project, rather than sharing feelings and processing a particular situation or event. As a result, men tend to require fewer friends than women do.

Like young adults, older adults nurture their friendships and feel a sense of loss when a friendship dissolves or becomes inactive. Poor health, new living arrangements, and loss in mobility frequently change the course of friendships and make sustaining them that much more difficult. As Kahn and Antonucci proposed in their "convoy of support,"[25] when maintaining relationships becomes too difficult to manage, older adults will break off some because they recognize they cannot reciprocate support. Instead, they choose to place their energy and resources into their most valued relationships, those with their closest family and friends.

Grandparenting   Grandparenting is a social role that many adults look forward to as their children mature. Because people are living longer, it is becoming common to see great-grandparents or even great-great-grandparents within families. The U.S. Census estimated that approximately one in four adults in the United States were grandparents in 2010.[41]

Grandparents generally welcome interactions with their grandchildren as a chance to relive their early years without balancing the stresses and responsibilities of caring for their own children the first time around. A new grandchild can be like a booster shot for some older couples, reawakening early days of marriage and the enthusiasm of early parenting.[24]

Not surprisingly, the role of grandparent is as varied as any other social role. Grandparents share multiple roles and responsibilities within families and as such can be described as one of five distinct types:[42]

- Distance figures (live far away and visit infrequently)
- Fun-seekers (provide and engage in exciting opportunities)
- Surrogate parents (take on a parenting role)
- Formal (as patriarch or matriarch of the family)
- Reservoirs of family wisdom (sources of knowledge and expertise)

Yet the role of grandparent is not static. The role of a grandparent today is generally responsive to the individual needs of the extended family. In the United States, one of the most important roles of a grandparent is that of a caregiver, in the broadest sense (**Figure 2-3**). Grandparents baby-sit, act as surrogate parents, pay educational costs, and sometimes provide the deposit for a new house. The toy industry especially likes grandparents because they purchase approximately 17% of all toys bought in the United States.[43]

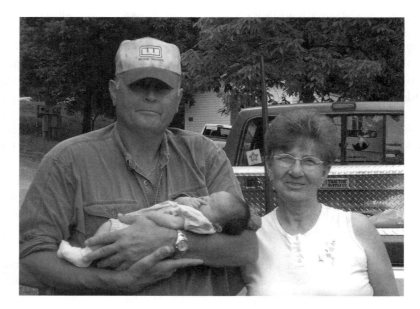

FIGURE 2-3   Grandparents often take on a caregiving role.
Source: Courtesy of Michelle Brossoie.

However, sometimes grandparents or adult children choose not to interact with each other and instead maintain a distance, not only physically but also emotionally. Having limited contact may be the result of personal priorities such as work or leisure or may stem from personal reasons based on unpleasant interactions in the past.[28]

The closeness felt between a grandparent and grandchild often correlates with how the grandparents saw their family members interact with their own grandparents. Healthy interactions between generations serve as positive role models for younger generations. Parents need to see grandparents spending quality time with their children to become good grandparents themselves.[28]

In addition to providing financial support, grandparents sometimes step in to take care of grandchildren when parents are abusive or addicted to drugs and are otherwise unable to parent. Grandparents also act as mediators when conflicts arise between a parent and child. Likewise, when parents divorce, grandparents can frequently offer support, comfort, consolation, and financial assistance to their child or grandchild, bringing the family closer together. Divorce, however, can also remove grandparents from their grandchild's life. In today's world of blended families and divorce, some grandparents find that they lose grandchildren as quickly as they welcome them into the family. In response, many have been fighting back for grandparent visitation rights so that they can maintain contact. Organizations that support grandparent rights are often state organizations because they address state-specific rights, although a few organizations, such as the Grandparents Rights Organization, are engaged at the national level.[44]

Arthur Kornhaber, MD, author of *The Grandparent Guide*, established the Foundation for Grandparenting to nurture and lobby for intergenerational relationships. This foundation even offers a summer camp and conference center where grandparents and grandchildren can build memories. Kornhaber's work has shown that children raised by grandparents tend to be more well-rounded and have a greater respect for the past. They are more likely to speak more than one language, perform better in school, and have a good sense of family and family values.[45]

Program developers for Road Scholar[46] and other adult adventure programs have also recognized the market for offering grandparent–grandchild vacation activities. Special summer programs are being offered in which both generations can share in a cultural or environmental experience. Spending time together provides an excellent opportunity to develop the grandparent–grandchild relationship without the distractions of daily life.

Recognition of the benefits and values of grandparenting has led to the creation of Adopt a Grandparent/Grandchild programs nationwide.[47] These programs provide excellent opportunities for kids without grandparents or older adults without grandchildren to engage and learn from each other's experiences. Similar programs provide older adults with the opportunity to become "foster grandparents" through youth centers or other community organizations.[48] No matter who is the focus of the program, experiencing the grandparent–grandchild relationship can be rewarding and fulfilling to everyone involved.

SOCIAL INFLUENCES ON AGING

INCOME AND FINANCIAL RESOURCES

The importance of financial security later in life cannot be overemphasized. Most older men and women have worked a good portion of their lives to establish a retirement fund (or so-called nest egg) from which to draw during their later years. It should, therefore, come as no surprise that older adults signal a rallying cry at every mention of reducing Social Security or Medicare benefits.

A major source of income for older adults in the United States is Social Security. Ninety percent of older adults collected Social Security in 2004. The Social Security Act was signed into law by President Franklin D. Roosevelt in 1935.[49] Its original and intended purpose was and continues to be acting as a supplemental source of retirement income for older adults to help pay expenses incurred during late life when earning potential is minimal. It was never designed to be a major source of retirement income. However, nearly one-third of Social Security beneficiaries report that Social Security provided 90% of their income. Fifty-three percent of beneficiaries reported receiving income from assets, 42% received income from retirement plans/funds, and 26% received income from earnings.[50]

Even though growing numbers of older adults are achieving financial security, in 2010 about 3.5 million older adults in the United States lived below the federal poverty level.[51] This group accounted for 9.4% of older adults (about the same as the rate for persons ages 18 to 64, which was 10.8%). Unlike younger adults, as older persons exhaust their resources, they are generally unable to generate the additional income necessary to improve their economic status or to leave assistance programs. Besides having diminished employment opportunities, they are also least likely to benefit from inheritance. Therefore, many are often left to fend for themselves, living off retirement savings, pension, or Social Security benefits that are only marginally adjusted for inflation. Because poorer older adults have fewer resources and live off of fixed incomes, they tend to spend a much larger portion of their total income on health care and housing than do their younger low-income counterparts.[52] For minority groups living in the United States, African American elders, the largest ethnic minority (12.4% of total population), have always lagged behind whites (81.9% of total population) in terms of social and economic status.[51] Many must continue to work into old age because they lack the resources to retire, and generally receive limited Social Security benefits because of a low earnings history.

Like African Americans, Hispanic elders tend to be socioeconomically less well off than older whites and most other ethnic elders.[50] Older African American and Hispanic women who are not married or partnered have a more difficult time financially than do their white counterparts. In 2004, approximately 27% of African American women age 65 and older were living alone with household incomes at or below 100% of the federal poverty level.[51] Like most impoverished adults, their situation is the result of a lifetime of low-skill, low-paying jobs, inadequate educational opportunities, and discrimination in the labor market.

Older Asian Americans constitute a small but rapidly growing segment of the older adult population in the country. As a group, they tend to be somewhat better off, by most social indicators, than other minority groups are. This may be attributed to their collectivist lifestyle with a focus on family and emphasis on meeting the needs of the family or community before the needs of the individual. Engaging in this lifestyle is important because many immigrant elders are not covered by Social Security.[53]

WORK AND RETIREMENT

Workplace Discrimination   Extensive research has been conducted on social attitudes toward older workers. Many employers and employees inaccurately perceive older workers to be rigid, inflexible, incapable of learning new skills, unproductive, and overpaid. It should, therefore, come as no surprise that the most common type of economic discrimination against older adults is work-related.[5] Research indicates that 80% of adults believe that most employers discriminate against older workers in hiring or on the job, and 61% of employers admit doing so.[54] Discrimination against older workers ignores several overall advantages to hiring them, including low absentee rates, less turnover, low accident rates, less alcohol- and drug addiction–related issues, increased job satisfaction, and company loyalty.[5] Additionally, the experiences, knowledge, and insight older workers bring to the workplace are invaluable and cannot be easily replaced by a younger person with a limited work history who is working for lower wages.

Some employers believe that older workers are unable to keep pace with change and learn new technologies. For example, they may think that computers and computer software are far too difficult for older adults to learn to operate proficiently. Based on this assumption, employers are less likely to consider hiring older workers. However, evidence exists that older adults can and do learn new technological skills, including computer technology. Their learning strategies and styles may be different from younger adults, but they have the ability to learn and can become quite accomplished when given the opportunity to learn and study in a way that works for them.[55] Some employers are now viewing older workers as an untapped resource that can provide experience and share their expertise with younger workers. This can be done during a sort of "bridge employment," which can occur as the older worker transitions from full-time work to part-time work and then into full retirement.[57] Many businesses and professions, now facing skills shortages, are beginning to view the retention of older workers as making good business sense. Also, the retiring person takes with them valuable institutional memory, because they often have been with the company a long time. This is prompting some employers to seriously consider allowing loyal older workers to continue on a part-time basis at least as they transition into retirement.[57]

Work discrimination against older adults is most obvious when companies attempt to reduce costs by asking older workers to take early retirement, even seducing them into it by offering a tempting retirement package, a so-called golden parachute. The offer may initially appear to be a good financial move but may short-change the worker of retirement income if not invested and managed wisely.

Retirement   Before the industrial revolution, retirement as a phase of life did not exist. Individuals worked until they became either disabled or too frail or infirm to do otherwise. They generally died shortly afterward. If they did live a long life, they were usually supported by family or by some charitable organization such as the local church. It was only in 1889 that Chancellor Bismarck of Germany established retirement for individuals reaching age 65. He chose the age of 65 as the beginning of retirement by adding 20 years to the then-normal life expectancy of 45 years. Other European countries soon followed with similar retirement systems. In 1935, the United States was the first country to establish a nationalized pension system for people age 65 and older (Social Security).[49] Since then, other countries have followed suit, and today most offer a national pension to adults age 65 and older. Variations in the age of eligibility range about 5 years, with most notable differences between males and females.[56]

Until 1967, retirement was compulsory for workers in the United States who reached age 65, regardless of their health status or abilities. Here again we see another myth of aging that implies there is a general loss of ability that begins around age 65 or even earlier. However, in typically aging adults there exists no sudden or general loss of ability at age 65 or at any other age.[5] Any losses that may occur generally do so gradually over many years. Even some disorders considered inevitable as we age (such as visual and hearing impairments) are now reversible or at least amenable to treatment. Because of better health status, today's retirees can potentially spend 20 or more years in retirement.[56]

Older adults, like most groups of individuals, are incredibly diverse. Ken Dychtwald, president of Age Wave Inc., states, "No age group is more varied in personal background, physical abilities, personal styles, social needs, or financial capabilities than today's older population. While some older people are dreadfully sick and waiting for death, some are fit and training for marathons. Some wait in breadlines for a warm meal. Others have condos in Vail and yachts in Tahiti."[35] Additionally, many continue working in the same or some new capacity, even after reaching retirement age. In sum, retirement is a stage of life that for some begins with a change in employment status.

Preparing for retirement is not a task that should be taken lightly or without preparation. Retirement requires planning, planning, and more planning. And despite what the television commercials may say, it is not all about finances. Important considerations in the retirement decision-making process include the following:

- Financial and social resources
- Spouse's/partner's retirement plans
- Desire to continue working part-time

- Need to remain active in current profession
- Desire to start a new career
- Desire to volunteer
- Desire to remain living in the same community

Prior to retirement, some older adults begin developing hobbies or spare-time occupations to engage in during retirement. Many daydream about being able to putter around their home and spend considerable time in their gardens. Although generally good ideas, hobbies and household activities are generally not intensive enough to fill the hours in a day.[57] As many older adults with a few years of retirement behind them frequently offer, you cannot just retire, you have to retire to something. Some older adults are determined to challenge themselves in pursuit of some activity that few, regardless of age, would choose to follow. Mary Harper, a 79-year-old great-grandmother, is one person who rose to such a challenge. In 1994, she became the oldest person to sail across the Atlantic single-handedly. Although she broke a rib in severe weather, she later said, "The whole trip was worth it just to see the waves." In answer to why she did it alone, she explained that "it was something I wanted to do . . . but didn't want to be responsible for a crew."[58] Another older adult who has refused to settle down to "quiet old age" is Corena Leslie, who completed a sky dive jump 3 days before her 90th birthday.[59] Some individuals reinvent themselves by returning to a youthful passion. Such was the case for David Morrison of Milgrove, Ontario, Canada, who earlier in life performed folk music in local coffeehouses with friends Judy Lanza and the now-famous actor Eugene Levy. A year prior to retirement, Morrison bought a new guitar and took up singing lessons. Three weeks after retiring as vice president of executive development for TD Bank, Morrison was on the verge of becoming a public performer again.[59]

For some older adults, engaging in lifelong learning activities helps them keep their minds active and alert. Special program topics offered at local community centers, senior centers, and colleges provide numerous opportunities for older adults to explore topics that pique their interest. Road Scholar is a not-for-profit global program that provides learning experiences for older adults on topics including history, culture, nature, music, outdoor activities, crafts, and study cruises.[46] Participants are able to explore their interests with leading scholars and researchers in the field while sailing on cruises, walking through national parks, and visiting culturally diverse areas.

Many older adults believe that successful aging starts with mental stimulation. At the Plymouth Harbor Retirement Community in Sarasota, Florida, the longevity among residents is greater than the national average. This unique community encourages individuals to get involved in a myriad of activities, which include electing representatives from each apartment cluster to serve on the board of residents that governs Plymouth Harbor. Residents also pool their resources in supplying volunteer lecturers on just about every topic imaginable. People at Plymouth Harbor appear more involved, interested, and perhaps *more alive* than the stereotypical portrayal of retirees.[60] As Ralph Waldo Emerson once wrote, "It is not length of life but depth of life."

Many adults take up new hobbies and activities that combine mental and physical fitness, such as tai chi or square dancing (**Figure 2-4**). Both provide retirees with the opportunity to exercise their bodies and keep a sharp mental focus. Square dance clubs travel frequently to dance with other groups, providing abundant opportunities for socializing on and off the dance floor.

Many older adults have the desire to give back to their communities and devote many hours to volunteering each week, sharing their lifetime of experiences and insights. Their skills, knowledge, resources, and abilities can affect changes and make a difference in the lives of people of all ages. The **Senior Volunteer Corps** is an umbrella organization for three programs connecting adults age 55 and older to nonprofit, faith-based, and community organizations such as the Retired Senior Volunteer Program (RSVP), Foster Grandparents, and Senior Companions. Since the 1960s, communities have eagerly tapped into this source of people power to alleviate a number of community challenges.[61]

The image of the "wise old person" can be hard for those of us in the West to conceive, but in eastern and indigenous cultures this is commonplace. West African teacher and author Malidoma Somé told an interviewer the following: "An elder is a repository for wisdom of the ancestors, the culture and the tribe. He or she is familiar with the various

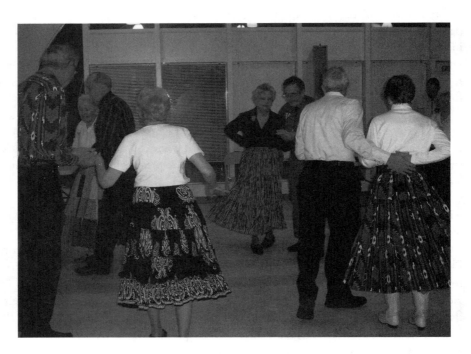

FIGURE 2-4   Square dancing helps maintain physical strength, coordination, and mental agility.
Source: Courtesy of Theodore N. Brossoie.

protocols for maintaining relationships with the other world and is keeper of the various 'recipes' that sustain the soul and spirit of the community. When elders are absent there is chaos and instability. The young are in charge but don't know where they are going."[62] Perhaps we in the West can listen and learn from our elders as these other cultures do.

ADVOCACY GROUPS FOR OLDER ADULTS

Advocating for the rights and needs of older adults at the local, state, and national levels can be a daunting task. However, as the baby boom generation ages and more individuals reach the age of 65, the voices of advocates are becoming louder and stronger. This should come as no surprise because older baby boomers fought for the rights of disempowered groups in the 1960s and 1970s. Their involvement in civil rights, gay rights, and the feminist movement was generation shaping.

Several advocacy groups that help represent the needs of older adults are profiled in this section. The most recognizable organization that has demonstrated considerable success in representing the needs of adults age 50 and older is **AARP**, a nonprofit, non-partisan organization. It was founded in 1958 as the American Association for Retired Persons with the agenda of addressing the social needs of retirees. Today, AARP has expanded its scope of interests to include all aspects of life. In 2006, it boasted a membership of more than 37 million people. The mission of AARP is simple: "To enhance the quality of life for all of us as we age." AARP advocates for social change through information, advocacy, and service as it represents adults of all ethnicities and cultures within the United States. All of its publications (magazine, bulletins, and website) are instilled with the attitude that age is merely a number and life is what you make of it. Together with the AARP Foundation, research on topics of current interest including prescription drug costs, grandparents raising grandchildren, and civic participation is funded to generate information that can be used to promote positive social change.[63]

The Gray Panthers was founded in 1970 by Maggie Kuhn and six other women who came together to discuss and address the issue of forced retirement at age 65. However, the first issue taken on by the fledgling organization was not age discrimination, but rather opposition to the war in Vietnam. This was because the Gray Panthers did not want to be perceived as an organization that was only dedicated to fighting ageism. The Panthers believed philosophically that "gray power" should be on the cutting edge of social change by working with other organizations. Today, the Gray Panthers' mission is "work for social and economic justice and peace for all people." Armed with intergenerational support and organizational values that include honoring maturity, unifying generations, active engagement, and participatory democracy, the Gray Panthers now proudly identify themselves as **Gray Panthers**, to "create a humane society that puts the needs of people over profits, responsibility over power, and democracy over institutions."[64]

A third organization founded to address workplace and retirement issues is **Senior Service America (SSA)**, once known as the National Council of Senior Citizens and founded by the American Federation of Labor and Congress of Industrial Organizations (AFL-CIO) in 1961. Today, the organization's fundamental purpose is broader than the scope of retirement because the group advocates for political and legislative issues that affect older adults. Legislative issues that received the organization's attention in past years have included the Older Americans Act, Medicare, Medicaid, and employment training opportunities. Today, the SSA updates members through newsletters that report on how Congress is addressing the needs of older adults. The SSA and its partner organizations also provide employment and training opportunities to more than 10,000 adults nationwide.[65]

HEALTH, WELLNESS, AND HEALTH CARE

Today, older adults are living longer and healthier, thanks to improvements in healthcare technology and lifestyles that incorporate healthy diets and exercise. Multiple studies conducted through the National Institute on Aging have revealed that many of the health problems found in old age are not caused by age itself but rather by improper care of and use of the body over time. If the body has been subjected to overeating, exposure to toxins (such as cigarette smoke and alcohol), lack of adequate exercise, and poor nutrition, it should come as no surprise that medical problems will be greater in old age.

Teaching older adults how to manage their health conditions and educating them about their conditions requires an approach different from activities designed for patients of other ages. Older adults tend to learn more effectively in small groups that foster discussion in an informal setting. Older adults are generally more concrete learners rather than theoretical learners, and they learn best when the subject matter has direct practical application. All information presented should be developed using plain language that clearly communicates the intended message at all literacy levels.

HEALTH PROMOTION AND DISEASE PREVENTION

Healthy People 2020 is a strategic plan set forth by the U.S. Department of Health and Human Services, the Healthy People Consortium, and other federal agencies to focus on preventable health threats (including disability and death) that affect citizens of all ages. The initiative challenges individuals, communities, and professionals to join together to improve the health of all citizens.[66] The objectives in Healthy People 2020 fall under four overarching goals:

- Attain high-quality, longer lives free of preventable disease, disability, injury, and premature death.
- Achieve health equity, eliminate disparities, and improve the health of all groups.

- Create social and physical environments that promote good health for all.
- Promote quality of life, healthy development, and healthy behaviors across all life stages.[66]

Healthy People 2020 emphasizes the need for vitality and independence with aging and uses a health-oriented rather than disease-oriented approach. Objectives take a true gerontological approach, accounting for socioeconomic, lifestyle, and other non-medical-related influences on personal health.[66]

Common complaints frequently associated with old age include joint stiffness, weight gain, fatigue, loss of bone mass, and loneliness. These conditions can be slowed, prevented, or eliminated by health promotion and disease prevention activities[67] such as exercise, stress management, nutrition, and substance abuse control.

Exercise   The old adage "use it or lose it" is applicable when it comes to making a case for older persons to exercise regularly. Abundant studies have demonstrated the benefits of exercise throughout the life span. Exercise helps maintain fitness, stimulates and quickens the mind, helps establish social contacts, prevents and/or slows progression of some diseases, and generally improves quality of life. Inactivity leads to muscle wasting and weakening of the bones. A number of chronic conditions such as heart disease, arthritis, osteoporosis, diabetes, obesity, and depression show improvement, or at least a slowing of progression, with regular physical activity.[68]

The ideal exercise program for individuals older than age 60 should emphasize exercises that increase strength, flexibility, and endurance and should be initiated only after consultation with a medical specialist.[68] Low-impact activities such as walking, swimming, or bike riding are ideally suited for most older adults. Exercise should be preceded by stretching and should be increased in gradual increments. An exercise "prescription" from a physician is a good way to begin, especially for those who have been away from exercise for any length of time. Additionally, older participants in fitness programs need to be reminded not to exceed their ability level and to respect pain. Exercise programs specifically tailored for older adults and staffed by fitness professionals are frequently offered through hospitals, colleges, and community organizations.

Stress Management   Much has been written on the relationship between stress and disease. Stress can increase the risk of, or worsen, heart disease, cancer, or other chronic conditions. It can also dampen the immune response. Stress tends to originate from three sources: the environment, our bodies, and our minds.[4] Environmental stressors such as the weather, crime, and crowds are usually beyond one's control, whereas physical and mental stressors, although sometimes seemingly insurmountable, can often be controlled by changing behaviors or thought patterns. There are numerous stress management techniques such as exercise, diet, muscle relaxation, meditation, deep breathing, visualization, desensitization, and biofeedback.[68] Any individual interested in finding a stress reduction technique needs to select one that is well suited to his or her lifestyle and temperament.

Nutrition   Although we purport to be a nation of plenty, 25% of persons older than age 65 may be malnourished.[69] Poverty—although the major cause of malnutrition—is not the only factor. It is estimated that one-third of all nursing home residents are malnourished.[70] This, in large measure, is because few doctors are trained to recognize malnutrition in older adults. In addition to poverty, additional reasons for malnutrition in older adults include depression, limited access to buying food, unbalanced diet, problems with chewing or swallowing, chronic illness, and medications that suppress appetite or interact with nutrients. The resulting lack of physical ability and energy to cook and eat naturally compounds the problem. Poor nutrition also contributes to the progressive decline of several body functions that manifest later in life, including bone density loss, atherosclerotic lesions, opacification of eye lenses, and a blunted immune system.[71]

Substance Abuse Control   Substance abuse can become a major source of problems for older adults. Because older adults generally have less lean body mass and a lower volume of body water, substances such as alcohol, recreational drugs, and medications are absorbed at higher levels into the body and retained for longer periods of time than experienced at a younger age. The presence of alcohol and drugs increases the risk for injuries and/or accidents. Additionally, alcohol and other drugs can have an adverse effect on sleep and can sometimes mask the symptoms of underlying diseases.

Once substance abuse has been identified in an older individual, a management plan should be established. This first involves an initial screening to assess the impact of alcohol or drug abuse both physically and psychologically. Then, a treatment plan, which includes education and promotes self-responsibility, must be established.

Sometimes substance abuse problems develop as a result of **polypharmacy**[72]; that is, the interactions of multiple medications prescribed for multiple conditions create new disabling medical conditions in the older adult, including adverse drug reactions and addictions. Polypharmacy problems generally occur when more than one medical provider is involved in the care of an older adult. To avoid problems, the older adult should make certain that each provider is aware of what the other is prescribing. Likewise, to stem problems arising from polypharmacy issues, providers and family members should attempt to identify the source of new health problems as they arise and work together with healthcare providers to make sure unnecessary medications are not prescribed.

HEALTHCARE FINANCES

The increased cost of health care and the aging population go hand in hand, and have assumed a position on the central stage of the national policy debate. The cost of public healthcare programs has risen to staggering levels. The proportion of the U.S. gross domestic product (GDP) for national health programs (i.e., Medicare, Medicaid, veterans' medical care) has increased from 0.4% in 1962 to approximately 5.4% in 2008.[73] Note, however, that although national health programs were at 5.4% of GDP, as stated, overall healthcare expenditures in the United States were determined to be 17.9% of GDP in 2011, which is among the highest percentages in the world.[73]

Not surprisingly, older adults with declining health spend more money on long-term institutionalized care than on any other type of health care. Most elders, however, cannot meet these overwhelming costs on their own, and Medicare coverage is limited. As of 2011, the average daily cost of $239 (over $87,000 annually) for a semiprivate room in a nursing home is forcing many older adults to watch their lifetime savings evaporate within a few years.[74] By 2030, the cost of institutional care is projected to increase to $190,600 per year, a sum few will be able to afford.[75]

Long-term care insurance is one method of affording nursing home care, at least for those who can afford to buy the insurance. This form of insurance has become the fastest-growing type of health insurance sold in recent years, and it promises to continue its growth in the coming years. By 2003, 13% of full-time workers in private industry were offered long-term care insurance, and 19% of full-time workers in large private establishments (100 or more workers) were offered this benefit.[76] Although it is still not routinely offered or included in regular health benefit plans, some health policy analysts believe that its availability will increase as the aging population grows in numbers.

SUMMARY

The aging process begins the moment we are born. Over the years our bodies and minds grow, develop, change, and mature. Gerontology is the scientific study of aging that examines the biological, psychological, and sociological (biopsychosocial) factors associated with old age and aging.

Ageism, a systematic stereotyping of and discrimination against people who are old, fosters the notion that older adults are not useful or valued. Ageism is fueled by numerous myths regarding aging and older adults as well as by language that conjures negative images of old persons. Ageism limits opportunities (employment and workplace discrimination) and access to health care, and in its worst form can lead to elder abuse, mistreatment, and neglect.

Research has shown that healthcare professionals are significantly more negative in their attitudes toward older patients than they are toward younger patients.[5] To avoid, even inadvertently, making ageist comments and remarks, it is important to recognize and explore your own feelings and attitudes as a healthcare professional. Stopping the spread of ageism is everyone's responsibility, and starts at the individual level.

The media regularly perpetuate the stereotypes of older adults through inaccurate and sometimes demeaning portrayals of older adults in print, advertising, and entertainment.

This is puzzling considering that older adults have the ability to purchase the advertisers' products that sponsor these media activities. Nonetheless, limited efforts continue to be made to accurately depict the daily lives of older adults through the media.

Social roles continue to be important in later life. However, relationships are sometimes dissolved as a result of poor health, limited mobility, and the inability to reciprocate support. Relationships with close family and friends are maintained before others because they are the source of most support. Some couples find later life to be a time of closeness, after weathering life's storms together. Others choose to separate and go their own ways, while others remain single and seek support from fictive kin. Relationships between aging parents and adult children tend to be as varied and challenging as spousal relationships, yet can generally be counted on to provide support. Maintaining friendships continues to promote psychological well-being well into old age. Grandparenting has been, and remains, a rewarding and fulfilling experience in later life.

Attitudes toward retirement vary greatly, as do lifestyles of older adults. For some, retirement heralds the chance to pursue a special interest or hobby they never had time to do while working. Others see it as an opportunity to travel or return to school to pursue a second career. Others view it with a bit of disappointment, especially if they previously held an influential position. For most people, however, retirement is a time of relaxation to be spent with spouse, children, grandchildren, and/or friends.

Financial security is extremely important to older adults. Social Security was a source of income for 87% of older adults in 2009, with one-third counting it as 90% of their entire income. Unfortunately, in 2010, 3.5 million adults lived below the federal poverty level. A great many impoverished individuals include single women who are African American or Hispanic.

Several organizations advocate for the rights and needs of older adults at the local, state, and national levels: AARP, Gray Panthers: Age and Youth in Action, and Senior Service America. All three organizations were founded more than 40 years ago with the mission of bringing about social change for older adults.

As a result of improvements in health care, better diet, and more emphasis on exercise, Americans are entering later life healthier than ever before. Healthy People 2020 is a strategic plan focusing on health prevention efforts. It emphasizes vitality and independence among older adults and uses a health-oriented rather than a disease-oriented approach. The plan addresses topics such as exercise, stress management, nutrition, and substance abuse.

One of the greatest problems facing our aging society is healthcare finances. The costs of financing the federal health programs including Medicare and Medicaid continue to rise. In response to rising costs, some older adults are buying long-term healthcare insurance.

It is important for everyone working with older adults to understand that social factors affect our aging society. By developing an appreciation for the diverse backgrounds of older adults, healthcare professionals can better serve their needs. Additionally, this should help us in our own personal approach to coping with aging family members and our own aging processes.

Review Questions

1. Gerontologists take into account the _____ forces that influence the aging process.
   A. Organic, synthetic, and supernatural
   B. Biennial, perennial, and annual
   C. Biological, psychological, and sociological
   D. Infantile, adolescent, and middle-aged

2. Ageism is
   A. The systematic stereotyping of and discrimination against people who are old
   B. Pretending to be older than you really are
   C. Pretending to be younger than you really are
   D. Another term for racism

3. Which of the following explains some of the negative comments made by healthcare workers about older adults?
   A. A need to justify why the medical needs of the older adult were not addressed
   B. Provides a feeling of satisfaction for managing the demands of the job
   C. Contributes to their ability to save or cure a patient's medical problems
   D. Explains a general unawareness of their own life and mortality

4. Work discrimination against older adults is a form of
   A. Bigotry
   B. Ageism
   C. Socialism
   D. None of the above

5. Social roles are important ways of _____ members of every society.
   A. Selecting and eliminating
   B. Categorizing and sorting
   C. Identifying and validating
   D. Discovering and isolating

Learning Activities

1. Role-play with a partner examples of ageism found in the workplace, in a healthcare setting, in social situations, and in the family.
2. Record television commercials or shows, or find YouTube videos featuring older adults. Review the items for how older adults are represented. Play these for your classmates and generate a discussion.
3. Establish a fictitious advocacy group representing older adults. Develop a mission, vision statement, goals, and objectives. Describe how you might use the group to effect changes to improve the lives of older adults.

4. With a partner, role-play some of the issues and concerns of an older caregiver faced with providing care for an ailing spouse.
5. Create a retirement plan for a fictitious couple that takes into account their financial resources, their family relationships, their personal interests, and their desire to work.
6. Design a health promotion/disease prevention course or workshop for older adults.

CASE STUDIES

CASE 1: John and Jason are both 68 years old and have been an exclusive couple for 33 years. Their lives are inextricably interwoven, although many people are not aware of their relationship—only a handful of close friends know. John is a banker and commutes daily into the city to work. Jason is an instructor at a local community college, and generally walks to his office. They have kept their relationship relatively secret because they fear that others will "out" them, which they fear will force them to leave the careers they adore. One day Jason suffers a severe stroke, and their carefully constructed world begins to unravel. As gay men, neither is provided the rights of a spouse in terms of overseeing medical care, and John is quickly pushed aside at the hospital as staff ask who next of kin is. As the days go by, John remains at Jason's side, and one nurse in particular repeatedly makes comments about the two old gay guys and how they don't deserve her time or care. A doctor pulls John aside and advises him to start looking for a nursing home for Jason. The thought of losing Jason and placing him in a nursing home is more than John can bear. He believes the nursing home staff would be no different than hospital staff and would not accept the men's relationship. John decides to quit his job to care for Jason at home. When his boss asks him why he is leaving, John lies and says his mother's health is failing and she needs him. The first 3 months of care go relatively well, but as Jason's health declines, John recognizes he needs help and a break from the care, but feels he has no one to turn to.

How are John and Jason's challenges in providing Jason with care different from the challenges faced by a heterosexual couple? What challenges do healthcare professionals face in providing care to same-sex couples? What can healthcare professionals do to help couples like John and Jason successfully manage their healthcare challenges?

CASE 2: Barbara, age 42, is a lucky woman, or at least that is what everyone tells her. She has an adoring husband, smart children, a career as a store manager, and impeccable taste in fashion. Barbara has always been an excellent multitasker and has successfully balanced her marriage, family, and career for 20 years. She makes every task look effortless. So, when her mother started having health problems, Barbara was sure to set aside the time needed to help. She always assumed she would be the best one to help her mother, even though she lived 200 miles away, because she was reliable and dependable. Barbara has a brother and sister who could probably help, but they have their own careers and families and they are just fine letting Barbara take over. They trust Barbara. After a few months, Barbara thought that being a long-distance caregiver was not that hard. She struggled a bit at first, but soon organized all the information she needed about her mother's health problems and care. She was in touch with doctors on a regular basis and authorized whatever care was needed. Soon she started managing her mother's finances. It didn't cross Barbara's mind to call her siblings to update them, and they didn't think to call her. Barbara was pleased that she could provide for her mother from a distance. Although long-distance caregiving was not convenient and often forced her to change her plans, she couldn't imagine not being available for her mom. One day Barbara received a call that her mother had been hospitalized. She called her sister and they agreed to meet at their mother's home and travel together to the hospital. Secretly, Barbara was glad to meet with her sister because she was getting tired of having the extra burden of her mother's life on her shoulders alone. Last week at work, the regional manager told her that her enthusiasm and work performance had started to slip. Even her husband had made a few comments that she didn't seem to have the time for him anymore. Barbara knew things needed to change, but just wasn't sure what to do.

What should Barbara do? What is the best way to get family members to work together to care for a parent? What steps does Barbara need to take to ensure her own needs are being cared for?

REFERENCES

1. Associated Press. Elders' knowledge of the oceans spares Thai "sea gypsies" from tsunami disaster. Retrieved January 19, 2013, from http://www.freerepublic.com/focus/f-news/1311910/posts
2. Butler, RM. Ageism: Another form of bigotry. *Gerontologist*, 1969;9:243–246.
3. Butler, RM. *The Longevity Revolution*. New York: Public Affairs, 2008.
4. Tagliareni, E, Waters, V. The aging experience. In MA Anderson, JV Braun (Eds.), *Caring for the Elderly Client*. Philadelphia: F. A. Davis, 1995, pages 2–15.
5. Palmore, EB. *Ageism: Negative and Positive*. New York: Springer, 1990.
6. Alliance for Aging Research. *Ageism: How Healthcare Fails the Elderly*. New York: Alliance for Aging Research, March 2003.
7. Simkins, CL. Ageism's influence on health care delivery and nursing practice. *Journal of Student Nursing*, 2007;1:24–28.
8. Anti-Ageism Task Force. What is ageism? In *Ageism in America*. New York: International Longevity Center; 2006. Retrieved January 19, 2013, from http://www.graypanthersmetrodetroit.org/Ageism_In_America_-_ILC_Book_2006.pdf
9. Kleyman, P. Media Ageism: The Link Between Newsrooms and Advertising Suites. Aging Today (2001 March/April). Retrieved April 25, 2008, from http://www.asaging.org/at/at-218/Media.html
10. Ferraro, KF. Aging and role transitions. In RH Binstock, LK George (Eds.), *Handbook of Aging and the Social Sciences*. 5th ed. San Diego: Academic Press, 2001.
11. Wang, M. Profiling retirees in the retirement transition and adjustment process: Examining the longitudinal change patterns of retirees' psychological well-being. *Journal of Applied Psychology*, 2007;92:455–474.
12. National Alliance for Caregiving. Caregiving in the U.S. 2005. Retrieved January 19, 2013, from http://assets.aarp.org/rgcenter/il/us_caregiving_1.pdf
13. Suitor, JJ, Pillmer, K, Keeton, S, Robison, J. Aged parents and aging children: Determinants of relationship quality. In R Blieszner, VH Bedford (Eds.), *Aging and the Family*. Westport, CT: Praeger, 1996.

14. U.S. Census Bureau. Facts for Features: Grandparent's Day 2012. July 31, 2012. Retrieved January 19, 2013, from http://www.census.gov/newsroom/releases/archives/facts_for_features_special_editions/cb12-ff17.html

15. Shapiro, ME. *Asian Culture Brief: India*. Vol. 2(4). Honolulu: National Technical Assistance Center, n.d.

16. Shapiro, ME. *Asian Culture Brief: Philippines*. Vol. 2(3). Honolulu: National Technical Assistance Center, n.d.

17. Shapiro, ME. *Asian Culture Brief: Vietnam*. Vol. 2(5). Honolulu: National Technical Assistance Center, n.d.

18. Wallis, V. *Two Old Women: An Alaska Legend of Betrayal, Courage and Survival*. Seattle, WA: Epicenter Press, 1993.

19. Kim-Rupnow, WS. *Asian Culture Brief: Korea*. Vol. 2(1). Honolulu: National Technical Assistance Center, n.d.

20. Brightman, J, Subedi, LA. *AAPI Culture Brief: Hawai'i*. Vol. 2(7). Honolulu: National Technical Assistance Center, 2007.

21. U.S. Census Bureau. The Hispanic Population: 2010. May 2011. Retrieved January 19, 2013, from http://www.census.gov/prod/cen2010/briefs/c2010br-04.pdf

22. Garcia, EC. Parenting in Mexican American families. In NB Webb (Ed.), *Culturally Diverse Parent–Child and Family Relationships: A Guide for Social Workers and Other Practitioners*. New York: Columbia University Press, 2001.

23. Carstensen, LL. Evidence for a life-span theory of socioemotional selectivity. *Current Directions in Psychological Science*, 1995;4:151–156.

24. Berkman, L, Breslow, L. *Health and Ways of Living: The Alameda County Study*. New York: Oxford University Press, 1983.

25. Kahn, R, Antonucci, T. Convoys over the life course: Attachment, roles, and social support. In P Baltes, OG Brim (Eds.), *Life-Span Development and Behavior*. New York: Academic Press, 1980.

26. Bargh, JA, McKenna, KYA. The Internet and social life. *Annual Review of Psychology*, 2004;55:573–590.

27. U.S. Census Bureau. Age and Sex Composition: 2010. May 2011. Retrieved January 19, 2013 from http://www.census.gov/prod/cen2010/briefs/c2010br-03.pdf

28. Silverstone, B, Hyman, H. *Growing Older Together*. New York: Pantheon Books, 1992.

29. Tournier, P. *Learn to Grow Old*. New York: Harper and Row, 1972.

30. Meisner, BA, Hynie, M. Ageism with heterosexism: Self-perceptions, identity, and psychological health in older gay and lesbian adults. *Gay and Lesbian Issues and Psychology Review*, 2009:5; 51–58.

31. National Resource Center on LGBT Aging. For Aging Providers: Creating LGBT-Affirming Environments. Retrieved January 19, 2013, from http://www.lgbtagingcenter.org/resources/index.cfm?a=1

32. Mancini, JA (Ed.). *Aging Parents and Adult Children*. Washington, DC: Lexington Books, 1989.

33. Dunham, CC. A link between generations: Intergenerational relations and depression in aging parents. *Journal of Family Issues*, 1995; 16:450–465.

34. MetLife and National Alliance for Caregiving. Since You Care: Long Distance Caregiving. 2008. Retrieved January 19, 2013, from http://www.metlife.com/assets/cao/mmi/publications/since-you-care-guides/mmi-long-distance-caregiving.pdf

35. Dychtwald, K. *Age Wave*. New York: Bantam Books, 1990.

36. Tamborinia, C. The never-married in old age: Projections and concerns for the future. *Social Security Bulletin*, 2007;67:25–40.

37. Connidis, IA, McMullin, JA. To have or not to have: Parent status and the subjective well-being of older men and women. *Gerontologist*, 1993;33:630–636.

38. Jordan-Marsh, M, Harden, JT. Fictive kin: Friends as family supporting older adults as they age. *Journal of Gerontological Nursing*, 2005;31:2.

39. Blieszner, R, Adams, RG. *Adult Friendship*. Newbury Park, CA: Sage, 1992.

40. Antonucci, TC. Social relations: An examination of social networks, social support, and sense of control. In JE Birren, KW Schaie (Eds.), *Handbook of the Psychology of Aging*. San Diego, CA: Academic Press, 2001.

41. MetLife Mature Market Institute. The MetLife Report on American Grandparents. July 2011.

Retrieved January 19, 2013, from https://www.metlife.com/assets/cao/mmi/publications/studies/2011/mmi-american-grandparents.pdf

42. Neugarten, BL, Weinstein, KK. The changing American grandparent. *Journal of Marriage and the Family*, 1964;26:199–204.

43. Dhjama, T. Grandparents offer an expanding market niche. *TD Monthly*. 2003. Retrieved January 18, 2013, from http://www.toydirectory.com/monthly/Aug2003/Special_Grandparents.asp

44. Grandparents Rights Organization. Home Page. Retrieved January 19, 2013, from http://www.grandparentsrights.org

45. Foundation for Grandparenting. Home Page. Retrieved January 19, 2013, from http://www.grandparenting.org

46. Road Scholar. Intergenerational Programs Page. Retrieved January 19, 2013, from http://www.roadscholar.org/programs/search_res.asp?keyword=grandchild

47. Adopt-a-Grandparent Program. Home Page. Retrieved January 25, 2013, from http://www.adoptagrandparent.org

48. Corporation for National and Community Service. Foster Grandparent Program. Retrieved January 25, 2013, from http://www.seniorcorps.gov/about/programs/fg.asp

49. Social Security Administration. Traditional Sources of Economic Security. Retrieved April 25, 2008, from http://www.ssa.gov/history/briefhistory3.html

50. Social Security Administration. *Income of the Aged Chartbook, 2004*. Washington, DC: Office of Research, Evaluation, and Statistics, 2006.

51. U.S. Census Bureau. Historical Poverty Tables. Retrieved April 25, 2008, from http://www.census.gov/hhes/www/poverty/data/histor

52. Koellin, K, et al. Vulnerable elderly households: Expenditures on necessities by older Americans. *Social Science Quarterly*, 1995;76:619–632.

53. Maddox, G (Ed.). *Encyclopedia of Aging*. New York: Springer, 1987.

54. U.S. Senate Special Committee on Aging, American Association of Retired Persons, Federal Council on the Aging, and U.S. Administration on Aging. *Aging America, Trends and Projections*. Washington, DC: U.S. Department of Health and Human Services, 1991.

55. Zemke, R, Zemke, S. 30 things we know for sure about adult learning. *Innovation Abstracts*, 1984;6:8.

56. AARP International. Global Aging. Retrieved July 16, 2013, from http://www.aarpinternational.org/explore-by-region

57. Allison, R. Easy steps to tone up retirement. *Advertising Age*, 1996;67(45):32.

58. Bennett, D. Great grandmother goes solo. *Cruising World*, 1994;19(12):8–9.

59. Clements, M. What we say about aging. *Parade Magazine*, December 12, 1993:4–5.

60. Plymouth Harbor at Sarasota Bay. About Us. Retrieved April 25, 2008, from http://www.plymouthharbor.org/about.html

61. Seniorcorp. Home Page. Retrieved April 25, 2008, from http://www.seniorcorps.com

62. Goodman, L. Between two worlds: Malidoma Somé on rites of passage. *Sun Magazine,* 2010;415

63. AARP. Home Page. Retrieved April 25, 2008, from http://www.aarp.org

64. Gray Panthers: Age and Youth in Action. Home Page. Retrieved April 25, 2008, from http://www.graypanthers.org

65. Senior Service America. Home Page. Retrieved April 25, 2008, from http://www.seniorserviceamerica.org

66. U.S. Department of Health and Human Services. Healthy People 2020. Retrieved December 2, 2010, from http://www.healthypeople.gov

67. Haber, D. *Health Promotion and Aging: Practical Applications for Health Professionals*. 4th ed. New York: Springer, 2007.

68. Anderson, M, Braun, J. *Caring for the Elderly Client*. Philadelphia: FA Davis, 1995.

69. Burrell, C. Malnutrition is common among older Americans. *Maine Sunday Telegram, Health Resources Guide*, October 13, 1996.

70. Burger, SG, Kayser-Jones, J, Prince, J. *Malnutrition and Dehydration in Nursing Homes: Key Issues in Prevention and Treatment*. Washington, DC: National Citizens' Coalition for Nursing Home Reform, The Commonwealth Fund, July 2000.

71. Ahmed, F. Effect of nutrition on the health of the elderly. *Journal of the American Dietetic Association*, 1992;92:1102–1108.

72. Wick, JY. Avoiding polypharmacy pitfalls: It's all in your approach. *Pharmacy Times,*

2006. Retrieved July 15, 2013, from http://www.pharmacytimes.com/publications/issue/2006/2006-01/2006-01-5144

73. World Health Organization. Health Expenditure, Total (% of GDP). Retrieved May 12, 2013, from http://data.worldbank.org/indicator/SH.XPD.TOTL.ZS

74. U.S. Government Printing Office. Outlays for Health Programs: 1962–2010. Retrieved April 25, 2008, from http://www.gpoaccess.gov/usbudget/fy06/sheets/hist16z1.xls

75. MetLife Mature Market Institute and LifePlans, Inc. *The MetLife Market Survey of Nursing Home and Home Care Costs*. Westport, CT: MetLife Market Institute, 2006.

76. Pfuntner, J, Dietz, F. Long-Term Care Insurance Gains Prominence. Retrieved April 25, 2008, from http://www.bls.gov/opub/cwc/cm20040123ar01p1.htm

THE PHYSIOLOGY AND PATHOLOGY OF AGING

CHARLES J. GREGORY, PhD and DAVID A. SANDMIRE, MD

It is frustrating that in a time when humans have gone into and returned from outer space and can manipulate DNA, they have not conquered death. Death, indeed, remains the last "sacred" enemy.
—Paola S. Timiras, *Physiological Basis of Aging and Geriatrics*[1]

Chapter Outline

Behavioral Objectives

Upon completion of this chapter, the reader will be able to:

1. Compare and contrast the concepts of aging as a "disease" and aging as a "process."
2. Compare and contrast preventive medicine and curative medicine.

3. Explain the difference between average life expectancy and maximum life span potential, and describe the determinants of each.
4. Compare and contrast the genetic and environmental theories of aging.
5. Explain the possible role of free radical formation in the aging process.
6. Explain the effects of aging on the various organ systems of the body.
7. Understand the concept of homeostasis—the maintenance of a stable internal environment in the body in the face of an ever-changing external environment.
8. Appreciate the interdependence among the body's organ systems and the ways in which these systems compensate for disturbances in homeostasis.
9. Describe how the compensatory capabilities of the body change with advancing age.
10. Understand the concept of *illness* as an inability of the body to adequately compensate for disturbances in homeostasis.

Key Terms

Alveoli	Heat stroke
Anemia	Homeostasis
Aneurysm	Hyposmia
Atherosclerosis	Hypothalamus
Autoimmune disease	Lipofuscin
Average life expectancy	Maximum life span potential
Benign prostatic hypertrophy	Myocardial infarction
Cataract	Non-insulin-dependent diabetes mellitus
Chronic bronchitis	Osteoarthritis
Chronic obstructive pulmonary disease	Osteoporosis
Dementia	Peptic ulcer
Diabetes mellitus	Pituitary gland
Diaphragm	Postural (orthostatic) hypotension
Diverticulosis	Presbycusis
Dysphagia	Presbyopia
Embolism	Senescence
Emphysema	Stroke
Fecal incontinence	Thrombus
Free radical	Urinary incontinence
Gastritis	Xerostomia

Whether death is seen as "our last sacred enemy" or as a necessity to conserve earth's resources, death certainly remains one of the great mysteries of our existence. How one deals with death, and the aging process that leads to it, is in large part dictated by cultural, technological, and even political beliefs.

Culture not only influences personal perspectives and family living arrangements, but also the way that scientists approach changes associated with aging (often called **senescence**) and death. Scientific enterprise is a mirror of culture, and vice versa. If society views the physiologic changes associated with aging as "diseases," researchers will do likewise. Indeed, Western medicine, with its greater emphasis on curative rather than preventive medicine, seems to favor the disease model of aging. We expend more time and resources curing cancer and treating heart attack victims than we do promoting healthful living. According to a report by the American Public Health Association, only 3% of all U.S. healthcare dollars in 2011 were spent on preventative measures,[3] and curative medicine continues to dominate our healthcare landscape. Curative medicine and the disease model of aging, in turn, help us rationalize the placement of older adults in nursing homes and other extended-care settings. If, instead, we accept senescence as a process that can be attenuated, we are likely to focus more on healthful living and preventive medicine throughout life than on a costly quick fix at the end of life.

From a strictly scientific standpoint, however, the distinction between aging and disease is, at best, a blurry one. Consider atherosclerosis, a pervasive affliction of older adults that predisposes them to hypertension, heart attacks, and strokes. Do the fatty plaques that develop in arteries result from degenerative changes that are inevitable with the passage of time or from specific injuries to the blood vessels, perhaps caused by turbulent blood flow or microbial infection? Do low-fat diets and exercise regimens merely slow down this unavoidable "phenomenon of aging"? Or is it more accurate to view healthy lifestyle habits as measures that prevent the "disease" atherosclerosis? Paola S. Timiras suggests the following distinctions be made between aging and disease:[4]

- Aging is a universal process, shared by all living organisms, whereas disease is a selective process, varying with species, organ, tissue, cell, and molecule.
- Aging is intrinsic, dependent on genetic factors, whereas disease is intrinsic and extrinsic, dependent on both genetic and environmental factors.
- Aging is always progressive, whereas disease may be discontinuous and may progress, regress, or be arrested entirely.
- Aging is always deleterious and likely to reduce functional competence, whereas disease is occasionally deleterious, often causing damage that is reversible.
- Aging is irreversible, whereas disease may be treatable and often has a known cause.

Whether you agree with these descriptors or not, there is good reason to continue refining definitions and conceptions of aging. Consider the following statistic: the **average life expectancy** in the United States has risen from about 45 years in 1900 to 78 years in 2010, an increase largely attributed to improvements in sanitation, food, and water supply and to the advent of antibiotics and vaccinations.[5–8] But during this period there has been no change in the **maximum life span potential** (MLP, that is, the oldest age reached by an individual in a population) of Americans, estimated to be about

120 years (**Figure 3-1**).[9–11] Thus, although improvements in our standard of living have helped spare us from several causes of premature death, such as cholera, tuberculosis, and influenza, they have done nothing to slow down the inherent aging process. In fact, any medical intervention that claims to slow down human aging must be shown to increase the maximum life span potential, and, to date, none have done so.

Our unchanging maximum life span potential in the face of an ever-increasing life expectancy suggests two things to those who ponder growing old. First, it supports the notion of distinguishing disease from aging. One of the most important chapters in the history of medicine has been the eradication of smallpox from the face of the earth by using vaccines. But although the child who is immunized to smallpox has been spared a devastating infectious disease, he or she is not likely to age more slowly than a nonimmunized child will. Second, a maximum life span potential that probably has not changed in centuries suggests that there exists some "biological clock" that predetermines our length of life. No such clock has been discovered, and it is perhaps an oversimplification of human physiology to suggest that one single mechanism in the body is responsible for aging. Nonetheless, it certainly appears that there are relatively fixed limits on how long the human body lasts.

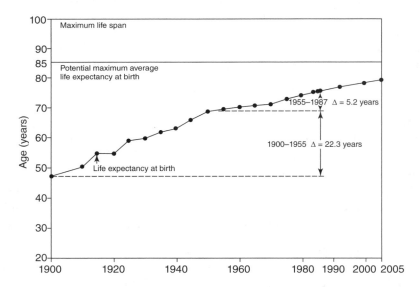

FIGURE 3-1 Life expectancy at birth and estimated maximum life span potential in the United States since 1990.
Source: Adapted from Harman, D. The aging process: major risk factors for disease and death. The Proceedings of the National Academy of Sciences, 1991;88:5362. And U.S. Department of Health and Human Services. Health: United States, 2007, Table 27, p. 192. Retrieved March 2, 2009, from http://www.cdc.gov/nchs/data/hus/hus07.pdf#027.

A fixed life span, however, does not necessarily sentence us to pain and suffering in our twilight years. Many of the physiologic changes associated with aging can be slowed to some extent with a healthy diet and consistent regimen of moderate exercise, and many of the chronic diseases prevalent in older adults are either preventable or modifiable with healthy lifestyle habits (**Table 3-1**). Reduction of dietary fat (especially saturated fats and cholesterol) lowers one's risk of coronary artery disease and stroke[12] as well as breast and colon cancer.[13,14] A program of increased physical activity increases one's resting and maximum cardiac output (the amount of blood pumped out of the heart per minute) while decreasing one's chance of developing hypertension.[4,15] To the extent

TABLE 3-1   Common Chronic Diseases of Aging Potentially Modifiable in Middle Age Through Personal Changes in Lifestyle

Disorder	Preventive Strategy
Hypertension	Reduction of dietary sodium Reduction of body weight
Atherosclerotic cardiovascular disease	Treatment of hypertension Cessation of cigarette smoking Reduction of excess body weight Reduction of dietary saturated fat and cholesterol Increased aerobic exercise
Cancers	Cessation of cigarette smoking Reduction of dietary fat Reduction of salt- or smoke-cured food intake Minimization of radiation exposure Minimization of sun exposure Minimization of environmental hazards
Chronic obstructive pulmonary disease	Cessation of cigarette smoking
Diabetes mellitus (type 2)	Reduction of excess body weight Diet consistent with atherosclerosis prevention
Osteoarthritis	Reduction of body weight
Osteoporosis	Maintenance of dietary calcium Regular exercise Cessation of cigarette smoking Avoidance of alcohol excess
Cholelithiasis (i.e., gallstones)	Reduction of body weight

Source: Reproduced from Bierman, EL, Hazzard, WP. Preventive gerontology: Strategies for attentuation of the chronic diseases of aging. In Hazzard, WR, et al. (Eds.), *Principles of Geriatric Medicine and Gerontology*, 3rd ed. New York: McGraw-Hill; 1994: 188.

that exercise helps prevent obesity, it also decreases the likelihood that one will develop osteoarthritis and non-insulin-dependent diabetes mellitus or suffer from a heart attack.[13] Regular exercise, coupled with sufficient dietary calcium intake, lowers one's risk of osteoporosis and its complications, such as broken hips and slipped intervertebral disks.[5] Along with these physical benefits, exercise appears to have psychological benefits as well, lifting one's spirits and alleviating loneliness and depression.[16] On the other hand, sedentary lifestyles and, in particular, extended bed rest increase the chance of thromboembolic disease, respiratory infection, and decubitus ulcers (bed sores). Perhaps the most important lifestyle choice one can make is to not smoke cigarettes. Indeed, cigarette smoking is the most common preventable cause of disease and death in the United States. It leads to chronic obstructive pulmonary disease (COPD, e.g., emphysema, chronic bronchitis) and lung cancer and is a major cause of other cancers of the upper respiratory and digestive tracts.[13,17] In addition, cigarette smoking enhances one's chance of developing atherosclerosis and its complications—heart attacks and strokes. In all, cigarette smoking decreases one's life expectancy by 7 years and one's disease-free years by 14.[18]

Clearly, there are many ways to enhance our health as we age, but such modifications to lifestyle, activity level, and diet must occur in early or middle life to have the maximum effect. One of the difficulties in convincing young people to adopt these measures is that, generally speaking, they already feel healthy. Persuading a teenager to quit smoking or a 40-year-old business executive to take her blood pressure medication is difficult when doing so offers them no immediate reward—delayed gratification is not something our society seems to value highly. But the tide appears to be turning, at least on some fronts, as evidenced by the growing popularity of aerobic exercise over the past three decades and the legislative effort to limit the public areas where smoking is allowed. Perhaps these societal changes will accomplish what gerontologists call the compression of morbidity—that is, decreasing the period and severity of illness experienced toward the end of life.

Human aging, in its pure form, is a process that runs a fairly predictable course from infancy to senescence. Superimposed on that developmental sequence, however, are lifestyle choices and environmental insults that influence how far we are able to travel along life's course and how well we feel along the journey. In fact, genetic makeup may account for only 25% of the variation in human longevity, with much of our health and well-being determined by environmental factors.[19] Although we may not be able to extend our maximum life span potential, we can certainly reduce the morbidity associated with aging on our way to the 12th decade. In addition, healthy lifestyles may help us accomplish what epidemiologists call a rectangularization of the survival curve—a condition where nearly everyone in a population reaches the maximum life span potential (**Figure 3-2**). Perhaps there is some truth to the observation by comedian George Burns that you can never live to be 100 if you stop living at 65.[5] Burns lived to enjoy his 100th birthday.

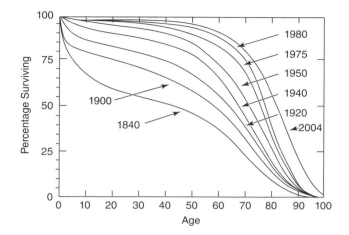

FIGURE 3-2   Specific mortality survival curve, illustrating the rectangularization occurring over the past 150 years.

Source: Adapted from Cassel, CK, Brody, JA. Demography, epidemiology, and aging. In CK Cassel (Ed.). *Geriatric Medicine.* 2nd ed. New York: Springer-Verlag, 1990, p. 17; *National Vital Statistics Reports*, 2007;56(9):6.

THEORIES OF BIOLOGICAL AGING

Although research on the aging process has proceeded for decades, we now seem as far away from the fountain of youth as we ever were. One of the stumbling blocks in senescence research is the lack of a true biological marker of aging (with the arguable exception of lipofuscin accumulation in cells, discussed later in this chapter). There is no single identifiable molecular, cellular, tissue, or organ change in the body that correlates closely with age.[20,21] Senescence appears to be a multifactorial process whose rate depends on both genetic (programmed) and environmental (damage or error) phenomena.[22–24] The following sections briefly review some of the theories of biological aging. The intent is not to suggest that any single theory explains the aging process, but rather to recognize that aging is a complex phenomenon orchestrated by events at several organizational levels in the body.

GENETIC THEORIES OF AGING

Because the stages of cellular, tissue, organ, and body development are, for the most part, controlled by our genetic machinery (i.e., programmed), many theories of aging have focused on the role of DNA (deoxyribonucleic acid), RNA (ribonucleic acid), and the proteins made from these nucleic acid "blueprints."

One such theory is that senescence results from the gradual accumulation of random mutations (alterations in the DNA) in somatic cells of the body.[25,26] According to this *somatic mutation theory*, radiation and other environmental mutagens alter the structure of the genetic code and thus change the sequence of amino acids found in enzymes and other proteins. Over time, such minor alterations could, in turn, accumulate and have damaging effects on protein function and thus on body functions. Differences in longevity among individuals might result from varying rates of mutagenesis and varying proficiencies of DNA repair. Studies have shown that longer-lived species tend to have more effective mechanisms for repairing molecular damage than do shorter-lived species.[27,28] However, although the number of DNA mutations increases with age,[29,30] proving that such changes are the cause, rather than the result, of aging has been more difficult.

Two other program-based theories, endocrine and immunological, focus on a gradual biological decline over time. In the former, biological clocks and hormone regulation control the rate of aging. In the latter, the immune system is "coded" to erode over time, thus enhancing the body's susceptibility to disease and death.

ENVIRONMENTAL THEORIES OF AGING

The *wear-and-tear theory* of aging proposes that aging is inevitable as cells, tissues, and organs, much like machines, gradually wear out from continued use. The machine analogy is not a perfect one because cells, unlike machines, have several mechanisms to repair their injuries. But with the passage of time, the damage resulting from wear and tear might accumulate to a point at which it overcomes the body's capacity for maintenance and repair. Cells (and therefore organisms) with higher rates of metabolism might "wear out" more quickly than do those with lower metabolic rates, thus aging more quickly and dying sooner.

The inverse correlation between basal metabolic rate and longevity across a wide number of species has led some experimental gerontologists to reformulate the wear-and-tear hypothesis into a rate-of-living theory of aging, which attributes interspecies variation in life span to varying metabolic rates per gram of metabolizing tissue.[31] Every organism, then, is endowed with the ability to burn up a fixed number of calories in its lifetime, after which the accumulation of wear and tear results in the organism's death. Members of a species with a higher metabolic rate would burn up their fixed number of total calories more quickly, suffer from accumulated wear and tear more rapidly, and die sooner than those of a species with a lower metabolic rate.

The well-documented effect of *caloric restriction* (i.e., limiting food intake) to increase average life expectancy seems on the surface to support the rate-of-living theory of aging.[32–37] Furthermore, a multitude of studies has shown that caloric restriction not only increases average life expectancy, but also diminishes many of the physiologic changes associated with increasing age, such as rising serum cholesterol levels,[38] decreasing bone mass,[39] and deteriorating immune system function.[40] Nonetheless, it does not appear that caloric restriction has a significant effect on an organism's specific basal metabolic rate.[41,42] The basis for its effect must therefore lie elsewhere. Furthermore, the rate-of-living theory itself has been called into question by studies that have found exceptions to the generalization that animals with lower metabolic rates live longer than those with higher metabolic rates.[43,44]

The rate-of-living theory of aging has helped focus experimental gerontology on another promising theory, the *free radical theory of aging*, which is a specific version of the wear-and-tear theory that attributes cellular (and therefore organismal) aging to random accumulating damage of macromolecules by the highly reactive by-products of oxidative metabolism known as **free radicals**.[45–50] Free radicals are molecules that contain at least one unpaired electron in their outer valence shells. Free radicals most notably form in the mitochondria of cells, the site of aerobic respiration (the "burning up of food" for energy), where electrons are stripped from temporary carrier molecules and passed down a chain of membrane-bound protein carriers to be accepted by oxygen.[51,52] Free radicals are relatively rare in nature because they are chemically unstable. When formed, they usually bind with other free radicals to create more stable molecules. However, when free radicals form in cells, they can initiate chain reactions that consume oxygen and randomly damage lipid molecules, enzymes, and nucleic acids.

One part of a cell's structure that is particularly vulnerable to chemical attack by free radicals is the lipid membrane, which bounds the cell and many of its internal organelles, such as the mitochondria, endoplasmic reticulum, and Golgi apparatus. The polyunsaturated fatty acids embedded in these membranes are major targets for free radicals. But cells have specific defenses against this lipid peroxidation, such as vitamin E (alpha-tocopherol), vitamin C (ascorbic acid), and several enzymes that arrest free radical chain reactions.[53]

If the levels of free radical "scavengers" such as vitamins E and C are depleted, however, damage to lipid membranes may be more permanent. Repeated peroxidation of unsaturated lipids can cause inappropriate cross-linking of lipids to proteins and nucleic acids.[54] The cross-linking of lipids with proteins leads to the formation of **lipofuscin** (pronounced lip-uh-*fuhs*-en; also known as age pigment). Granules of this yellowish-brown pigment are found in the cytoplasm of aged cells (**Figure 3-3**). Interestingly, the slow, predictable accumulation of lipofuscin is considered to be the most reliable marker of chronological age in cells, and it has been found in nearly every eukaryotic organism (those having cells with nuclei) studied thus far.[55,56]

Although evidence for the age-related accumulation of lipofuscin and other types of free radical–mediated cell damage is widespread, proving that free radical damage is the primary determinant of aging has been more difficult; lipofuscin accumulation, it appears, is a result, rather than a cause, of aging.[57] Recall that any intervention that truly slows down the aging process must be shown to increase the maximum life span potential of a species. And although studies in which organisms were given supplements of vitamin E throughout life revealed that the rate of lipofuscin accumulation decreased and the average life expectancy often increased, none showed a change in the maximum life span potential.[58–63]

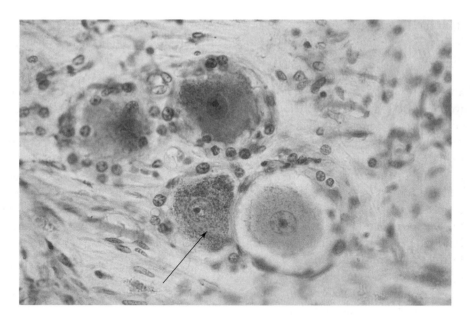

FIGURE 3-3 **Light micrograph of a dorsal root ganglion cell illustrating the accumulation of lipofuscin.**
Source: Courtesy of Allen Bell, University of New England.

Nonetheless, the potential importance of free radical–mediated destruction in aging cells should not be ignored, especially when you consider its role in disease. Consider cigarette smoking, the most common preventable cause of disease and death in the United States. The smoke from cigarettes contains free radicals whose presence can alter or destroy important biological molecules such as DNA and enzymes.[64,65] Damage to DNA, in turn, may play a role in the etiology of lung cancer, whereas damage to enzymes, such as alpha-1 antitrypsin, may cause the progressive and irreversible destruction of lung tissue in patients with emphysema (see the section titled "Respiratory System" later in this chapter). Thus, smoking may accelerate the aging process by enhancing the free radical mechanism, a process that some researchers claim is at the heart of the natural aging process.[44] You can see how the distinction between disease and pure aging becomes less clear at the cellular level.

As you can quickly realize from this review of the theories of aging, no one particular explanation for aging is completely satisfactory. As noted earlier, it is most likely that aging is a complex phenomenon orchestrated by events at several organizational levels in the body. Research efforts aimed at limiting the effects of aging will likely have to occur at multiple levels, from the molecular and cellular to the environmental. Although the causes of aging remain elusive, the effects of aging on the body are more readily apparent.

The next section focuses on the actual physiologic and pathologic changes that occur in the organ systems as we grow older.

AGE-RELATED CHANGES OF THE ORGAN SYSTEMS

INTEGUMENTARY SYSTEM

The integumentary system consists of the skin and all of its accessory structures, such as hair, nails, sebaceous (oil) glands, and eccrine (sweat) glands. From outermost in, skin consists of three major layers: the epidermis, dermis, and subcutaneous layers. Because the skin covers our bodies, changes in its appearance are the most visibly noticeable of all aging phenomena. This section focuses on the particular changes that occur in the epidermis, dermis, and subcutaneous layers with age and the consequences of those changes for the structure and function of the integumentary system (**Figure 3-4**).

The *epidermis* is a multilayered sheet of epithelial cells called keratinocytes, which are named for their production of keratin, a fibrous protein that gives this layer its strength. Interspersed among the keratinocytes are smaller numbers of melanocytes, which produce the melanin pigment that browns the skin, and dendritic (or Langerhans) cells, which

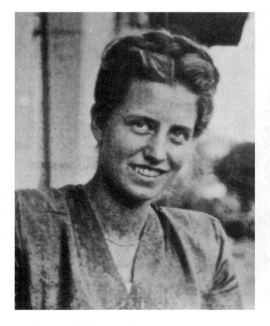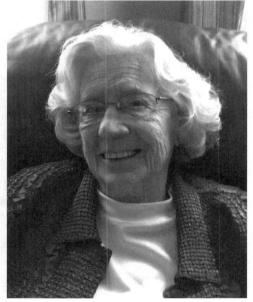

FIGURE 3-4   Change in appearance of skin with aging. The same woman is shown at (left) age 19 and (right) age 90.

play a role in the immune response, preventing the development of skin cancers, ingesting microorganisms, and in the process, stimulating white blood cells called lymphocytes.[66] The epidermal cells rest on a thin layer of protein called the basement membrane, which separates the epidermis from the underlying dermis. This membrane is normally undulated, which helps hold the two layers together. However, with age it flattens out, making the skin more vulnerable to shearing forces, abrasion, and blister formation (**Figure 3-5**).[67] Because of the everyday wear and tear on the skin, the epidermal cells must be continuously replaced with new cells that divide by mitosis in the deepest layers. The new cells slowly get pushed up through the epidermis and ultimately are shed from the skin, a process that takes about 28 days. Thus, our epidermis is completely replaced every month. The turnover rate, however, decreases by 30–50% between ages 20 and 70, which increases the time during which individual epidermal cells are exposed to carcinogens (i.e., cancer-causing agents) such as ultraviolet light from the sun.[68,69] Furthermore, the number of melanocytes, and therefore the amount of protective melanin pigment, decreases with age, making ultraviolet light more dangerous. Combined with the fact that the number of macrophage-like dendritic cells also declines with age, it becomes clear why older adults are particularly prone to developing skin cancer.

The *dermis* is a thick layer of loose connective tissue that is well supplied with blood vessels, lymphatic vessels, nerves, and accessory organs such as sweat glands, sebaceous glands, and hair follicles. The predominant cells found in the dermis are fibroblasts, mast cells, and macrophages. Fibroblasts produce and release collagen and elastin into the extracellular matrix, which gives skin its strength and elasticity. Mast cells release substances that mediate the inflammatory response following injury to the skin. The rich

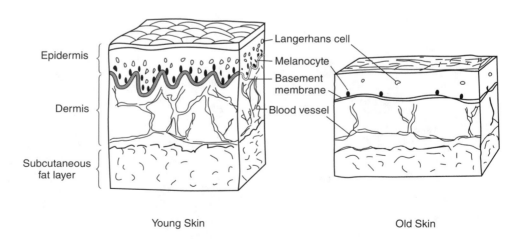

Young Skin   Old Skin

FIGURE 3-5   Changes in the structure of skin with aging. Note that older skin has: (1) a thinner epidermis, (2) a flatter basement membrane, (3) fewer melanocytes and Langerhans cells, (4) a diminished dermal blood supply, and (5) a thinner subcutaneous fat layer.

supply of blood vessels in the dermis provides oxygen and nutrients as well as an efficient mechanism for regulation of body temperature. When the body is overheated, blood flow to the dermis increases so that heat can be radiated through the skin. This, together with the action of sweat glands, allows for the release of large amounts of heat in a short period of time.

The amount of collagen and elastin in the dermis decreases as we age, accounting for the thinning and wrinkling of the skin in older adults. Loss of collagen makes the skin more susceptible to wear and tear, while loss of elastin causes skin to lose its resilience over time. The density of the dermal blood supply also decreases with age, blunting the outward signs of inflammation in elderly skin. This is particularly important to realize because older adults often lack some of the early warning signs of tissue injury (e.g., redness and swelling) from, for example, sunburn, bacterial infection, or skin cancer. The diminished blood flow to the dermis also impairs wound healing and, together with the gradual loss of functioning sweat glands, makes older adults especially vulnerable to over-heating syndromes such as **heat stroke**. The dermis contains sensory receptors called lamellated (Pacinian) and tactile (Meissner) corpuscles, which make the skin sensitive to vibration, pressure, and light touch. The gradual loss of these receptors with age decreases the *tactile sensitivity* of the skin and probably increases the threshold for pain stimuli.

The *subcutaneous layer* of the skin is largely adipose (i.e., fat) and loose connective tissue. This fat layer provides cushioning and thus protection to the underlying tissues. It also serves to insulate the body from rapid heat loss or gain. With age comes a thinning (or atrophy) of this layer, particularly in the face, backs of the hands, and soles of the feet. Loss of this fat pad on the soles can increase the physical trauma of walking and thus exacerbate other foot conditions in older adults.

Perhaps the most striking age-related changes to the integumentary system are the graying, thinning, and loss of hair. Hair follicles are specialized epidermal cells packed into cylinders rooted in the dermis. Hair growth is made possible by mitotic cell divisions at the base of the follicle, and hair color is dependent on varying amounts of melanin pigment within the specialized cells. Blonde, brown, and black hair have successively higher concentrations of melanin. With advancing years, the number of hair follicles decreases, and those follicles that remain grow at slower rates and have lower concentra-tions of melanin (because of declining numbers of melanocytes at the base of the hair follicles), causing the hair to become thin and white. Such changes over the scalp hamper hair's ability to screen the skin on the scalp from the damaging effects of sunlight.

Chronic exposure to sunlight, in fact, is the biggest scourge of aging skin. It is to the skin what cigarette smoking is to the internal organs and is largely responsible for the wrinkling, yellowing, coarseness, and irregular pigmentation of the skin with advancing years. It is also implicated in the development of several benign dermatologic lesions, such as skin tags, seborrheic keratoses, and sebaceous nevi. More important, the ultraviolet component of sunlight predisposes people to the three major forms of skin cancer: malig-nant melanoma, basal cell carcinoma, and squamous cell carcinoma. The latter two comprise more than 50% of all malignancies in the United States; malignant melanoma is the most lethal of the three and is the sixth highest in incidence among aggressive types of cancer.[70,71] Taken together, these sun-induced changes in the skin resemble an accelerated form of skin aging. Yet, despite all of the damaging effects of *photoaging*, the vanity of our youth often directs us to cultivate the "great tan" rather than to protect our skin. Again, the rewards of a great tan are immediate, whereas the benefits of skin protection come decades later. Nonetheless, if you still want to look great at 80, the use of protective hats and clothing, along with sunscreens of sun protection factor 15 (SPF-15) strength or higher, is in order.

Whereas excessive exposure to sunlight has adverse effects on the skin, some exposure is still needed to stimulate the production of vitamin D in the skin. This vitamin is needed to stimulate sufficient absorption of calcium from the small intestines into the bloodstream. The ultraviolet (UV) B radiation in sunlight stimulates the conversion of 7-dehydrocholesterol to previtamin D_3, which is further chemically converted to vitamin D. Approximately 5 to 30 minutes of sun exposure to the face, arms, legs, or back without sunscreen between 10 a.m. and 3 p.m. twice a week stimulates sufficient vitamin D production.[72] However, UV-B light exposure decreases the farther a person lives from the equator. Individuals living more than 42° of latitude north or south of the equator do not receive sufficient sunlight during the winter months to produce vitamin D.[73] Although vitamin D can be stored in adipose tissue, such individuals must nonetheless be sure that they have adequate dietary intake of vitamin D during those months. It is not currently known whether there is a minimal amount of sun exposure that stimulates sufficient vitamin D production without increasing the risk of skin cancer.[74]

NERVOUS SYSTEM

The nervous system is the principal regulatory system of the body. An intact nervous system, therefore, is requisite to the proper functioning of all the other systems. The central nervous system (CNS), consisting of the brain, brain stem, and spinal cord, regulates and monitors peripheral activities via the nerves, the communication networks that form the peripheral nervous system (PNS). The *neuron* is the functional unit of the nervous system, capable of transmitting electrochemical impulses (or messages) over its cell body and cell extensions (the axon and dendrites). (See **Figure 3-6**.) Neurons form functional boundaries, or *synapses*, with other neurons and with target structures such as muscles and glands. In response to electrochemical impulses, signaling chemicals called *neurotransmitters* are released from neurons at these synapses to bind with and activate (or inhibit) the next cell in the sequence. The number of neurons in the nervous system is relatively fixed early in life because most mature neurons lack the ability to divide. Although there is evidence to the contrary,[75] the continued development of the nervous system throughout life (to make possible learning and memory formation, for example) is not attributed to an increase in the number of cells, but most likely to an increase in

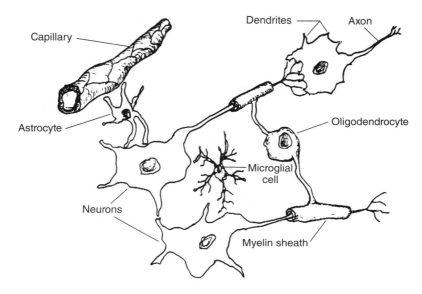

FIGURE 3-6   Neurons and related neuroglial cells.

the complexity of neuronal circuits (resulting from axonal sprouting) and to intracellular modifications. More than 100 billion neurons are distributed throughout the nervous system, and any single neuron can synapse with several hundred other neurons. The neurons are supported by an even larger number of *neuroglial cells* (e.g., astrocytes, microglial cells, and oligodendrocytes) that help nourish, protect, and myelinate the neurons. Given these considerations, you can understand the claim that the human nervous system is the most complex functioning system in nature.

Because of its complexity and relative inaccessibility to study, the nervous system is probably the least understood of all body systems. Thus, we know relatively little about the effects of aging on the central nervous system. Furthermore, the age-related microscopic structural alterations to this system are typically unobservable until autopsy. And even at autopsy, it is often difficult to distinguish disease-related changes from changes resulting from normal aging. Our meager progress in understanding the brain is reflected in the fact that CNS disorders remain one of the most common causes of disability in older adults, accounting for almost 50% of disability in those older than 65 years.[76] Nonetheless, some generalizations can be made concerning the appearance of the aged brain. Whereas the total number of neurons does not change much during healthy aging, certain parts of the nervous system such as the hippocampus, cerebellum, raphe nucleus, locus ceruleus, and nucleus basalis show decreases in neuron numbers. Interestingly, Alzheimer's disease, a condition whose incidence rises as people grow older, is also marked by a loss of neurons in the locus ceruleus and nucleus basalis, though this loss is far greater than that in the normal, aging brain. Parkinson's disease, like Alzheimer's disease, rises in incidence with age and is also marked by local loss of neurons, primarily in the substantia nigra.[77]

Important structural and functional alterations in neurons occur as people age. *Axons* in some parts of the nervous system lose moderate amounts of myelin (a lipid wrapping around the axon that increases the speed of the nerve impulse) or become swollen with age. These changes may contribute to the 10% decrease in nerve impulse conduction velocity noted with aging, a phenomenon that is partly responsible for the slowed reaction time and speed of mental processing in older adults.[78,79] The degree of branching of *dendrites* decreases with age, whereas the number of synapses between neurons remains fairly stable. There appears to be a decline in function of the neurotransmitter signaling mechanisms as well. These changes probably impair communication throughout the nervous system.

The nervous system utilizes several different neurotransmitters, some of which are excitatory and some of which are inhibitory. The more well-characterized neurotransmitters include acetylcholine, dopamine, gamma-aminobutyric acid (GABA), serotonin, and glycine. Individual neurons may store and release more than one type of neurotransmitter. The smooth functioning of the nervous system appears to rely on the appropriate balance in activity among the various neurotransmitters. The neurotransmitter dysfunction that occurs with aging has more to do with a loss of this balance than with an absolute loss of any one particular neurotransmitter.

Like any other organ system, the nervous system is vulnerable to the effects of atherosclerosis with advancing age. As fatty plaques narrow cerebral arteries, blood flow to the brain diminishes. Blood clots (thrombi) developing in these narrowed arteries can block off the blood supply completely. Within minutes, brain tissue deprived of oxygen can be irreversibly damaged, resulting in infarction of tissue. The symptoms of this particular type of stroke depend on which area of the brain has been damaged. Repeated episodes of cerebral infarction can lead to multi-infarct dementia, which accounts for 8–29% of all cases of dementia in older adults, surpassed in frequency only by Alzheimer's disease, which accounts for about 50–80% of the total.[80,81] Interestingly, the risk for developing this vascular dementia appears to be 100 times greater than normal in individuals with prematurely shortened telomeres, those protective end segments of DNA whose length appears to dictate the number of times that a cell will be able to divide.[82] **Dementia** should be distinguished from the memory loss that typically occurs with age. Although most mental functions do not decline with age, mild loss of memory for recent events is quite common, whereas long-term memory remains intact in most cases. Dementia, on the other hand, is less common.

Aspects of one's intelligence appear to change with aging. *Crystallized intelligence* refers to transfer-of-learning skills, or one's ability to apply previously learned concepts to new tasks, whereas *fluid intelligence* is the ability to organize information in new ways and generate novel ideas or hypotheses about phenomena. Although our overall intelligence quotient (IQ) remains fairly stable throughout adult life, the subcomponents of intelligence do change as we age. Crystallized intelligence increases with age, perhaps because a lifetime of experiences and the cumulative exposure to ideas gives older adults a broader knowledge base to apply to problems. In contrast, fluid intelligence decreases with age, and older adults frequently score lower on timed tests of cognitive performance because they require more decision-making time and favor a slow, deliberate approach to tasks.[83]

Gradual impairment of *locomotor function* is an important contributor to disability in older adults. Chief among these symptoms are a slowing of fine motor tasks, diminished postural reflexes, and alteration of the gait, or pattern of walking. The confident, long stride of youth changes to a more hesitant, broad-based gait as people age. Such deficiencies in motor skills have been attributed primarily to an overall decrease in function of motor control centers in the brain, such as the basal nuclei, cerebellum, and cerebral cortex. However, they result in part from diminished sensory input to these areas as well as diminished *proprioception* (sense of body position), *vestibular sensation* (sense of head movement), and *kinesthetic sensation* (sense of body movement). These may all decrease slightly in typical aging. Interestingly, many of the characteristics of the elderly stride, such as the tentative, shuffling steps and stooped posture, are similar to those seen in individuals with Parkinson's disease, the only difference being those with the disease show more severe impairments. These changes in balance and movement place older adults at risk for falls.

Finally, the aging process brings about notable changes in the pattern and quality of *sleep* one gets. The total amount of time spent sleeping changes little over the course of a lifetime, but as one ages, episodes of sleep are shorter and more frequent. The proportion of stages 3 and 4 sleep decreases with advancing years. These are the deepest levels of sleep and are thought to be, physiologically speaking, the most rejuvenating forms of slumber. Indeed, about one-third of the elderly population complains of insomnia.[84]

SPECIAL SENSES

Vision   All of the special sensory systems undergo changes with aging. The changes in vision result from alterations in the structure of a number of the components of the visual system (**Figure 3-7**). The cornea and the lens are the principal focusing structures in the eye; they refract (or bend) incoming light rays so that images can be brought into focus on the retina in the back of the eye. Both the cornea and lens undergo predictable changes. The convex *cornea* is the thin and transparent anterior border of the eye. With advancing years, it becomes thicker and more opaque. The biconvex *lens* is transparent, consisting of several layers of crystallin lens protein. Its attachment to the surrounding sphincter-shaped ciliary muscle allows us to regulate its curvature. To focus on near objects, the ciliary muscle contracts, causing the lens to become rounder (a process called *accommodation*). Conversely, to focus on distant objects, the ciliary muscle relaxes and the lens flattens out.

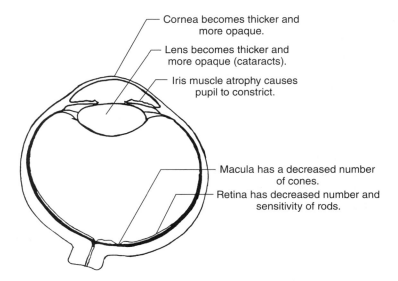

Cornea becomes thicker and more opaque.

Lens becomes thicker and more opaque (cataracts).

Iris muscle atrophy causes pupil to constrict.

Macula has a decreased number of cones.

Retina has decreased number and sensitivity of rods.

FIGURE 3-7   The structure of the eye and its age-related changes.

With age, the lens increases in anterior–posterior diameter as successive layers of crystallin protein are laid down. It also becomes more opaque as its proteins become increasingly oxidized, glycosylated, and cross-linked (see earlier theories of aging)—severe degrees of which cause **cataracts**. These molecular changes render the lens less elastic and more rigid, which significantly impairs accommodation and thus the ability to focus on near objects, a condition called **presbyopia**. This change is so universal that nearly everyone older than 55 needs corrective convex lenses to read.[85]

The *iris* is a pigmented ring of tissue whose opening, or pupil, regulates the amount of light entering the eye. Two sets of smooth muscle, the dilator (radial) and constrictor (circular) muscles, regulate the diameter of the pupil. Over time, the dilator muscle atrophies to a greater extent than the constrictor muscle, causing the average diameter of the pupil to decrease. The *retina* is the photoreceptive surface in the back of the eye. It is covered with highly sensitive *rods* (which detect white light) and less sensitive *cones* (which detect colored light). With aging comes increased lipofuscin accumulation in these photoreceptive cells, a change that might cause cell death.[86] Both the number and photosensitivity of the rods decrease with age, which, coupled with the inability to completely dilate the pupils, makes night vision more difficult for the elderly. There is also a gradual loss of cones, which are normally densely packed in the *macula* of the retina. This may contribute to the decreased visual acuity common with aging. Possibly related to these changes is age-related macular degeneration, one of the most common causes of blindness among older adults in the United States.[87]

Hearing   As with vision, impairment of hearing is common in older adults, affecting about 40% of those older than 63 years and 64% of those age 80 and older; it is the third most common chronic disease in the elderly.[88,89] We normally hear and interpret sounds through a multistep process that converts sound waves (air pressure) into nerve impulses (**Figure 3-8**). The sound waves travel through the external auditory canal and set the *tympanic membrane* (eardrum) into vibration, which in turn causes the lever-like *ossicles* (middle ear bones) to vibrate, all at the same frequency as the original sound. The smallest ossicle "taps" on the oval window, which creates a fluid pressure wave that travels through the *cochlea* of the inner ear. Specialized cochlear *hair cells* sense this wave and generate nerve impulses that travel via the auditory nerve to the brain stem and brain. Hair cells at the base of the spiral-shaped cochlea are sensitive to high-pitched sounds, whereas hair cells at the apex are sensitive to low-pitched sounds. Hearing impairment related to problems of the outer ear canal (e.g., excessive wax) or middle ear (e.g., damage to the ossicles or middle ear infection) is called conductive hearing loss, whereas difficulty hearing caused by alteration of the inner ear or auditory nerve function (e.g., Meniere's disease or acoustic neuroma) is called sensorineural hearing loss.

With aging comes a gradual, progressive hearing loss called **presbycusis**. Presbycusis is the most common form of sensorineural hearing loss in adults. Men are affected more than women, and urban dwellers suffer greater losses than those living in rural areas (suggesting a role played by chronic exposure to environmental noise). The degree of loss is more severe for high-frequency sounds than for low-frequency sounds. This selectivity suggests that the origin of the problem is in the inner ear and/or the nerve pathways to and through the brain. Cochlear hair cells near the base of the cochlea, for example, accumulate lipofuscin in proportion to the degree of high-frequency loss. Other likely mechanisms for age-related damage include altered mechanical function of the basilar membrane (on which the hair cells sit), damage to the neurons in the auditory nerve, and diminished blood flow to the cochlea. The selective loss of high-frequency hearing makes

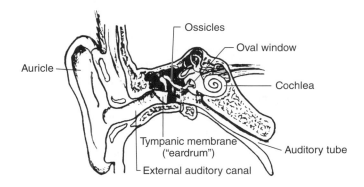

FIGURE 3-8   The auditory system.

it especially difficult for the elderly to hear consonants. Vowel sounds, on the other hand, are lower pitched and can still be heard fairly well. Overall, these changes cause speech to sound muffled. Many elderly compensate for this loss by lip-reading, which is easier to do for consonant sounds than for vowel sounds. Hearing conversations in a crowded room can be difficult for an elderly person, not only because of the presbycusis, but also because older adults have a diminished ability to localize sound and to ignore those sounds that are deemed less important.

Taste   There appears to be a decline in sensitivity to taste with age as well. Our ability to taste results from the activation of taste cells, which are clustered together in the taste buds on our tongue and other regions of the oral cavity. Nerves transmit this information to the brain stem and on to higher centers in the brain. Taste buds have been classically described as being of five types—sweet, sour, bitter, salty, and umami (oo-mom'-ee)—which are regionally distributed over the tongue. The degree of taste impairment with age seems to vary from taste to taste, being least profound for sweet and most profound for salt.[90] The decline in taste is consistent with the age-related loss in the number of taste buds on the tongue, but may also be caused by the decreased production of saliva and resultant dry mouth older adults experience with aging. Older adults also have more difficulty gauging the intensities of tastes and identifying individual tastes, such as salty, in a mixture of flavors. This impairment may cause older individuals to add excessive amounts of salt to foods, which could be detrimental, particularly if they have hypertension or congestive heart failure.

Smell   Another functional decline with important ramifications is the impairment of the ability to smell, a condition known as **hyposmia**. Similar to taste, the degree of impairment varies with the particular odor, and the ability to identify individual odors in a mixture is gradually lost with age. Interestingly, men are more profoundly affected than women are. Smell is made possible by the activation of sensory cells in the upper mucosal surface of the nasal cavity, which pass the sensory information through the bony roof into the *olfactory bulb* at the base of the frontal lobe. From there, the information is processed and relayed through the *olfactory tract* to higher brain centers. As you might expect, there is an age-related decline in the numbers of mucosal sensory cells and olfactory bulb relay cells, accounting for the decreased sensitivity to smell.

Because of the crucial role played by smell in distinguishing the tastes of different foods, hyposmia makes foods less desirable, causing a decreased appetite and irregular eating habits with subsequent weight loss and malnutrition in the elderly. In addition, the inability to smell can have dire consequences if a person fails to notice a poison gas leak or other toxic inhalant. Older adults, for example, have a 10 times higher threshold than younger individuals for the smell of ethyl mercaptan, an odiferous substance added to propane gas to warn individuals of gas leakage.[91] Clearly, the sense of smell has protective value.

MUSCULOSKELETAL SYSTEM

Musculoskeletal dysfunction is a major cause of disability in older adults, altering mobility, fine motor control, and the mechanics of respiration. As a result, older adults are more prone to falls (and thus fractures), respiratory infections, and the general physiologic decline that accompanies an increasingly sedentary lifestyle. One of the most significant changes in the aging skeleton is **osteoporosis**. Defined as a reduction in bone mass and bone density, this condition predisposes an individual to fractures, especially in the vertebrae, proximal femur, and distal radius. In the United States, an estimated 10 million people over the age of 50 have osteoporosis, and another 34 million have lower than normal bone mass. About 1.6 million fractures per year result from osteoporosis, the morbidity of which accounts for about $22 billion in healthcare costs annually.[92–94] The average lifetime cost for the care of an individual's hip fracture is about $81,000. Clearly, with the shifting demographics of the U.S. population and the aging of the baby boomer generation, these costs will rise further over the next few years.[93] Important risk factors for osteoporosis include estrogen depletion (in postmenopausal women), calcium deficiency (exacerbated in older adults because of decreased intestinal absorption of calcium), decreased bone mass at the end of development, physical inactivity, testosterone depletion (in males), alcoholism, and cigarette smoking. The loss of bone mass in the vertebrae and the thinning of the intervertebral disks account for a gradual decrease in height of about 2 inches between ages 20 and 70.[95] Collapse or severe wedging of the vertebrae cause the characteristic appearance of kyphosis, an exaggerated convex curvature of the upper spine leading to a "hunch-backed" posture. Concomitant deformity of the rib cage can alter the normal mechanics of breathing. At about age 40, the rate of bone resorption surpasses the rate of new bone formation, with a subsequent loss of about 40% of total bone mass in women and 30% in men over the course of the life span.[96] Bone resorption is most extreme in the inner spongy bone at the enlarged ends (epiphyses) and along the inside rim of long bones, making older bones more vulnerable to fractures from both compression and lateral impact.

Osteoarthritis, also called degenerative joint disease, is the second most common cause of disability in this country, affecting more than 27 million Americans.[97,98] Its incidence increases with age, affecting about 30% of those between the ages of 45 to 64, 50% of those older than 65 years, and 85% of those older than 75 years.[99] It is estimated that almost 10% of men and 18% of women aged 60 and older worldwide have symptoms related to osteoarthritis.[100] So common is this disease in older adults that, for many years, it was believed to be a normal aspect of aging. More recent histological studies, however, have revealed clear differences in joint and cartilage structure between the healthy aged and those with osteoarthritis. Osteoarthritis is marked by ulceration and destruction of joint cartilage, leading eventually to exposure and destruction of underlying bone. The normal cushioning effect of cartilage is lost, causing bone to rub on bone. As you might guess, the weight-bearing joints are the most commonly affected (e.g., knee and hip joints), and obesity is a major risk factor. Osteoarthritis is the most common cause of total knee and hip replacements,[101] but other highly used, freely movable joints, such as the proximal and distal interphalangeal joints of the fingers, are also commonly affected. Inflamed joints are marked by pain, swelling, and decreased range of motion. Other less common forms of arthritis that increase in incidence with age include rheumatoid arthritis, gout, pseudogout, and polymyalgia rheumatica.

Skeletal muscle undergoes changes with aging as well. Overall, the number of skeletal muscle fibers (cells) decreases with age,[102] although the rate of decline varies from muscle to muscle. For example, little change is noted in the diaphragm, the primary breathing muscle that never relaxes for more than a few seconds; muscles used less frequently, such as those of the extremities, exhibit greater rates of muscle fiber loss. Other microscopic changes in aging skeletal muscle include a variable decrease in muscle fiber size (atrophy) and capillary supply, an increase in deposition of lipofuscin and adipose (fat) cells, and a spotty loss of the motor neuron innervation. These microscopic changes result in a gradual decline in muscle strength and efficiency over time, although this too varies from one muscle group to the next. It cannot be overemphasized, however, that regular physical training can improve muscle strength and endurance, even in the very old.[103] This fact, coupled with the benefits of exercise in maintaining bone strength and cardiovascular fitness, argues for a cautioned exercise regimen for almost everyone.

CARDIOVASCULAR SYSTEM

The cardiovascular system consists of the *heart* and *blood vessels*. It is responsible for the circulation of blood that allows for delivery of oxygen and nutrients to, and removal of waste products from, all parts of the body. Damage to this system, therefore, can have negative implications for the entire body. The *ventricles* of the heart generate pressure that propels blood through arteries, arterioles, capillaries (the site of nutrient and waste exchange), venules, and finally veins, the blood vessels that return blood to the *atria* of the heart. The left ventricle has the thickest muscular wall and pumps blood out to the body systems (via higher pressure *systemic circulation*) while the right ventricle pumps blood to the lungs (via lower pressure *pulmonic circulation*). (See **Figure 3-9.**)

The significance of cardiovascular disease in middle-aged and elderly adults cannot be overemphasized. It is the most common cause of death worldwide. Although mortality resulting from cardiovascular disease has been decreasing in the United States since the late 1960s, probably as a result of healthier diets, increased exercise, less smoking, and better control of hypertension (high blood pressure), it is nonetheless still a major killer.

Although the heart may increase in size considerably as a result of chronic congestive heart failure, its size and weight change little with age in healthy individuals. Nevertheless, the heart exhibits several structural alterations with advancing years. Lipofuscin is deposited at a regular rate and mitochondrial DNA is damaged in cardiac muscle cells. Adipose tissue accumulates in and around the heart. The inner lining, or endocardium, undergoes

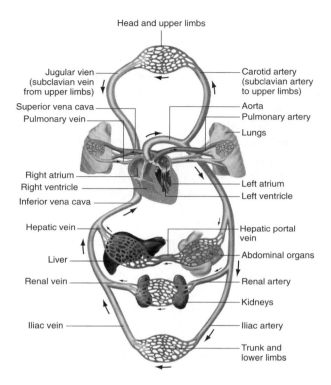

FIGURE 3-9   The cardiovascular system.
Note: The arrows indicate the direction of blood.

fibrosis (i.e., scarring), and there is a gradual loss of specialized conduction cells (auto-rhythmic cells) that coordinate events of the cardiac conduction system.

Coinciding with these changes are important functional alterations. The resting *cardiac output*, defined as the total volume of blood pumped out of the heart in 1 minute while at rest, decreases by 1% per year after age 30.[95] To understand the reasons for this, you must be familiar with the determinants of cardiac output, which is computed by multiplying *heart rate* (in beats per minute) by *stroke volume* (the volume of blood pumped out of the ventricle in one contraction). A decline in resting cardiac output with age is primarily caused by a decrease in stroke volume. This decrease is caused in part by a decreased efficiency of cardiac muscle as well as a decreased responsiveness of the heart to the sympathetic nervous system, the branch of the nervous system whose effect is normally to increase the strength of the heart's contraction, or *contractility*.

Other factors influencing stroke volume, and therefore cardiac output, are preload and afterload work requirements placed on the heart. *Preload* is a measure of the amount of blood filling the ventricles just prior to contraction. When the volume of blood filling the ventricles increases, the heart responds by contracting more strongly, pumping out more blood to keep pace. Conversely, a decreased preload causes a weaker contraction. This phenomenon, known as *Starling's law of the heart*, ensures that blood does not get backed up in the venous circulation. However, with aging comes change in the elasticity and smooth muscle of venous walls and subsequent dilations, or varicosities, of veins. This increases the capacity of veins to hold blood and decreases the rate of venous return to the heart, ultimately causing a decreased preload and cardiac output. Afterload is a measure of pressure against which ventricles must pump to force blood out into arteries. All other things being equal, the greater the afterload, the smaller the stroke volume, and therefore cardiac output. Systemic hypertension is defined as a resting blood pressure greater than 140 mmHg/90 mmHg on three separate occasions or the condition of being treated with antihypertensive medications. Hypertension is more prevalent in the aged population. In the United States, more than 70% of men and women aged 75 and older have hypertension.[104]

Hypertension increases afterload and thus reduces cardiac output. Successful treatment of high blood pressure, therefore, reduces the workload placed on the heart and thus the severity of heart disease. It has become clear in the past 15 years that for those people in their 50s and older, an elevated systolic blood pressure (i.e., the higher number in the blood pressure measurement) is an even more significant risk factor for strokes and other hypertension-related complications than is an elevated diastolic blood pressure (i.e., the lower number).[105] Thus, much emphasis has been placed in the healthcare arena on treatment of isolated systolic hypertension in older adults.

Despite cardiovascular changes associated with aging, cardiac output generally remains sufficient for the body's resting needs well into old age. It is during physical exertion that the decreased work capacity of the heart becomes more evident. During exercise, heart rate and stroke volume normally rise to meet the body's increased metabolic needs. These changes, which are part of the so-called fight-or-flight response to stress, occur largely under the direction of the sympathetic nervous system. At the same time that the heart is working harder, the sympathetic nervous system preferentially redirects blood flow to skeletal muscles, the brain, and heart muscle while limiting blood flow to "less vital" organs of the digestive, reproductive, and urinary systems. But these normal responses to exercise are dampened as we age, largely because of decreased sympathetic nervous system activity. The maximum heart rate during exercise, calculated roughly as 220 minus one's age, decreases with advancing years. Thus, during exercise, older adults become short of breath (*dyspnea*) and tire more quickly than do younger individuals. A related problem, probably also caused in part by insufficient sympathetic nervous system activity, is **postural**, or **orthostatic**, **hypotension**, which is a fall in systemic blood pressure upon rising from a supine to a standing position (usually too quickly). It can cause lightheadedness when a person stands up and can thus increase the risk of falling.

These age-related changes in heart structure and function may result from aging per se or from an increasingly sedentary lifestyle or a combination of both. Because regular exercise improves cardiac functioning in the young and middle-aged, it is likely to have similar benefits in older adults, provided the regimen is safe and commensurate with an individual's abilities. In fact, one study found that healthy 60- to 71-year-old subjects improved their maximal oxygen consumption (a measure of physical fitness) in response to regular exercise to the same relative extent as younger individuals did, independent of initial level of fitness.[106] In another study, a meta-analysis of 13 studies, individuals older than age 60 experienced an 8.4% decline in resting heart rate following an endurance training regimen.[107]

The predominant change that occurs in blood vessels with age is **atherosclerosis**, defined as the development of fatty plaques and proliferation of connective tissue in the walls of arteries. Slow destruction of the arterial wall can lead to blockage of the artery, particularly when a blood clot develops on its damaged surface. So prevalent is this condition that one may argue it is an inevitable phenomenon of aging. And although the clinical consequences of atherosclerosis are often sudden and life-threatening (e.g., heart attacks and strokes) and come toward the end of life, it has become clear in recent years that the earliest evidence of fatty accumulation is detectable in the first decade of life, and that lesions progress throughout life.

Knowledge of the normal structure of the artery wall is necessary to understand the changes of atherosclerosis. The three major layers of arteries, from the innermost out, are the intima, media, and externa (**Figure 3-10A**). The *intima* is a thin layer of connective

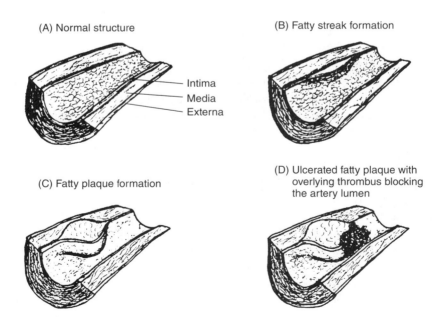

(A) Normal structure

(B) Fatty streak formation

Intima
Media
Externa

(C) Fatty plaque formation

(D) Ulcerated fatty plaque with overlying thrombus blocking the artery lumen

FIGURE 3-10 The progressive changes in arteries resulting from atherosclerosis.

tissue covered on the inner surface by endothelial cells. The *media* is primarily smooth muscle, bounded on its inner and outer surfaces by elastic connective tissue. The *externa* is a connective tissue layer containing tiny blood vessels (vasa vasorum) that nourish the outer half of the arterial wall. The inner half of an artery wall receives its nutrients by direct diffusion from blood in the lumen of an artery.

According to one widely held theory of atherogenesis (fatty plaque formation), white blood cells called monocytes adhere to the surface of the intima in areas where microscopic damage has occurred (e.g., because of turbulent blood flow). These cells transform into macrophages and begin to ingest lipids from the bloodstream. Lipids and proteins from blood begin to accumulate in the intra- and extracellular spaces of the intima and media as endothelial, smooth muscle, and macrophage cells begin to proliferate. As lipid deposits enlarge, they become visible as *fatty streaks*, which form as early as the first decade of life (**Figure 3-10B**). As fatty deposits grow and the arterial wall thickens, cells of the intima and media are forced farther away from their nutrient supplies and ultimately die and disintegrate, leaving behind a fatty paste, or *atheroma*. In an effort to contain the damage, fibroblasts form a fibrous connective tissue capsule around the atheroma. The encapsulated lesion, referred to as a *fibrous* (or *fatty*) *plaque*, appears as early as the second decade of life (**Figure 3-10C**).

Fatty plaques create several problems for us as we age. First, enlargement of fatty deposits may partially or completely block blood flow through the artery. Second, thickening of artery walls makes them more rigid, which in turn can raise systolic blood pressure and increase the afterload work requirement of the heart. Third, destruction of the inner layers of the artery wall can weaken it and cause it to balloon out under the force of blood pressure. These dilations, called **aneurysms**, are prone to rupturing and causing severe internal bleeding. Finally, breaks in the fibrous capsule of fatty plaques can cause ulcerations, leaving underlying fat deposits exposed to the bloodstream. This is ominous because such ulcerations attract platelets from the bloodstream, which clump and release substances that stimulate formation of a blood clot, or **thrombus** (**Figure 3-10D**). Enlarging thrombi can quickly occlude arteries, or break off and travel farther down the bloodstream to lodge in a smaller vessel, a phenomenon known as **embolism**.

Complications of atherosclerosis begin as early as the fourth decade of life and increase in frequency with each succeeding decade. Particular consequences of the disease depend on the artery or arteries involved. Blockage of coronary arteries can cause **myocardial infarction** (heart attack), whereas occlusion or rupture of a cerebral artery can result in a **stroke**. The development of fatty plaques in the renal arteries can cause hypertension and kidney failure, whereas blockage of an artery in the leg can cause peripheral vascular disease marked by severe pain (called claudication) and ulcerations of the skin. Although nearly everyone is prone to some degree of atherosclerosis, there are several risk factors that seem to accelerate the disease process. They include age, genetic predisposition, hypertension, diabetes mellitus, high blood cholesterol level, cigarette smoking, obesity, poor physical fitness, and "type A" personality. The confluence of many of these risk factors in older adults makes complications of atherosclerosis more prevalent in this age group. Heart attacks are more common in individuals older than age 50, and the coronary artery disease that causes heart attacks is the number one killer of people in the United States.[108] Worldwide, cardiovascular disease accounts for about 30% of all deaths.[109] Unfortunately, warning signs of an impending heart attack are not always as obvious in the elderly population and those with diabetes mellitus, making immediate treatment less likely. Peripheral vascular disease, by some estimates, affects more than 30% of individuals older than 80.[110] And although the lifetime risk of stroke at age 65 has decreased over the past 40 years, it is still high (14.5% in men and 16.1% in women).[111] Given the increased risk of atherosclerosis in older adults, it makes good sense for everyone, young or old, to eat right, exercise, keep trim, avoid cigarettes, and comply with any prescribed blood pressure medications. Indeed, as is true of most preventive health measures, these interventions are more effective if initiated early in life.

RESPIRATORY SYSTEM

The function of the respiratory system is to transport oxygen to and remove carbon dioxide from the bloodstream. The air breathed in is warmed, humidified, and cleansed as it passes successively through the mouth and nasal cavities, pharynx, larynx, trachea, and bronchi to reach the lungs (**Figure 3-11**). In the lungs, inhaled air continues through

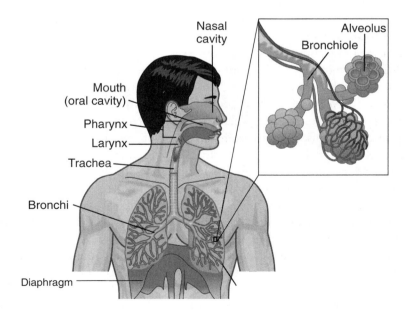

FIGURE 3-11 The respiratory system.

smaller bronchi, bronchioles, and alveolar ducts to finally reach **alveoli**, the tiny, thin-walled air sacs covered by capillaries that are the major site of gas exchange between air and the bloodstream. The 300 million alveoli in the lungs account for most of the lung volume and provide about 75 square meters of surface area for gas transport to and from the blood. The lungs, located in the thoracic cavity (or thorax), are enclosed by the rib cage and **diaphragm**, a dome-shaped skeletal muscle located beneath the lungs. During inhalation, the diaphragm contracts, lowering the floor of the thorax while external inter-costal muscles between the ribs contract to swing the ribs forward and upward. Both of these actions help expand the thorax, creating a vacuum-like effect that draws air into the respiratory tract and lungs. The lungs expand passively during this process because of their adherence to the inner thorax wall. Exhalation is normally a passive process whereby the relaxation of breathing muscles causes the thorax to contract down to a smaller volume, largely by elastic recoiling of the rib cage and lung tissue. The elastic recoiling (and lower-ing of volume) of lungs during exhalation results from two factors (**Figure 3-12A**):

- The tendency of individual alveoli to become smaller at lower air pressures because of the surface tension generated by a watery inner alveolar lining
- The recoiling of elastic tissue around respiratory airways that was stretched out during inhalation

Elastic tissue in the lungs is tethered between alveoli and bronchioles in a way that actually prevents bronchioles from completely collapsing during exhalation. Elastic recoil-ing of the rib cage and lungs decreases thoracic volume, thus increasing air pressure in the thorax and creating a necessary pressure gradient to force much of the air back out of the respiratory system.

A major indicator of pulmonary fitness is *forced vital capacity (FVC)*, defined as the maximal volume of air breathed out during one forced exhalation after maximal inhala-tion. The normal FVC in adults is 3 to 4 L in women and 4.5 to 5.5 L in men. FVC increases with growth of the body during childhood, adolescence, and early adulthood, reaching a peak at about age 25. Thereafter, FVC declines at a steady rate of about 21 mL/year, primarily because of changes in soft tissue of the lungs.[112] As we age, elastin fibers in the lungs are altered, probably by both excessive cross-linking between fibers and break-age of individual fibers. As a result, the lungs, as a whole, lose some of their elastic recoil, and the small bronchioles tend to partially or completely collapse during exhalation, causing obstruction of airflow and trapping of air in the alveoli (**Figure 3-12B**). Air trap-ping decreases the rate of oxygen delivery to and carbon dioxide delivery from the blood-stream. In addition, air trapping in alveoli increases *residual volume*, which is the volume of air remaining in the lungs after a forced exhalation. Because *total lung capacity* (or maximum volume of air that the lungs can hold) changes little in a healthy aging person, any increase in residual volume comes at the expense of decreasing FVC. Further hamper-ing of gas exchange occurs with age as a result of a gradual loss of alveolar wall surface area, estimated to be a 4% decline per decade after age 30.[113] These changes in lung

(A) Normal elastic recoil of the alveoli and unobstructed bronchiolar airflow in healthy lungs.

(B) Decreased elastic recoil of alveoli and obstructed bronchiolar airflow noted with emphysema.

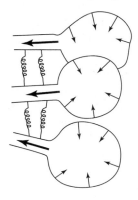 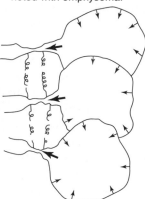

FIGURE 3-12   Elastic recoiling.

elasticity and alveolar surface area are similar to, but smaller in scale than, the changes that occur in emphysema.

Coupled with changes in lung tissue are changes in mechanical properties of the thorax wall. As we grow older, the rib cage stiffens largely because of calcification of cartilage between ribs and vertebrae, and the exaggerated curvature of the thoracic spine (kyphosis). These skeletal changes limit mobility of the rib cage, making it difficult for external intercostal muscles (as well as the accessory muscles of inhalation, such as the sternocleidomastoid and pectoralis major and minor) to expand the rib cage. Although a healthy elderly person might breathe adequately to meet the body's needs at rest, the previously described changes may limit his or her tolerance for exercise, especially when coupled with the age-related decrease in cardiac output described earlier in this chapter. Thus, it is not surprising that older adults, in general, experience shortness of breath (dyspnea) more quickly during exercise than do younger individuals.

Superimposed on the normal age-related changes to the respiratory system are certain diseases that increase in frequency from the fifth decade of life onward. They include emphysema, chronic bronchitis, pneumonia, and lung cancer. Together, the first two are referred to as **chronic obstructive pulmonary disease** (COPD), and along with lung cancer, are caused primarily by cigarette smoking or chronic exposure to unhealthy air. The steps leading to **emphysema** begin when cigarette smoke irritates the respiratory tract, stimulating proliferation of white blood cells called macrophages. These macrophages release chemicals that attract large numbers of another type of white blood cell, neutrophils, to the inflamed area. Neutrophils, in turn, release protease enzymes, one of which, called elastase, can damage elastin proteins found in elastic tissue of the lungs. The effects of elastase are limited by a protective enzyme called alpha-1 antitrypsin, which inactivates elastase. However, alpha-1 antitrypsin is damaged by the free radicals produced from cigarette smoke. Thus, elastase is free to destroy lung tissue. The stage is then set for a slow, irreversible loss of functional elastic tissue in the lungs, resulting in the loss of alveolar wall surface area and premature collapsing of small bronchioles during exhalation (hence, the "obstructive" in chronic obstructive pulmonary disease).[114-118] As more air gets "trapped" distal to the bronchiolar obstruction, the lung volume increases, creating the classic "barrel chest" appearance. In the end stages of emphysema, destruction of alveolar walls can be so extreme that large, visible air pockets form in the lungs. Collapsed bronchiolar airways are more difficult to reopen on inhalation. Thus, emphysema increases the work of breathing so that an individual must use the accessory muscles of inhalation to supplement the activity of the diaphragm and external intercostal muscles. Because of the diminished rate of gas transport and increased work of breathing, the sufferer of emphysema is short of breath and cannot tolerate rigorous exercise well.

Chronic bronchitis, like emphysema, is more common in the elderly, especially in those with a long history of cigarette smoking. It is clinically defined as a chronic cough ("smoker's cough") productive of sputum, occurring on most days for at least 3 months' duration over at least 2 consecutive years. Whereas emphysema primarily affects the smallest airways, chronic bronchitis is inflammation of the larger bronchi, brought about by the irritating effects of cigarette smoke or other environmental inhalants. The inflammatory process causes excessive mucus production, which is difficult to clear from the lungs not only because of its abundance, but also because the tiny, beating cilia covering the bronchi that normally help move the mucus upward are damaged by smoking. The pooling of excessive mucus can block bronchi (additional "obstructive" in chronic obstructive pulmonary disease) and provide a nutrient-rich environment for bacterial infection. When you consider that the elderly immune system is not as efficient, and the cough reflex that helps clear excess mucus and aspirated food from the respiratory tract does not work as well, you can easily understand why an older smoker with chronic bronchitis is at increased risk for spreading inflammation and infection to the bronchioles and alveoli—the development of *pneumonia*. Collectively, the number of people who die each year of respiratory illnesses is considerable. COPD and other chronic lower respiratory tract diseases (e.g., asthma) represent the fourth leading cause of death in the United States; pneumonia and influenza collectively rank seventh on the list.[119] The World Health Organization estimates that 300 million people worldwide have been diagnosed with asthma and an additional 210 million have chronic obstructive pulmonary disease.[120]

HEMATOLOGIC SYSTEM

The hematologic system consists of those organs and tissues in the body that contribute red blood cells (RBCs), white blood cells (WBCs), and platelets to the bloodstream. Production of these cells from precursor stem cells, a process called *hematopoiesis*, occurs primarily in the bone marrow. The WBCs, or *leukocytes*, protect the body from infectious organisms and cancer cells, coordinate the events of the inflammatory and allergic responses, and participate in tissue and organ transplant rejection. Following their production in the bone marrow, WBCs travel through blood and lymphatic vessels to "seed" other organs, such as the spleen, tonsils, and lymph nodes, where they provide a continuous supply for life. Their role in aging is discussed in the next section. Platelets, or *thrombocytes*, are really cell fragments produced by the disintegration of large megakaryocyte cells in the bone marrow. They play a role in hemostasis (i.e., the stoppage of bleeding) by clumping together and releasing chemicals that stimulate blood clot formation in damaged blood vessels.

This section focuses on RBCs, called *erythrocytes*, which are flexible, disk-shaped cells filled with hemoglobin, an iron-containing protein that reversibly binds to and helps transport oxygen and carbon dioxide through the bloodstream. The life span of an RBC is relatively short, lasting only about 120 days. This is because RBCs undergo significant wear and tear as they are repeatedly squeezed through the small capillaries of the circulation. In addition, mature RBCs lack a nucleus (it is extruded from the RBCs during their final stage of development) and thus cannot repair themselves when damaged. For these reasons, RBCs must be produced at the astonishing rate of more than 2 million per second in healthy bone marrow (a process called *erythropoiesis*). They are broken down by macrophages at the same rate in the spleen. When the rate of erythropoiesis is equal to the rate of RBC destruction, there is no net change in the oxygen-carrying capacity of the blood over time. This capacity is often gauged by measuring the *hematocrit*, defined as the percentage of total blood volume taken up by red blood cells. The healthy range for hematocrit is 42–54% for men and 37–47% for women.[121]

A major hematologic concern in geriatric medicine is the high prevalence of **anemia** (defined as a lower than normal oxygen-carrying capacity of blood) in older adults, particularly those older individuals in acute hospital and long-term care settings. Anemia, however, is not a single disease, but rather a syndrome that has several different causes. Individuals with anemia often have pale skin, shortness of breath, and fatigue as a result of subnormal hematocrit. A majority of the blood's oxygen is carried in RBCs, and anemias are caused by inadequate production or premature destruction of these RBCs. It has become clear in recent years that the high incidence of anemia in the elderly is not caused by aging per se, but rather a high frequency of other age-related illnesses that can cause anemia. In healthy elderly individuals, there is no significant decline in the rate of erythropoiesis under normal conditions. However, when the body is stressed in ways that require an increase in erythropoiesis (e.g., chronic bleeding), aged bone marrow has a more difficult time keeping up than does young bone marrow.

The most common category of anemia diagnosed in older adults is *hypoproliferative anemia*, anemia resulting from a lower rate of RBC production than would be expected for the degree of hematocrit decline. The most common cause of hypoproliferative anemia in older adults is an inadequate supply of iron to make hemoglobin in RBCs. However, the problem in most cases is not insufficient iron in the diet, but rather excessive loss of iron and/or the inability to recycle iron that collects in macrophages from broken-down RBCs. Excessive loss of iron is caused by acute or chronic bleeding, which in older adults occurs most frequently in the digestive tract (e.g., from ulcers, diverticulitis, or colon cancer). Another type of hypoproliferative anemia, anemia of inflammation, affects those individuals undergoing inflammatory responses as a result of conditions such as infection, tissue damage, or cancer. Extensive inflammation hampers the recycling of iron from macrophages in the spleen and liver. Thus, as older RBCs are continuously broken down, the supply of iron available for erythropoiesis in the bone marrow is inadequate. Chronic diseases such as rheumatoid arthritis and inflammatory bowel disease (e.g., ulcerative colitis and Crohn's disease) have a similar effect. These anemias can be exacerbated by protein and caloric malnutrition, which appears to decrease levels of the protein erythropoietin, a hormone produced by the kidneys, whose normal effect is to stimulate erythropoiesis in bone marrow.

Other types of anemia that can afflict older adults fall under the category of *ineffective erythropoiesis*, defined as a group of anemias that result from destruction of developing RBCs while they are still in the bone marrow or immediately after they are released into circulation. Anemia resulting from vitamin B_{12} deficiency is an example of ineffective erythropoiesis often diagnosed in older adults. Vitamin B_{12} is a coenzyme required for DNA production. When levels of this vitamin are deficient, RBCs develop abnormally in the bone marrow. Specifically, the cells cannot divide efficiently, and maturation of the cell nucleus lags behind maturation of the cytoplasm. The large, nucleated RBC precursors called megaloblasts (hence, the disease's alternative name, megaloblastic anemia) that form are often destroyed in the bone marrow before they can be released into the bloodstream. The cause of vitamin B_{12} deficiency may be:

- Insufficient dietary intake (particularly in those who consume excess alcohol)
- Inflammation or destruction of the ileum, the terminal portion of the small intestine, where vitamin B_{12} is absorbed
- Inflammation or destruction of the stomach lining (e.g., because of an autoimmune disorder called pernicious anemia) and thus the cells that produce intrinsic factor, a glycoprotein required for successful vitamin B_{12} absorption in the ileum

Having just reviewed the cardiovascular, respiratory, and hematologic systems, it becomes clear that all three of these systems are required to ensure adequate delivery of oxygen to the tissues. An age-related decline in the function of one or two of these systems will exacerbate any physiologic dysfunction present in the others. The presence of anemia in someone with congestive heart failure would be much more detrimental than it would be in an otherwise healthy individual. If that person with anemia and congestive heart failure also had emphysema, the disruption to the body would be still more extreme. It is this interdependence of our organ systems that, on the one hand, allows for appropriate compensatory adjustments to homeostatic disturbances in younger, healthy individuals but, on the other hand, can create a chain reaction of dysfunction in older, less healthy persons with decreased physiologic functional reserve.

IMMUNE SYSTEM

The ability of our bodies to remain free of infections and cancer requires that the WBCs in our immune system are able to distinguish "self" cells (i.e., our own healthy cells) from "nonself" cells (i.e., invading microorganisms and parasites or structurally altered cancer cells). To appreciate the enormity of this task, think about the thousands of different types of organisms that can invade the body, each of which must be specifically recognized by the immune system as foreign and destroyed without damaging the integrity of our own tissues in the process. Similarly, imagine the countless number of precancerous cell types, each of which may differ from normal cells in only subtle ways, that are recognized and destroyed by the immune system on a regular basis. Indeed, in its prime, the immune system is to be marveled at for its accuracy. But, as is true of most systems, age takes its toll. A discussion of the most important aspects of the immune response is followed by a review of those age-related changes in immunity that have implications for our health and well-being.

To be immune to an infection implies being protected from it. The development of immunity to a particular infectious organism, however, usually requires initial exposure to it, which in turn often causes mild illness. Nonetheless, on recovery from the sickness, the individual is immune to subsequent infection and illness from that organism; the body has developed an "immunological memory" (sometimes called adaptive immunity) so that it can act more swiftly and effectively the next time it is exposed to the same invader. The development of this immunological memory occurs by one of two general processes, called the humoral-mediated and cell-mediated immune responses. The former process produces proteins called antibodies, which circulate through the blood (or "humor") and specifically bind to the foreign organism; the latter process activates white blood cells called killer T-lymphocyte cells, which directly destroy the invading organism. Lymphocytes play a critical role in the development of immunity to infections and cancer. Unfortunately, it is these lymphocytes whose function most noticeably diminishes with age.

The age-related decline of immune system functioning gives rise to three general categories of illness that preferentially afflict the elderly: infections, cancer, and autoimmune disease.

The overall incidence of *infectious disease* rises in late adulthood. Particularly prevalent among the aged are influenza, pneumonia, tuberculosis, meningitis, and urinary tract infections. Deficiencies in both humoral- and cell-mediated immunity have been implicated in the increased incidence of infections as well as the decreased immune response to vaccines in older adults.[122] Utsuyama and colleagues studied human blood from individuals ranging from newborn to 102 years old and found that numbers of both B and

T cells remain somewhat stable between the third and seventh decades of life, but decline thereafter.[123] The age-related decreases in the numbers and activities of various clones of T cells may be caused by a slow, postpubertal destruction of the thymus gland, an organ that stimulates development of T-helper and T-killer cells by releasing various hormone-like chemicals. Another possible reason for diminished functioning of T cells is the derangement of precursor stem cell development in bone marrow. Regardless of the cause, it is important to bear in mind that any decline in T-helper cell function will have widespread repercussions for our health because this cell is the catalyst for both humoral- and cell-mediated immunity. It is, incidentally, destruction of these cells by the human immunodeficiency virus (HIV) that makes acquired immune deficiency syndrome (AIDS) such a devastating disease. There appears to be an age-related decline in the number and function of different B cell clones as well. Thus, there is a general decline in the body's ability to generate antibody responses to certain infections.

Cancer increases in prevalence with age as well, particularly leukemia and lung, prostate, breast, stomach, and pancreatic cancer. This rise may be caused in part by altered immune surveillance of precancerous and cancer cells that comes with age. Several components of the immune system play roles in cancer protection, including the previously mentioned natural killer cells. Both the number and function of natural killer cells in animals decline with aging. If this is the case in humans, it may partly explain the rising incidence of cancer in older adults.

Autoimmune diseases also are more common in older adults. These diseases are marked by the mistaken immunological destruction of the body's own cells. In such diseases, the body loses the ability to distinguish self from nonself. Prominent examples of autoimmune diseases affecting the elderly are rheumatoid arthritis, Hashimoto's thyroiditis, lupus, and chronic hepatitis. Tolerance to our own tissues develops early in life (during development of the immune system), when the thymus gland selects out and eliminates those clones of T cells programmed to destroy our own tissues—a process called *clonal deletion*. However, with the slow, age-related destruction of the thymus gland, the body may lose the ability to detect and destroy these potentially self-harming T cells. Indeed, with aging comes increased levels of autoantibodies.

DIGESTIVE SYSTEM

One major function of the digestive system is to process incoming food so that nutrients can be absorbed into the body. The primary structural feature of this system is the digestive tract, made up of the mouth, pharynx, stomach, small intestine, large intestine (or colon), rectum, and anus (**Figure 3-13**). This canal works like an assembly line, with each part having a specialized function in digestion. Attached to the digestive tract are exocrine glands, such as salivary glands, pancreas, and liver, which secrete substances to aid in digestion and absorption. Although aging in an otherwise healthy individual has minimal

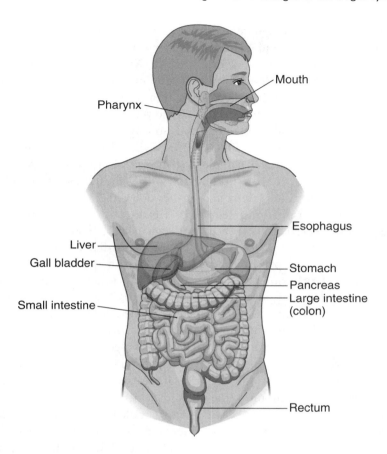

FIGURE 3-13 The digestive system.

effects on the digestive system, many specific diseases of this system increase in frequency with advancing years. The age-related alterations in structure and function are discussed in descending order, starting with the mouth and proceeding to the rectum.

Food entering the *mouth* undergoes the initial stages of mechanical digestion (via chewing) and chemical digestion (via release of salivary amylase enzyme). In the mouth, teeth undergo perhaps the most visible changes with age, becoming yellowish-brown (because of exposure to coffee, cigarette smoke, and other staining agents) and worn on the surface (because of years of chewing, night grinding, and jaw clenching). Osteoporotic changes of the jaw bones (maxilla and mandible) can cause teeth to loosen from their sockets. This change, coupled with the recession of gums (*periodontal disease*), can cause loss of teeth in older adults. Indeed, one-fourth of U.S. adults age 65 and older have lost all of their teeth.[124] Although dental caries (cavities) are not an inevitable result of aging, the diminished strength and dexterity of older adults can make teeth brushing difficult, thus increasing the likelihood of dental caries. **Xerostomia**, or dry mouth, is another problem of aging and has several causes, including decreased saliva production, cigarette smoking, and medication side effects (e.g., from certain blood pressure medications).

Once sufficiently chewed, food is swallowed by complex coordination of several muscles of the tongue, palate, pharynx, and esophagus. In this regard, a common problem in the elderly is **dysphagia**, or difficulty swallowing. This may be caused by weakness of the tongue muscles, improper nervous system control of the swallowing reflex, or unco-ordinated muscular action of the pharynx or esophagus. Severe dysphagia can cause aspiration of food into the larynx and farther down the respiratory tract, which in turn puts one at risk for aspiration pneumonia. Treatment of more severe cases of dysphagia may require the expertise of a speech and language pathologist.

In the *stomach*, the swallowed food is chemically digested by virtue of hydrochloric acid (gastric acid) and pepsin enzyme secretion, and is mechanically digested by the stomach's muscular churning action. The rate of gastric acid secretion decreases with age, whereas the incidence of **peptic ulcers** and **gastritis** (i.e., inflammation of the stomach lining) increases. The latter two phenomena may be a result of an increased incidence of *Helicobacter pylori* bacterial infection in older adults, drug ingestion (e.g., aspirin, caffeine, alcohol), or genetically programmed changes with age. Chronic bleeding from a peptic ulcer or gastritis can result in iron-deficiency anemia, whereas acute bleeding can place severe stress on the elderly individual's cardiovascular system. *Carcinoma* (or cancer) of the stomach is most common in the old and carries a poor prognosis for survival.

The initial section of the *small intestine*, called the *duodenum*, receives partially digested food (or chyme) from the stomach and continues the process of digestion with the help of secretions from the liver and gallbladder (bile) and from the pancreas (diges-tive enzymes and bicarbonate-rich fluid). As chyme is further digested, nutrient molecules become small enough to be absorbed through the small intestine wall, a process that occurs primarily in the more distal parts of the small intestine (*jejunum* and *ileum*). Move-ment of chyme through the small intestine by peristaltic contractions of the muscular wall is fairly slow to allow sufficient time for nutrient absorption. Aging has surprisingly little effect on the small intestine's digestive function and smooth muscle contractility. In addition, with the possible exceptions of calcium, vitamin D, and iron, most nutrients are absorbed efficiently in the small intestine in healthy older adults. The decreased calcium and vitamin D absorption may contribute to increased incidence of osteoporosis in older adults.

The *liver* has several functions, some related to digestion and others not. It produces bile that is stored below in the gallbladder until its release into the duodenum. Bile is required for emulsification of fats in chyme. Without bile, fats would pass through the digestive tract without being absorbed, a condition called *steatorrhea*. Storage of bile in the gallbladder can lead to its precipitation into solid stones, or *gallstones*, a phenomenon that is increasingly likely as we age. Gallstones, in turn, can get lodged in the ducts that

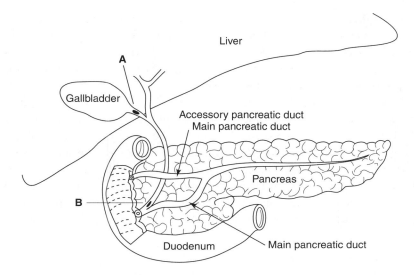

Liver

A

Gallbladder

Accessory pancreatic duct
Main pancreatic duct

Pancreas

B

Duodenum

Main pancreatic duct

FIGURE 3-14 Hepatobiliary tree with gallstone lodged in (A) the cystic duct and (B) the common bile duct.

normally convey the bile to the duodenum, resulting at times in obstructive jaundice, inflammation of the gallbladder (*cholecystitis*) or pancreas (*pancreatitis*), and steatorrhea (**Figure 3-14**).

The liver also detoxifies many foreign and potentially damaging chemicals that enter or are produced within the body. Indeed, many medications given for disease and illness are broken down by the liver and are released either through the bile or in the bloodstream to be eliminated by the kidneys in urine. But with age, this detoxifying ability is diminished. This is particularly important to realize because it means that many drugs given to older adults remain in the body for longer periods of time. Thus, recommended dosages of many drugs for older adults are smaller than they would be for younger individuals. Failure to consider this leads to dangerous overdosing of medications for older adults.

The remainder of the small intestinal contents (largely water and indigestible fiber) enters the *large intestine* (or *colon*), an area of the digestive tract that is heavily colonized by a normal bacterial flora. The large intestine reabsorbs much of the remaining water and stores the feces until defecation. One common problem in the elderly is **diverticulosis**, which is a development of small sacs where the large intestinal lining has herniated through the intestinal muscular wall. These herniations usually result from muscular spasms and increased intracolonic pressure associated with diets low in fiber. These pockets, or diverticuli, can become impacted with feces, resulting in ulceration and inflammation of the mucosal lining (*diverticulitis*). Also with age comes decreased motility of smooth muscle in the large intestinal wall, prolonging the time that feces are stored in the colon and rectum. This, in turn, causes excessive water reabsorption and hardening of feces, leading to *constipation* and, in extreme cases, intestinal obstruction. On the other end of the spectrum, older adults may suffer from **fecal incontinence** (the inability to voluntarily control defecation), largely because of the weakening of the external anal sphincter muscle. This can be exacerbated when there is a simultaneous increase in intra-rectal pressure caused by episodes of *diarrhea*.

The small and large intestines, like most other parts of the body, are vulnerable to the ravages of atherosclerosis. Blockage of mesenteric arteries supplying the intestines can result in *ischemia* (reversible tissue damage caused by oxygen depletion) and, ultimately, *infarction* (tissue death and breakdown). In the latter case, perforations can develop in the intestinal wall, allowing bacteria-laden feces to spill out into the normally sterile peritoneal cavity, causing severe inflammation (*peritonitis*), a life-threatening condition. Finally, the large intestine is susceptible to cancer as well. In fact, in those people 70 and older, colon cancer is the second most common malignancy (behind lung cancer).[125]

GENITOURINARY SYSTEM

The paired *kidneys* serve two principal, and somewhat overlapping, functions:

- Excretion of certain waste products from the body
- Maintenance of **homeostasis** (stability) in the fluid compartments of the body, such as plasma and interstitial fluid

The fact that these two fairly small organs (each weighing only 5 ounces) receive about 20% of the cardiac output illustrates their importance in carrying out these tasks. Failure to perform these functions can result in a buildup of nitrogenous waste products (e.g., urea) in the bloodstream and in imbalanced levels of water, electrolytes, or acids in the body, any of which can in turn alter normal physiologic processes. One would expect organs of such importance to have considerable functional reserve so that they could make necessary compensations when damaged in any way. For the most part, this is true. Consider the *nephrons*, the microscopically sized functional units of the kidneys that filter blood and then "choose" which substances of the filtered fluid to excrete and which substances to place back in the bloodstream. At age 25, there are approximately 1 million nephrons in each kidney. By age 85, 30% to 40% of them have been lost, yet an otherwise healthy 85-year-old can still maintain homeostasis under normal circumstances.[95]

Nonetheless, because of the loss of nephrons and the less efficient functioning of those that remain, the kidneys of older adults have a more difficult time responding to any added metabolic stressor on the body. Thus, as is true of the other organs discussed, older kidneys work well under normal conditions but have reduced tolerance for disease processes, whether originating from the kidneys themselves or from other organs. This is why, compared with younger individuals, older adults more commonly suffer from *acute* and *chronic renal failure*, conditions in which toxic metabolites build up in the body because of an inability of the kidneys to remove them at a sufficient rate. It is also important for healthcare providers to understand that the kidneys, like the liver, help eliminate drugs and their breakdown products from the body. The decreased functional reserve capacity that comes with age makes it more difficult for the kidneys to efficiently excrete drugs. Thus, to prevent overdosing of medications, older adults typically require smaller drug dosages than do younger individuals.

One of the major roles of the kidneys is to maintain water balance in the body. Indeed, the amount of water in fluid compartments such as blood, interstitial fluid, and intracellular fluid is a major determinant of the concentrations of all substances dissolved in those fluid compartments. Therefore, to maintain levels of sodium, potassium, calcium, and other vital components within the appropriate narrow concentration ranges, the kidneys must regulate the rate of water removal from the body. Severe dehydration (e.g., resulting from excessive sweating or inadequate fluid intake) might increase the concentration of dissolved substances in the body to dangerously high levels, if not for the ability of the kidneys to respond by producing smaller volumes of highly concentrated urine, thus minimizing the amount of water lost. On the other hand, when someone is overhydrated, the kidneys respond by producing large volumes of dilute urine. But this ability to regulate the concentration according to the body's needs diminishes with age. For this reason, older adults are more likely to become dehydrated, especially when confusion, immobility, or fear of urinary incontinence (discussed later) prevents them from drinking adequate amounts of liquids. This dehydration may be exacerbated by the overdosing of diuretics, medications used for congestive heart failure and hypertension, whose effect is to increase urinary output.

Other age-related changes in the genitourinary system pertain to the structures required for urinary collection and removal—that is, the *ureters, urinary bladder*, and *urethra* (**Figure 3-15**). Normally, urine produced by the kidneys flows continuously through the ureters to be temporarily stored in the urinary bladder. As the urinary bladder fills with urine, its walls stretch out, initiating a reflexive contraction of the bladder wall. The expanding urinary bladder compresses the ureteral openings, preventing a reflux of urine in the bladder back into the ureters. In addition, a smooth muscle sphincter at the urethral opening (internal urethral sphincter) prevents urine in the bladder from entering the urethra. Nonetheless, as fluid pressure in the bladder rises, the internal urethral sphincter opens up and urine enters the proximal urethra. However, a more distal, voluntary, skeletal muscle sphincter (the external urethral sphincter, located in the pelvic floor) must relax before urine can exit through the urethra. Thus, although the release of urine, called micturition, is made possible by an involuntary reflex, we nonetheless have voluntary control over it under normal conditions.

The loss of this voluntary control of micturition, called **urinary incontinence**, is a common problem in the older population. Indeed, 50–60% of those living in institutions may have this embarrassing and distressing condition.[126] Postmenopausal women are prone to this problem because lowered estrogen levels cause skeletal muscles of the pelvic floor and smooth muscles of the urethra to weaken. Women who have had multiple

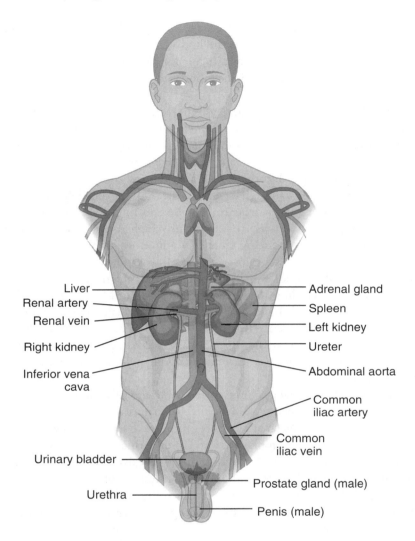

Liver

Renal artery

Renal vein

Right kidney

Inferior vena cava

Urinary bladder

Urethra

Adrenal gland

Spleen

Left kidney

Ureter

Abdominal aorta

Common iliac artery

Common iliac vein

Prostate gland (male)

Penis (male)

FIGURE 3-15 The urinary system.

pregnancies are particularly susceptible and may involuntarily urinate whenever intra-abdominal pressure rises, for example, when coughing, sneezing, or laughing. This is called stress incontinence. In elderly men, urinary incontinence is often caused by an enlarged *prostate gland*. The prostate gland, which produces some components of semen, is wrapped around the beginning of the urethra. It undergoes enlargement as a man ages, which can, in turn, partially or completely obstruct the urethra. This enlargement is either benign (**benign prostatic hypertrophy** [BPH]) or malignant (*prostate cancer*). In either case, the urinary bladder must contract more forcefully to eliminate urine. Over time, the bladder can become distended (a condition called *urinary retention*) and its muscular wall can weaken, leading to a lack of coordination of micturition and, in turn, incontinence. As a result, urinary retention increases the chance of *urinary tract infection* and kidney damage (caused by a buildup of fluid pressure). To avoid these complications, surgery is often performed to remove that part of the prostate gland blocking the urethra (a procedure called transurethral resection of the prostate [TURP]).

ENDOCRINE SYSTEM

Like the nervous system, the endocrine system is a principal regulatory system in the body. It helps control several aspects of our physiology, such as body temperature; basal metabolic rate; growth rate; carbohydrate, lipid, and protein metabolism; stress responses; and reproductive events. Clearly, dysfunction of this system could have widespread ramifications for one's health and well-being. Only a few of the many age-related changes to this system are highlighted here.

The endocrine system is a collection of glands that produce and secrete into the bloodstream chemical messengers called *hormones* that have physiologic effects on various *target organs* throughout the body. The cells of target organs have protein *receptors* that specifically bind to the hormone in question. This binding initiates a cascade of metabolic events within the target cell that mediate the hormone's effects.

Although the endocrine glands are spread throughout the body, there is a hierarchical control of the release of most hormones, which begins in the central nervous system (CNS) (**Figure 3-16**). Neural activity from higher centers in the CNS is relayed to the **hypothalamus**, a small but extremely important structure that, in turn, controls activity of the **pituitary gland** by releasing hormones that stimulate or inhibit its hormonal production and release. The pituitary gland, under the influence of these higher control centers, releases a battery of tropic hormones that have selective stimulatory effects on glands such as the thyroid, adrenal gland, and gonads (ovaries and testes). It should be emphasized, however, that even the structures at the top of this endocrine hierarchy are influenced by "lower" events. For example, the thyroid gland is stimulated to release thyroid hormone in response to the sequential release of thyrotropin-releasing hormone (TRH) from the hypothalamus and thyroid-stimulating hormone (TSH) from the pituitary gland. But as its level in the blood increases, thyroid hormone "turns off" further production of TRH and TSH in the higher centers in a negative feedback fashion—in effect, the endocrine system operates under a system of checks and balances so that under normal conditions the appropriate levels of all hormones are maintained.

The *thyroid hormone* released from the *thyroid gland* has many physiologic effects, such as regulation of tissue growth and development (particularly of the skeletal and nervous systems), regulation of the basal metabolic rate (BMR) by promoting oxygen consumption and heat production in most tissues (i.e., a calorigenic effect), enhancement of the effects of the sympathetic nervous system (or fight-or-flight response), increased mental alertness, and possibly regulation of cholesterol metabolism. As one ages, the level of thyroid hormone secretion declines. However, this decrease is matched by a decline in

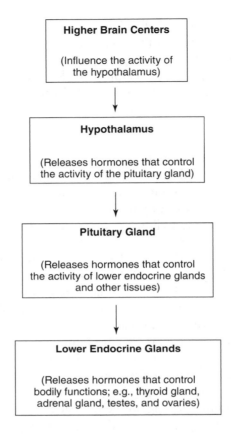

FIGURE 3-16 The hierarchy of control over the endocrine system.

its rate of removal from the bloodstream so that, overall, levels change little over the years. Furthermore, aging per se does not appreciably affect the increased release of TRH, TSH, or thyroid hormone required in times of greater need. However, several characteristics of older adults, such as a reduced metabolic rate, suboptimal regulation of body temperature, decreased effectiveness of the fight-or-flight response, reduced mental alertness, and increased incidence of cholesterol-related atherosclerosis, are also symptoms of reduced thyroid activity (hypothyroidism). Thus, it is possible that the age-related changes in thyroid function result from inadequate responses of target cells to the thyroid hormone rather than from direct damage to the thyroid gland.

The paired *adrenal glands* consist of an outer layer called the adrenal cortex and an inner section called the adrenal medulla (which, from a functional standpoint, is more aptly considered part of the sympathetic nervous system, and thus is not discussed here). The *adrenal cortex* produces a number of corticosteroid hormones, such as cortisol, which helps the body adapt to stress; aldosterone, which helps the body conserve sodium and thus water; androgens, which have masculinizing effects; and estrogens, which have feminizing effects. The latter two hormones, whose levels decline with age, supplement the action of testosterone and estrogen released from the testes and ovaries, respectively. The loss of estrogen production from postmenopausal ovaries appears to upset the androgen–estrogen balance in favor of androgens produced in the adrenal gland. This might explain the mild masculinization of a woman's physique as she ages.

Aldosterone levels also fall as one ages, impairing an important component of blood pressure regulation. Normally, this hormone stimulates the reabsorption of sodium ions from renal tubules back into the bloodstream, which osmotically draws water back in as well, thus increasing blood volume and therefore blood pressure when needed. Although the aldosterone mechanism is just one of many ways to increase blood pressure, its loss may bring the body one step closer to disruption of homeostasis.

Cortisol is the quintessential stress hormone, released into the bloodstream during prolonged periods of physical or psychological stress. It is a catabolic hormone whose function is to mobilize the body's energy reserves, increasing blood levels of glucose, fats, and amino acids during times of illness, physical injury, or emotional distress. In addition, baseline cortisol release (in conjunction with release of the hormone glucagon from the pancreas) in the absence of stress helps prevent blood glucose levels from falling dangerously low during sleep and in between meals.

As was true of thyroid hormone, cortisol levels remain normal well into old age because of a balance between the hormone's decreased production and its decreased excretion. In addition, stress-induced increases in cortisol release are not affected by aging. However, it appears to take older adults longer to reestablish normal blood cortisol levels following a stressful event, possibly as a result of a faulty negative feedback system in which the hypothalamus and pituitary gland fail to slow down the release of corticotropin-releasing hormone (CRH) and adrenocorticotropic hormone (ACTH) when cortisol levels are increased. A persistently elevated cortisol level may actually have a negative impact on the health of older adults. Some of the well-documented effects of chronically high blood cortisol levels include hyperglycemia (excessively high blood glucose level), hypertension (high blood pressure caused by the aldosterone-like effects of cortisol), and immunosuppression (increased susceptibility to infection and cancer). It is plausible, then, that elevated cortisol responses to stress might exacerbate concomitant diabetes mellitus, hypertension, and infectious disease in older adults.

Unlike in the thyroid gland, adrenal cortex, and gonads, control of hormone release from the endocrine cells of the *pancreas* is not primarily controlled by the hypothalamus and pituitary gland. Instead, the two major hormones produced by the pancreas, *insulin* (which decreases the blood glucose level) and *glucagon* (which increases the blood glucose level) are released at various rates based primarily on blood glucose levels. Deficient insulin action causes **diabetes mellitus** (DM), a condition marked by hyperglycemia and long-term complications such as blindness (resulting from cataracts and retinal damage), renal failure, nerve damage, atherosclerosis, and gangrenous infection often necessitating amputation of all or part of the leg. **Non-insulin-dependent diabetes mellitus** (NIDDM) is a type of diabetes mellitus that increases in frequency with age and accounts for about 90–95% of all cases. It appears to be caused by deficient target organ responses to the effects of insulin—the level of insulin itself is actually normal or increased. It is estimated that, in the United States, 25.8 million people (8.3% of the total population) have the diagnosis of diabetes, the vast majority having NIDDM.[127,128] Because it is so common in older adults, affecting approximately 27% of those aged 65 and older, non-insulin-dependent diabetes mellitus is of great interest to geriatric medicine.[129]

SUMMARY

It is clear that our health and well-being depend on the degree to which our organ systems can successfully work together to maintain homeostasis, or the body's internal stability. Diminished function in one organ system is minimized by appropriate compensatory mechanisms in other systems. An older individual with emphysema, and therefore less efficient ventilation of the lungs, often has an elevated hematocrit (i.e., a greater proportion of RBCs in the blood) to maintain adequate oxygen delivery to the bloodstream and tissues. An individual with systemic hypertension will have enlargement of muscle in the heart's left ventricle, generating a greater force of contraction to maintain adequate cardiac output in the face of increased afterload. A person's excessive exposure to sunlight not only stimulates increased production of protective melanin pigments in skin, but also may heighten immune surveillance for precancerous epidermal cells.

However, also apparent is the gradual impairment of these homeostatic mechanisms with age, most likely as a result of the linear decline that seems to characterize many physiologic functions such as cardiac output, forced vital capacity, the number of functioning nephrons, bone mass, and epidermal melanocyte density. What is gradually lost with age is the functional reserve capacity of our organ systems. A physiologic disturbance that is easily correctable at age 30 may cause significant illness at age 60 or death at age 90. Perhaps it should not be surprising that coinciding with the linear decline in physiologic functioning is a logarithmic increase in mortality.[5] It is as though our bodies function well during the younger years despite the accumulation of environmental and genetic insults. However, at some stage in life, we reach a "critical mass" of impairment, a point beyond which our homeostatic correction mechanisms are no longer able to keep pace. When this point is reached, the likelihood of illness, disease, and death rises exponentially.

We may take comfort in the fact that much of the illness and suffering that tends to come with old age can be delayed or at least modified by taking proper care of ourselves. The hallmarks of preventive medicine, such as eating right, exercising, and avoiding cigarettes, are most effective when initiated early in life. Although there may be wisdom in the adage "live for the day," it is equally wise, from a health perspective, to "live for tomorrow."

Review Questions

1. Which of the following statements is *correct*?
   A. Improvements in sanitation have helped to increase the maximum life span potential of U.S. citizens over the past 100 years.
   B. Most of the increase in average life expectancy over the past 100 years can be attributed to advances in medical technology.
   C. The percentage of U.S. citizens nearing the maximum life span potential is higher today than it was 100 years ago.
   D. In the effort to increase average life expectancy, curative medicine is more cost-effective than preventive medicine.
   E. Dietary practices such as vitamin intake and caloric restriction can prevent aging.

2. Match the following theories of aging with their most appropriate descriptions.
   _____ Rate of living theory
   _____ Free radical theory
   _____ Gene regulation theory
   _____ Somatic mutation theory
   _____ Wear-and-tear theory
   A. Aging results from accumulating damage to cells caused by molecules that have unpaired electrons in their outermost valence shells.
   B. Certain species live longer because they have lower metabolic rates.
   C. The random accumulation of DNA mutations and subsequent errors in protein production cause aging.
   D. Aging occurs along an intentional timeline dictated by the sequential expression of particular genes in cells.
   E. Cells and tissues are damaged by years of continuous use.

3. The skin gradually loses its brown tone with age as a result of a decrease in the number of _____ in the skin.
   A. Melanocytes
   B. Keratinocytes
   C. Fibroblasts
   D. Mast cells
   E. Langerhans cells

4. Which of the following is *not* a characteristic change in the nervous system as one ages?
   A. A decrease in nerve conduction velocity
   B. A loss of moderate amounts of myelin around some axons
   C. A generalized and substantial decrease in the number of neurons
   D. A decrease in the number of dendrites
   E. An increase in the size of fatty plaques in the cerebral arteries

5. Which of the following is *not* a risk factor for osteoporosis?
   A. Cigarette smoking
   B. Sedentary lifestyle
   C. Depletion of estrogen levels following menopause
   D. High blood pressure
   E. Calcium deficiency

Learning Activities

1. Compare and contrast aging and disease. How do the effects of cigarette smoking on the body illustrate the difficulty of distinguishing aging from disease?
2. A 76-year-old man with a long history of peptic ulcer disease has become increasingly fatigued and short of breath over the past 3 weeks. He complains of a dull pain below his sternum that is worse following meals. On physical examination, he looks pale and has a slightly elevated heart rate.
   A. What might be this man's diagnosis?
   B. Suggest some possible explanations for his
      i. Shortness of breath
      ii. Elevated heart rate
   C. From a physiologic standpoint, why might it be more difficult for this man to compensate for his current problem than it would be for a 30-year-old man? In your answer, explore possibilities from at least three different organ systems.

REFERENCES

1. Timiras, PS. Introduction: Aging as a stage in the life cycle. In PS Timiras (Ed.), *Physiological Basis of Aging and Geriatrics*. 2nd ed. Boca Raton, FL: CRC Press, 1994: 1.
2. Hayflick, L. Myths of aging. *Scientific American*, 1997;276:110.
3. Forsberg, V, Fichtenberg, C. The Prevention and Public Health Fund: A Critical Investment in Our Nation's Physical and Fiscal Health, 2012. Retrieved July 10, 2013, from http://www.apha.org/NR/rdonlyres/D1708E46-07E9-43E7-AB99-94A29437E4AF/0/PrevPubHealth2012_web.pdf
4. Schneider, EL. Aging research: Challenge of the twenty-first century. In AD Woodhead et al. (Eds.), *Molecular Biology of Aging*. New York: Plenum Press, 1985: 1.
5. Timiras, PS. Aging and disease. In PS Timiras (Ed.), *Physiological Basis of Aging and Geriatrics*. 2nd ed. Boca Raton, FL: CRC Press, 1994: 23.
6. National Center for Health Statistics. *Vital Statistics of the United States 1985*. PHS Publication No. 88-1104, Life Tables, Vol. 2, Sect 6. Hyattsville, MD: U.S. Department of Health and Human Services, 1988: 9.
7. National Center for Health Statistics. *National Vital Statistics Reports 2004*. United States Life Tables, Vol. 56, No. 9. Hyattsville, MD: U.S. Department of Health and Human Services, 2007: 3.
8. United Nations, Department of Economic and Social Affairs, Population Division. *World Population Prospects: The 2010 Revision, Highlights and Advance Tables*. Working Paper No. ESA/P/WP. 220. 2011.
9. Comfort, A. *The Biology of Senescence*. 3rd ed. New York: Elsevier, 1979: 81.
10. Finch, CE. *Longevity, Senescence, and the Genome*. Chicago: University of Chicago Press, 1990.
11. Gerontology Research Group. Verified Supercentenarians (Excludes Disputed Cases). Retrieved

June 14, 2013, from http://www.grg.org/Adams/B2.HTM

12. Spence, JD. Stroke prevention in the high-risk patient. *Expert Opinion on Pharmacotherapy*, 2007;8(12):1851–1859.

13. Bierman, EL, Hazzard, WR. Preventive gerontology: Strategies for attenuation of the chronic diseases of aging. In WR Hazzard et al. (Eds.), *Principles of Geriatric Medicine and Gerontology*. 3rd ed. New York: McGraw-Hill, 1994: 187.

14. Committee on Diet and Health, Food, and Nutrition Board, Commission on Life Sciences, National Research Council. *Diet and Health*. Washington, DC: National Academy Press, 1989.

15. Evans, W, Rosenberg, I. *Biomarkers*. New York: Simon & Schuster, 1991.

16. Ruuskanen, JM, Ruoppila, I. Physical activity and psychological well-being among people aged 65 to 84 years. *Age and Ageing*, 1995;24:292–296.

17. Wynder, EL. Etiology of lung cancer: Reflections on two decades of research. *Cancer*, 1972;30:1332.

18. Bernhard, D, et al. Cigarette smoke: An aging accelerator? *Experimental Gerontology*, 2007;42(3):160–165.

19. Cournil, A, Kirkwood, TBL. If you would live long, choose your parents well. *Trends in Genetics*, 2001;17:233–235.

20. Timiras, PS. Demographic, comparative, and differential aging. In PS Timiras (Ed.), *Physiological Basis of Aging and Geriatrics*. 2nd ed. Boca Raton, FL: CRC Press, 1994: 7.

21. Martin, GM. Interactions of aging and environmental agents: The gerontological perspective. In SR Baker, M Rogul (Eds.), *Environmental Toxicity and the Aging Process*. New York: Alan R Liss, 1987: 25.

22. Jin, K. Modern biological theories of aging. *Aging and Disease,* 2010;1:72.

23. Weinert, BT, Timiras, PS. Invited review: Theories of aging. *Journal of Applied Physiology,* 2003;95:1706.

24. Tosato, M, et al. The aging process and potential interventions to extend life expectancy. *Clinical Interventions in Aging*, 2007;2(3):401–412.

25. Failia, G. The aging process and cancerogenesis. *Annals of the New York Academy of Sciences*, 1958;71:1124.

26. Szilard, L. On the nature of the aging process. *Proceedings of the National Academy of Sciences USA*, 1959;45:30.

27. Ogburn, CE, et al. Exceptional cellular resistance to oxidative damage in long-lived birds requires active gene expression. *Journals of Gerontology. Series A, Biological Sciences and Medical Sciences*, 2001;56:B468–B474.

28. Burkle, A, et al. Poly(ADP-ribose) polymerase-1, DNA repair and mammalian longevity. *Experimental Gerontology*, 2002;37:1203–1205.

29. Martin, GM, et al. Increased chromosomal aberrations in first metaphases of cells isolated from the kidneys of aged mice. *Israel Journal of Medical Sciences*, 1985;21:296.

30. Curtis, HJ. Cellular processes involved in aging. *Federal Proceedings*, 1964;23:662.

31. Kirkwood, TBL. Evolution of ageing. *Nature*, 1977;270:301.

32. Pearl, R. *The Rate of Living*. London: University of London Press, 1928.

33. McCay, CM, Crowell, MF. Prolonging the life span. *Scientific Monthly*, 1934;39:405.

34. Barrows, CH, Kokkonen, GC. Relationship between nutrition and aging. *Advances in Nutritional Research*, 1977;1:253.

35. Bishop, NA, Guarente, L. Genetic links between diet and lifespan: Shared mechanisms from yeast to humans. *Nature Reviews Genetics*, 2007;8(11):835–844.

36. Dilova, I, et al. Calorie restriction and the nutrient signaling pathways. *Cellular and Molecular Life Sciences*, 2007;64(6):752–767.

37. Masoro, EJ. Overview of caloric restriction and aging. *Mechanisms of Aging and Development*, 2005;126:913.

38. Masoro, EJ, et al. Temporal and compositional dietary restrictions modulate age-related changes in serum lipids. *Journal of Nutrition*, 1983;113:880.

39. Kalu, DN, et al. Life-long food restriction prevents senile osteopenia and hyperparathyroidism in F344 rats. *Mechanisms of Ageing and Development*, 1984;26:103.

40. Weindruch, R, et al. Influence of controlled dietary restriction on immunologic function. *Federal Proceedings*, 1979;38:2007.

41. Masoro, EJ, et al. Action of food restriction in delaying the aging process. *Proceedings*

of the National Academy of Sciences USA, 1982;79:4239.

42. McCarter, R, et al. Does food restriction retard aging by reducing the metabolic rate? *American Journal of Physiology*, 1985;248:E488.

43. Austad, SN, Fischer, KE. Mammalian aging, metabolism, and ecology: Evidence from the bats and marsupials. *Journal of Gerontology*, 1991;46:B47.

44. de Magalhaes, JP, et al. An analysis of the relationship between metabolism, developmental schedules, and longevity using phylogenetic independent contrasts. *Journals of Gerontology A, Biological Sciences and Medical Sciences*, 2007;62:149.

45. Harman, D. The aging process: Major risk factor for disease and death. *Proceedings of the National Academy of Sciences USA*, 1991;88:5360.

46. Harman, D. Aging: A theory based on free radical and radiation chemistry. *Journal of Gerontology*, 1956;11:298.

47. Chance, B, et al. Hydrogen peroxide metabolism in mammalian organs. *Physiological Reviews*, 1979;59:527.

48. Finkel, T, Holbrook, NJ. Oxidants, oxidative stress and the biology of aging. *Nature*, 2000;408:239.

49. Mehlhorn, RJ. Oxidants and antioxidants in aging. In PS Timiras (Ed.), *Physiological Basis of Aging and Geriatrics*. 3rd ed. CRC Press, Boca Raton, FL: 61–83, 2003.

50. Von Zglinicki, T, et al. Stress, DNA damage and ageing: An integrative approach. *Experimental Gerontology*, 2001;36:1049–1062.

51. Nohl, H, Hegner, D. Do mitochondria produce oxygen radicals in vivo? *European Journal of Biochemistry*, 1978;82:563.

52. Lippman, RD. The prolongation of life: A comparison of antioxidants and geroprotectors versus superoxide in human mitochondria. *Journal of Gerontology*, 1981;36:550.

53. Leibovitz, BE, Siegel, BV. Aspects of free radical reactions in biological systems: Aging. *Journal of Gerontology*, 1980;35:45.

54. Pryor, WA. The formation of free radicals and the consequences of their reactions in vivo. *Photochemistry and Photobiology*, 1978;28:787.

55. Sohal, RS (Ed.). *Age Pigments*. Amsterdam: Elsevier/North-Holland, 1981.

56. Brunk, UT, Terman, A. Lipofuscin: Mechanisms of age-related accumulation and influence on cell function. *Free Radical Biology and Medicine*, 2002;33:611.

57. Timiras, PS. Degenerative changes in cells and cell death. In PS Timiras (Ed.), *Physiological Basis of Aging and Geriatrics*. 2nd ed. Boca Raton, FL: CRC Press, 1994: 47.

58. Berg, BN. Study of vitamin E supplements in relation to muscular dystrophy and other diseases in aging rats. *Journal of Gerontology*, 1959;14:174.

59. Porta, EA, et al. Effects of the type of dietary fat at two levels of vitamin E in Wistar male rats during development and aging. I. Life span, serum biochemical parameters and pathological changes. *Mechanisms of Ageing and Development*, 1980;13:1.

60. Blackett, AD, Hall, DA. Vitamin E: Its significance in mouse ageing. *Age and Ageing*, 1981;10:191.

61. Ledvina, M, Hodanova, M. The effect of simultaneous administration of tocopherol and sunflower oil on the life-span of female mice. *Experimental Gerontology*, 1980;15:67.

62. Tappel, AI. Lipid peroxidation damage to cell components. *Federal Proceedings*, 1973;32:1870.

63. Packer, L, Smith JR. Extension of the lifespan of cultured normal human diploid cells by vitamin E: A reevaluation. *Proceedings of the National Academy of Sciences USA*, 1977; 74:1640.

64. Nakayama, T, et al. Generation of hydrogen peroxide and superoxide anion radical from cigarette smoke. *Gann*, 1984;75:95.

65. Church, DF, Pryor, WA. Free radical chemistry of cigarette smoke and its toxicological implications. *Environmental Health Perspectives*, 1985;64:111.

66. Romani, N, et al. Epidermal Langerhans cells—changing views on their function in vivo. *Immunology Letters*, 2006;106(2):119–125.

67. Montagna, W, Carlisle, K. Structural changes in aging human skin. *Journal of Investigative Dermatology*, 1979;73:47.

68. Grove, GL, Kligman, AM. Age-associated changes in human epidermal cell renewal. *Journal of Gerontology*, 1983;38:137.

69. Leyden, JJ, et al. Age-related differences in the rate of desquamation of skin surface cells.

In RD Adelman et al. (Eds.), *Pharmacological Intervention of the Aging Process.* New York: Plenum Press, 1978: 297.

70. Kaminer, MS, Gilchrest, BA. Aging of the skin. In WR Hazzard et al. (Eds.), *Principles of Geriatric Medicine and Gerontology.* 3rd ed. New York: McGraw-Hill, 1994: 414.

71. U.S. Cancer Statistics Working Group. *United States Cancer Statistics: 1999–2004 Incidence and Mortality Web-Based Report.* Atlanta, GA: U.S. Department of Health and Human Services, Centers for Disease Control and Prevention, and National Cancer Institute, 2007.

72. Holick, MF. Vitamin D deficiency. *New England Journal of Medicine,* 2007;357(3):266–281.

73. Cranney, C, et al. *Effectiveness and Safety of Vitamin D.* Evidence Report/Technology Assessment No. 158 prepared by the University of Ottawa Evidence-Based Practice Center under Contract No. 290-02.0021. AHRQ Publication No. 07-E013. Rockville, MD: Agency for Healthcare Research and Quality, 2007.

74. Office of Dietary Supplements. *Dietary Supplement Fact Sheet: Vitamin D.* Bethesda, MD: National Institutes of Health, 2008. Retrieved January 20, 2009, from http://ods.od.nih.gov /factsheets/vitamind.asp

75. Eriksson, PS, et al. Neurogenesis in the adult human hippocampus. *Nature Medicine,* 1998;4(11):1313–1317.

76. Timiras, PS. Aging of the nervous system: Functional changes. In PS Timiras (Ed.), *Physiological Basis of Aging and Geriatrics.* 2nd ed. Boca Raton, FL: CRC Press, 1994: 103.

77. Palmer, AM, DeKosky, ST. The neurochemistry of ageing. In MSJ Pathy (Ed.), *Principles and Practice of Geriatric Medicine.* 3rd ed. Chichester, England: John Wiley and Sons, 1998: 65–76.

78. Shock, NW. The physiology of aging. *Scientific American,* 1962;206:100.

79. Ferro, JM, Madureira, S. Age-related white matter changes and cognitive impairment. *Journal of the Neurological Sciences,* 2002;15:221–225.

80. Alzheimer's Association. *Alzheimer's Disease Facts and Figures.* Chicago, IL: Author, 2008. Retrieved July 10, 2013 from http://www.alz .org/alzheimers_disease_what_is_alzheimers.asp

81. Jarvik, LF, et al. Dementia and delirium in old age. In JC Brocklehurst et al. (Eds.), *Textbook of Geriatric Medicine and Gerontology.* 4th ed. London: Churchill Livingstone, 1992: 332, 338.

82. Von Zglinicki, T, et al. Short telomeres in patients with vascular dementia: An indicator of low antioxidative capacity and a possible prognostic factor? *Laboratory Investigation,* 2000;80:1739–1747.

83. Szwabo, PA. Psychological aspects of aging. In MSJ Pathy et al. (Eds.), *Principles and Practice of Geriatric Medicine.* 4th ed. Chichester, England: John Wiley and Sons, 2006: 53–57.

84. Morgan, K. Sleep in normal and pathological aging. In JC Brocklehurst et al. (Eds.), *Textbook of Geriatric Medicine and Gerontology.* 4th ed. London: Churchill Livingstone, 1992: 122.

85. Pointer, JS. The burgeoning presbyopic population: An emerging 20th century phenomenon. *Ophthalmic and Physiological Optics,* 1998; 18(4):325–334.

86. Shamsi, FA, Boulton, M. Inhibition of RPE lysosomal and antioxidant activity by the age pigment lipofuscin. *Investigative Ophthalmology and Visual Science,* 2001;42:3041–3046.

87. Kevorkian, R. Physiology of aging. In MSJ Pathy et al. (Eds.), *Principles and Practice of Geriatric Medicine.* 4th ed. Chichester, England: John Wiley and Sons, 2006: 39.

88. Gates, GA, et al. Hearing in the elderly: The Framingham cohort, 1983–1985. *Ear Hear,* 1990;11:247.

89. Lewis, TJ. Hearing impairment. In RJ Ham, PD Sloane, GA Warshaw, MA Bernard, E Flaherty (Eds.), *Primary Care Geriatrics: A Case-Based Approach.* 5th ed. Philadelphia: Mosby, 2007: 334.

90. Stalworth, M, Sloane, PD. Clinical implications of normal aging. In RJ Ham, PD Sloane, GA Warshaw, MA Bernard, E Flaherty (Eds.), *Primary Care Geriatrics: A Case-Based Approach.* 5th ed. Philadelphia: Mosby, 2007: 23.

91. Stevens, JC, et al. Aging impairs the ability to detect gas odor. *Fire Technology,* 1987;23:198.

92. Berg, RL, Cassells, JS. *The Second Fifty Years: Promoting Health and Preventing Disability.* Washington, DC: National Academy Press, 1990: 76.

93. Office of the Surgeon General. *Bone Health and Osteoporosis: A Report of the Surgeon General.* Hyattsville, MD: U.S. Department of Health and Human Services, 2004.

94. Blume, SW, Curtis, JR. Medical costs of osteoporosis in the elderly Medicare population. *Osteoporosis Int*, 2011;22(6):1835–1844.

95. Kallenberg, GA, Beck, JC. Care of the geriatric patient. In RE Rakel (Ed.), *Textbook of Family Practice*. 3rd ed. Philadelphia: W. B. Saunders, 1984: 249.

96. Mazess, RB. On aging bone loss. *Clinical Orthopaedics and Related Research*, 1982;165:239–252.

97. Sorensen, LB. Rheumatology. In CK Cassel et al. (Eds.), *Geriatric Medicine*. 2nd ed. New York: Springer-Verlag, 1990: 185.

98. Arthritis Foundation. Osteoarthritis. Retrieved July 10, 2013, from http://www.arthritis.org/conditions-treatments/disease-center/osteoarthritis/

99. American Geriatrics Society Panel on Exercise and Osteoarthritis. Exercise prescription for older adults with osteoarthritis pain: Consensus practice recommendations. *Journal of the American Geriatrics Society*, 2001;49:808–823.

100. Centers for Disease Control and Prevention, 2013, Arthritis Related Statistics. Retrieved July 10, 2013, from http://www.cdc.gov/arthritis/data_statistics/arthritis_related_stats.htm

101. Felson, DT, et al. Osteoarthritis: New insights. Part 1: The disease and its risk factors. *Annals of Internal Medicine*, 2000;133:635–646.

102. Brunner, F, et al. Effects of aging on type II muscle fibers: A systematic review of the literature. *Journal of Aging and Physical Activity*, 2007;15(3):336–348.

103. Mian, OS, et al. The impact of physical training on locomotor function in older people. *Sports Medicine*, 2007;37(8):683–701.

104. Wolz, M, et al. Statement from the national high blood pressure education program: Prevalence of hypertension. *American Journal of Hypertension*, 2000;13:103–104.

105. Lewington, S, et al. Age-specific relevance of usual blood pressure to vascular mortality: A meta-analysis of individual data for one million adults in 61 prospective studies. *Lancet*, 2002;360:1903–1913.

106. Kohn, WM, et al. Effects of gender, age, and fitness level on response of VO_2 max to training in 60–71-year-olds. *Journal of Applied Physiology*, 1991;71:2004.

107. Huang, G, et al. Resting heart rate changes after endurance training in older adults: A meta-analysis. *Medicine and Science in Sports and Exercise*, 2005;37(8):1381–1386.

108. Johnson, D, Sandmire, D. *Medical Tests That Can Save Your Life: 21 Tests Your Doctor Won't Order Unless You Know to Ask*. New York: Rodale and St. Martin's Press, 2004: 68.

109. World Health Organization. Cardiovascular Diseases Fact Sheet. Retrieved July 10, 2013, from http://www.who.int/mediacentre/factsheets/fs317/en/index.html

110. Ness, J, et al. Risk factors for symptomatic peripheral arterial disease in older persons in an academic hospital based geriatrics practice. *Journal of the American Geriatrics Society*, 2000;48:312–314.

111. Carandang, R, et al. Trends in incidence, lifetime risk, severity, and 30-day mortality of stroke over the past 50 years. *Journal of the American Medical Association*, 2006;296(24):2939–2946.

112. Crapo, RO, et al. Reference spirometric values using techniques and equipment that meet ATS recommendations. *American Review of Respiratory Diseases*, 1981;123:659.

113. Timiras, PS. Aging of respiration: Erythrocytes, and the hematopoietic system. In PS Timiras (Ed.), *Physiological Basis of Aging and Geriatrics*. 2nd ed. Boca Raton, FL: CRC Press, 1994: 226.

114. Pryor, WA, et al. The inactivation of alpha-1-proteinase inhibitor by gas-phase cigarette smoke: Protection by antioxidants and reducing species. *Chemico-Biological Interactions*, 1986;57:271.

115. Weiss, SJ. Tissue destruction by neutrophils. *New England Journal of Medicine*, 1989; 320:365.

116. Travis, J, Salvesen, JS. Human plasma protease inhibitors. *Annual Review of Biochemistry*, 1983;52:655.

117. Janoff, A. Elastase in tissue injury. *Annual Review of Medicine*, 1985;36:207.

118. Boross, M, et al. Effect of smoking on different biological parameters in aging mice. *Z Gerontol*, 1991;24:76.

119. Anderson, RN, Smith, BL. Deaths: Leading causes for 2002. *National Vital Statistics Report*, 2005;53(17). Hyattsville, MD: U.S. Department of Health and Human Services: 7.

120. World Health Organization. Chronic Respiratory Diseases. World Health Organization, 2008. Retrieved January 20, 2009, from http://www.who.int/respiratory/en/

121. Marieb, EN. *Human Anatomy and Physiology*. 6th ed. San Francisco, CA: Benjamin Cummings, 2004: 1162.

122. Kovaiou, RD, et al. Age-related changes in immunity: Implications for vaccination in the elderly. *Expert Reviews in Molecular Medicine*, 2007;9(3):1–17.

123. Utsuyama, M, et al. Differential age-change in numbers of CD4+CD45RA+ and CD4+CD29+ T cell subsets in human peripheral blood. *Mechanisms of Ageing and Development*, 1992;63: 57–66.

124. Centers for Disease Control and Prevention. 2011. Oral Health. Preventing Cavities, Gum Disease, Tooth Loss, and Oral Cancers. At a Glance 2011. Retrieved July 10, 2013 from http://www.cdc.gov/chronicdisease/resources/publications/AAG/doh.htm

125. Nelson, JB, Castell, DO. Gastroenterology. In CK Cassel et al. (Eds.), *Geriatric Medicine*. 2nd ed. New York: Springer-Verlag, 1990: 356.

126. Herzog, AR, Fultz, NH. Prevalence and incidence of urinary incontinence in community dwelling populations. *Journal of the American Geriatrics Society*, 1990;38:273.

127. Centers for Disease Control and Prevention. *National Diabetes Fact Sheet: General Information and National Estimates on Diabetes in the United States, 2005*. Atlanta, GA: U.S. Department of Health and Human Services, Centers for Disease Control and Prevention, 2005.

128. American Diabetes Association. Diabetes Statistics 2011 National Diabetes Fact Sheet. Retrieved July 10, 2013 from http://www.diabetes.org/diabetes-basics/diabetes-statistics/

129. Goldberg, AP, Coon, PJ. Diabetes mellitus and glucose metabolism in the elderly. In WR Hazzard et al. (Eds.), *Principles of Geriatric Medicine and Gerontology*. 3rd ed. New York: McGraw-Hill, 1994: 826.

THE COGNITIVE AND PSYCHOLOGICAL CHANGES ASSOCIATED WITH AGING

REGULA H. ROBNETT, PhD, OTR/L, and
JESSICA J. BOLDUC, DrOT, MS, OTR/L

If your brain is a garden, new activities are mental manure: the fertilizer for new brain cells.
—Ken Budd, *AARP Magazine*[1]

Chapter Outline

Behavioral Objectives

Upon completion of this chapter, the reader will be able to:

1. List the three basic factors that cause cognitive impairments in older adults.
2. Describe how general (fluid and crystallized intelligence) and specific aspects of cognition (attention, orientation, memory, executive functioning, and learning) may change with the aging process.
3. Describe compensatory measures related to decreased or changed cognitive functioning.
4. List possible screens for use in detecting cognitive changes.
5. Compare and contrast signs of delirium, depression, and dementia.
6. Complete a screen for depression to make a referral for assistance.

7. List general guidelines for working with people who have dementia.
8. Describe the bereavement process, and state recommendations for healthcare professionals who are working with bereaved individuals.
9. Differentiate aspects of personality that may tend to change over time from those that may not, based on current research.
10. Describe factors believed to contribute to a positive quality of life in older people.

Key Terms

Age-associated memory impairment	Learned helplessness
Alzheimer's disease	Long-term memory
Anhedonia	Malnutrition
Attention	Mild cognitive impairment
Bereavement	Orientation
Cerebrovascular accident	Personality
Cognition	Primary memory
Crystallized intelligence	Procedural memory
Delirium	Prospective memory
Dementia	Quality of life
Depression	Self-efficacy
Episodic memory	Semantic memory
Failure to thrive	Short-term memory
Fluid intelligence	Stereotypes
Gerotranscendence	Suicide
Heterogeneous	Working memory

The aging process is often viewed through a distorted lens, although the truth is hard to see with absolute clarity. The trajectory of human performance has been determined to "develop" through young adulthood, reach a plateau through middle age, and "decline" in old age. For example, cognition from birth to maturity is seen as *development*, whereas the changes of cognition from the age of maturity onward have been viewed as the *decline* of aging. Development is described as a positive emerging state, whereas aging is viewed as a negative state moving toward the inevitable end of life.[2] The simple statement—cognition decreases with age—although widely accepted as hard-core fact, needs to be questioned.

This chapter explores human development throughout life in the typical aging process and juxtaposes it with the atypical, or abnormal, aging process with which it is sometimes confused. Although change is a constant in our lives and the aging process inevitably entails change, not all age-related changes are negative. We need to consider whether the negative physical and cognitive changes that do occur in older people result from the aging process alone or from the accumulation of poor lifestyle choices, the expectations of decline, or a combination of these two detrimental forces.

Not all behaviors undergo transformation over time. In working with older people, knowledge of the typical aging processes needs to be combined with an understanding of the importance of individuality within this heterogeneous population. This chapter demonstrates that chronological age is less a predictor of cognitive performance than other factors such as subjective and objective health status, personality traits, and lifestyle choices (especially as the impact of these choices accumulates over decades of time).

Levy, in conducting important research on the **stereotypes** associated with aging, concluded that aging stereotypes may become self-fulfilling prophecies actually leading to poorer performance among elders.[3] Bennett and Gaines purport that these stereotypes can be both negative and positive, but that in the United States, they tend to be negative.[4] Additionally, as we age, these stereotypes become ingrained in a person's self-perception, which can impact an older person's cognitive and functional well-being.[4] Levy suggests that we need to restructure our deep-seated views by focusing more on the positive changes of aging. By activating more affirmative stereotypes and increasing societal awareness of the strong impact of negative stereotypes (i.e., not actual changes of aging, but merely the associated expectations), we can promote a more realistic image of aging, improved health, and better performance over time.[3]

Aging, or just living life, does entail inevitable change, but when people age well, they become more aware of, and more determined to take advantage of, the positive changes they encounter (e.g., wisdom, maturity, increased self-esteem, increased level of confidence, increased ability to appreciate ambiguity). They also take actions to counteract the negative changes (potential declines in physical and cognitive realms). Older people deserve a hopeful and caring, positive attitude that we, as healthcare professionals, can share with them to promote an optimal, individualized aging process.

An important factor contributing to the current less-than-rosy outlook on the aging process is the increase in the prevalence of dementia, a condition that now touches nearly every extended family. Approximately 5.4 million people in the United States currently have **Alzheimer's disease**, the most common form of dementia, with 5.2 million being over the age of 65.[4] In the Aging, Demographics and Memory Study, researchers found that 13.9% of adults over the age of 71 had dementia.[5] Ironically, the disease is a gift associated with our vast scientific progress. As a greater proportion of the population lives longer, more people are getting dementia. The incidence of dementia increases with advancing age, although it never becomes an inevitable diagnosis even among the oldest-old. We are also more apt to hear about the "suffering" of old age (e.g., cancer, arthritis, stroke), not realizing that many people can still live well and happily even with health problems. A recent study of centenarians found that a significant proportion of the oldest-old has been living with chronic conditions (associated with the condition of "suffering") for decades. Yet the majority of older people do not suffer through life but rather learn to live well despite pain or bodily restrictions.[6]

Finally, because of the cumulative nature of lifestyle choices (e.g., in the realms of nutrition, self-neglect, or substance use or abuse) and the impact disabling conditions have on some older people but not others, elders tend to become more and more different from each other over time—they become a more **heterogeneous** group. Yet often those of an advanced age (age 60 or 65 and older) are lumped together into a single group, as if they were all more alike than different. Older people who have inherited the right genes, have made positive choices throughout life (e.g., with regard to exercise, nutrition, and managing stress), and perhaps have garnered a little luck may be able to function as well as or even better than when they were young, whereas others succumb to disease or functional decline or may even begin "dying by degrees" (described by an elder who felt he was experiencing this prior to his eventual death). As caring healthcare professionals, we can help older people live their best possible lives until they die and to "rage, rage against the dying of the light."[7]

COGNITION

Cognition includes thinking, learning, and memory.[9] Our brains control everything we do intentionally and much of our unintentional behavior as well. Normal aging has biological markers such as decreased brain mass. When this loss is found in the frontal lobes, it impacts cognition, such as executive function and memory.[10] A well-known assertion posits that cognition declines with older age. This premise is only partially true. Zec asserts that cognitive impairments in older adults are primarily caused by three factors[11]:

1. Disease
2. Disuse
3. Aging

Several disease processes affect cognition, and these diseases are more common in the elderly than in younger people. Diseases related to cognitive performance include the most common debilitating disease of old age, Alzheimer's disease (AD), and other dementias, as well as Parkinson's disease, diabetes mellitus, cardiac disease, and the sequelae of acquired brain injuries such as stroke. Those with an interest in the problems of aging related to specific diseases are encouraged to investigate these on their own because detailed information about individual disease processes is beyond the scope of this text. Only AD is considered in more depth because of its prevalence.

Often simple old age is implicated as the cause of cognitive declines, but variables such as education, innate intelligence, and sensory abilities impact cognitive aging.[11] More years of education, and intact audition and vision (corrected) are all associated with a slower rate of cognitive decline.[10]

Disuse may be as much to blame as the impact of just living a certain number of years. We have all heard the advice "use it or lose it" to keep our brains active and performing optimally. We explore optimal brain functioning later in the chapter. First, we delve into various aspects of cognition and how each aspect may change over the course of typical (i.e., healthy) aging. To simplify the presentation, cognition is divided into several sections. However, keep in mind that these cognitive components rarely have distinct boundaries. Given the vast interconnecting brain networks, each aspect of cognition influences many other aspects as we perform our daily tasks. In fact, it is rare for a person to have an isolated cognitive deficit because the human brain tends to work in a highly integrated fashion.

Table 4-1 gives a brief overview of the cognitive changes associated with advanced age, along with a few helpful hints for healthcare providers. An important caveat is that these hints just briefly scratch the surface. People need individualized (client-centered) care, and these ideas may occasionally help. A few areas are described in more depth in the body of the chapter.

ORIENTATION

People who are aging typically are generally alert and oriented in all realms (A&O × 3 or A&O × 4),* as described in Table 4-1. However, retirement—rather than a specific disease process—may contribute more to apparent disorientation to exact date or time of day. Without a planned schedule or daily appointments, one can easily lose track of the exact day and time. Therefore, when determining someone's level of **orientation**, allow a little flexibility and consider the potential influence of an unstructured lifestyle. A psychiatric disturbance is indicated when a person is alert but is not oriented at least to him- or herself. This is not a common occurrence among older people, except for those with severe dementia or another psychiatric illness or those who are currently delirious, perhaps under the influence of medication.

DELIRIUM

Delirium is a common occurrence for those who have been hospitalized, have undergone surgery, or who are overmedicated, but it is not common in a healthy aging population. However, up to 30% of those admitted to the hospital without delirium will develop it during their hospital stay.[12] Generally, delirium is a transient state of fluctuating cognitive abilities often characterized by hallucinations, decreased ability to focus, increased confusion, and poor memory. The symptoms of delirium can be difficult to recognize, and can be mistaken for dementia or depression.[13] A healthcare professional can ease the tense

---

*A&O × 1 = Alert and oriented to self only; A&O × 2 = Oriented to self and surroundings; A&O × 3 = Oriented to self, place, and time; and A&O × 4 = Oriented to self, place, time, and situation (not always used; therefore, A&O × 3 is considered "normal").

TABLE 4-1 The Cognitive Changes of Aging

Aspect of Cognition	Changes of Aging	Helpful Hints
Orientation—knowing who one is (A&O × 1), where one is (A&O × 2), and having an adequate understanding of time (A&O × 3). A&O × 4 may include situation as well.	In the typical aging process, orientation usually remains largely intact as part of crystallized intelligence.[a] As a result of retirement lifestyle, older adults may have more difficulty remembering the exact date or day.	Use calendars and orient person as needed. If the older adult is in an institution, be sure that the orienting information available is up-to-date. Questioning people about orienting information may be intimidating.
Attention—includes being able to sustain attention or focus on one task, alternating attention between two tasks, or dividing attention between two or more tasks (simultaneously). Selective attention involves paying attention to relevant stimuli while filtering out unimportant information.	Ability to sustain attention without distractions remains intact, although older adults tend to be less able to ignore distractions during tasks. Alternating and divided attention tasks may become more difficult, for example, in the task of driving.[b]	Limit distractions, especially when older adults are completing difficult tasks (such as driving) or when they are attending to crucial information (such as healthcare instructions).
Memory—the different types of memory are defined in the chapter.	A decline in memory acuity at older ages has been corroborated by a number of cross-sectional studies.[c] Older people tend to have more difficulty with short-term memory and remembering more recent episodes in their lives, including the source of information or the episode (e.g., where it happened, whom they already told).[d]	Repetition is important for learning. Writing lists and other memory aids can be helpful (and may be used more spontaneously by older adults than by younger people).[e] Do not assume just by telling someone something that he or she will remember and incorporate what you said.
Crystallized intelligence—includes both basic knowledge and skills that accumulate over the course of life.	In typical aging this remains intact or may even continue to improve, especially for overlearned material and individual work-related skills. Reading comprehension, for example, is maintained well into old age, at least until age 75 or beyond.[f] Elders may see themselves as more open-minded or able to better differentiate shades of gray (i.e., ambiguity), rather than just accepting concrete black/white "facts" as truth.[g]	This is related to the construct known as wisdom, and may relate to the ninth stage of life, "gerotranscendence."[h] Well older adults have the potential to gain wisdom through life experience and an increased universal knowledge base.[i] Plenty of older people have wisdom to share with others, including their healthcare providers.

TABLE 4-1   The Cognitive Changes of Aging *(continued)*

Aspect of Cognition	Changes of Aging	Helpful Hints
Fluid intelligence—"the ability to find meaning in confusion and solve new problems . . . [and] to draw inferences and understand the relationships of various concepts, independent of acquired knowledge."[j] Includes executive skills that involve judgment, awareness, and problem solving.	Declines with age to a degree; older adults tend to have more difficulty with more complex, multiple-step tasks.[k] Because fluid intelligence is crucial to the learning process,[l] learning may slow down but does not stop in typical older adults.	Fluid intelligence may improve through practice of tasks requiring executive skills such as self-monitoring performance, completing two tasks simultaneously, and inhibiting irrelevant stimulation. However, this finding was based on respondents mostly in their 20s.[l] Challenging (not frustrating) tasks, especially novel ones, may be crucial for maintaining brain health.[m]

[a] Perlmulter, M. Cognitive potential throughout life. In JE Birren, VL Bengston (Eds.), *Emergent Theories of Aging.* New York: Springer.

[b] Tun, PA, Wingfield, A. One voice too many: Adult age differences in language processing with different types of distracting sounds. *Journals of Gerontology Series B: Psychological Sciences and Social Sciences,* 1995;54B(5):P317–P327. West, R. Visual distraction, working memory, and aging. *Memory and Cognition,* 1999;27(6):1064–1072. Verhaeghen, P, Cerella, J. Aging, executive control, and attention: A review of meta-analyses. *Neuroscience and Behavioral Reviews,* 2002;26(7):849–857.

[c] Colsher, P, Wallace, R. Longitudinal application of cognitive function measures in a defined population of community-dwelling elders. *Annals of Epidemiology,* 1991;1:215–230. Hultsch, D, Hertzog, C, Small, B, McDonald-Miszcak, L, Dixon, R. Short-term longitudinal change in cognitive performance in later life. *Psychology and Aging,* 1991;7:571–584. Wheeler, MA. A comparison of forgetting rates in older and younger adults. *Aging, Neuropsychology, and Cognition,* 2000;7(3):179–193.

[d] Hoyer, WJ, Verhaeghen, P. Memory aging. In JE Birren, KW Schaie (Eds.), *Handbook of the Psychology of Aging.* Burlington, MA: Elsevier, 2006: 209–232.

[e] Baddeley, AD. The psychology of memory. In AD Baddeley, BA Wilson, FN Watts (Eds.), *The Handbook of Memory Disorders.* Chichester, UK: John Wiley and Sons, 1995.

[f] Schaie, KW. *Intellectual Development in Adulthood: The Seattle Longitudinal Study.* New York: Cambridge University Press, 1996. Salthouse, TA. Pressing issues in cognitive aging. In N Schwartz, D Park, B Knauper, S Sudman (Eds.), *Cognition, Aging and Self-Reports.* Philadelphia: Psychology Press.

[g] Erikson, EH, et al. *Vital Involvement in Old Age.* New York: W. W. Norton, 1989: 36.

[h] Erikson, EH, Erikson, JM. *The Life Cycle Completed.* New York: W. W. Norton, 1998.

[i] Ardelt, M. Intellectual versus wisdom related knowledge: The case for a different kind of learning in later years of life. *Educational Gerontology,* 2000;26:1–15.

[j] Cavanaugh, JC, Blanchard-Fields, F. *Adult Development and Aging.* 5th ed. Belmont, CA: Wadsworth Publishing/Thomson Learning, 2006.

[k] West, R. Visual distraction, working memory, and aging. *Memory and Cognition,* 1999;27(6):1064–1072.

[l] Jaeggi, SM, Buschkuehl, M, Jonides, J, Perrig, WJ. Improving fluid intelligence with training on working memory. Proc Natl Acad Sci USA105:6829–6833.

[m] Nussbaum, PD. *Brain Health and Wellness.* Tarentum, PA: Word Association Publishers, 2003.

Source: Adapted from Robnett, RH. Client factors and their effect on occupational performance in late life. In S Coppola, SJ Elliott, PE Toto (Eds.), *Strategies to Advance Gerontology Excellence.* Bethesda, MD: AOTA Press, 2008: 163–197.

situation experienced by families by explaining that the state of being delirious is generally temporary in nature and by educating the family about the side effects of the patient's current medical procedure or medication. Nonetheless, the development of delirium is associated with increased mortality, increased length of stay in the hospital, increased rate of discharge to long-term care facilities, and increased medical complications. Cognitive decline is also a risk for those who experience delirium as they age.[13]

Risk factors for delirium include age greater than 70 years, self-reported alcohol abuse, poor cognitive status, visual impairment, depression, poor functional status, malnutrition, metabolic abnormalities, infections, noncardiac thoracic surgery, or abdominal aneurysm surgery.[12,13] Any change in mental status should be reported to and addressed by the healthcare team. Postoperation delirium research is ongoing. Medical teams are looking for ways to reduce the incidence of delirium by developing better postoperation pathways to address the medications used for various reasons (e.g., to control pain, decrease nausea, address nutritional needs, resume pre-op medication routines [e.g., for Parkinson's], manage constipation, reduce post-op complications, and restore a healthy sleep cycle). In addition, the teams seek to provide needed equipment (glasses, hearing aids, dentures, etc.) and to reorient the person with familiar objects.[13] Furthermore, family collaboration is crucial if delirium is suspected, because the family can provide information regarding the older adult's baseline behavior and may be first to detect a change.[14] Prevention, detection, and management are the solutions for delirium, with prevention being the best line of defense.

ATTENTION

Being able to focus or concentrate on an activity does not seem to be affected specifically by age.[11] Simple, overlearned tasks do not usually become more difficult for older people. However, in a study by Tun and Wingfield,[15] older adults were questioned about their perceptions of their own abilities to complete 16 different divided-attention tasks, such as walking and talking, or driving and planning a schedule. The researchers determined that older people did not perceive routine tasks and those involving speech processing to become more challenging over time. Relative to younger adults, however, the older respondents reported increasing difficulties with simultaneous dual task performance on more demanding tasks. Therefore, it may be more difficult for older adults to divide their **attention** between two activities (e.g., driving and talking; cooking multiple courses at the same time). Objectively, older people do have more difficulty with divided-attention tasks, especially when the two or more tasks are complex (e.g., not simple or overlearned).[16]

MEMORY

Memory is not a simple, unidimensional construct. Although, generally speaking, memory does decline with age, it is worth taking the time to qualify exactly what the construct of memory entails and to explore the different aspects of memory in relation to the aging process. Recalling something out of the blue is a more complex task and is affected to a greater extent than recognition (in which one is given hints about the potential answer, for example, in multiple-choice answers). Recognition, which is simpler, may be retained to a high level throughout life.[17] Other basic memory tasks, such as those requiring procedural memory (i.e., motor patterns), basic cognitive skills (mathematics or use of vocabulary), or remembering facts that have been well-learned, are usually preserved throughout the typical aging process.

Several types of memory are described here, although these categories are not an exhaustive list. The description includes how aging is associated with the type of memory in question.

The following types of memory are based on temporal aspects of remembering:

- **Primary memory**: Primary memory has limited capacity and is based on incoming information that is either used or generally forgotten in a matter of seconds. Immediate recall of seven digits (plus or minus two) has been considered normal for adults since Miller's research in the 1950s.[18] Primary memory does not seem to be affected by aging. This type of memory involves sustained attention and is of extremely short duration (unless rehearsal takes place).
- **Short-term memory**: Short-term memory involves remembering information for a short duration. An example of normal short-term memory is being able to recall a seven-digit number (for example, a telephone number) for a few minutes. Although older people do show a decline in this type of memory, the decline is more pronounced as the information increases in length or complexity.[19]
- **Working memory**: Working memory refers to being able to actively use or manipulate the information from the brain's short-term storage base during a task. For example, it involves recalling a telephone number while dialing the number or retaining the steps of a new recipe while cooking (both without looking back). Age-related deficits, such as in reading and listening span, have been consistently significant.[19]
- **Prospective memory**: Prospective memory enables a person to remember to do something in the future (e.g., appointments, medications, meetings, chores). With regard to aging, older people may be better at spontaneously compensating for losses in prospective memory as they learn to adjust to memory losses gradually.[20] In naturalistic or real-life settings, older people often outperform their younger counterparts by incorporating compensatory strategies such as list making.[19]
- **Long-term memory**: Long-term memory is permanent or long-term storage, for example, autobiographical information, early life experiences, or repetitive information that involves "more durable encoding and storage systems."[21(p.479)] For well-learned knowledge, this type of memory is the least affected by age, although it may be difficult to conjure up the exact facts when needed.

The following types of memory are based on the type of information to be encoded:

- **Episodic memory**: Episodic memory is oriented toward the past and is what most people think of when they think of the global term *memory*. This type of declarative or conscious memory particularly involves remembering episodes or experiences in our lives (e.g., what we ate for lunch, our last birthday party) or as Bäckman, Small, and Wahlin state, it is the "acquisition and retrieval of information acquired in a particular place at a particular time."[22(p.354)] Episodic memory can be either short term, such as remembering that you just turned on the stove, or long term, such as remembering the very first day of school. Episodic memory is particularly vulnerable to the effects of aging.[19,23] When tested simultaneously, younger people tend to outperform older people on tests of episodic memory.[23,24]

  An analogy involving episodic memory is to imagine a bucket that holds just a certain amount (**Figure 4-1**). As time goes by, the bucket is filled by memories of life's events. As the bucket nears capacity, more of the potential memories get sloshed out. Although this analogy has limited direct scientific basis, it can explain the increased difficulty of retaining additional information as we grow older. (If only we

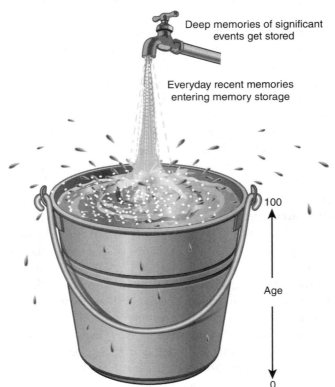

FIGURE 4-1 Episodic memory: hypothetical bucket. Everyday memories hold little significance and therefore easily "splash out" (i.e., are forgotten).

could delete unimportant information to make room for additional incoming data of significance.) Another explanation for declining episodic memory skills could be disuse caused by less environmental stimulation (e.g., during retirement, especially if the older person is homebound, or has a decrease in vision or hearing).

- **Semantic memory**: Semantic memory involves a cumulative knowledge base about the world in general (e.g., language, including the meaning of words and the relationship of words, mathematical facts, symbols and formulas, vocational information learned during one's career, and recall of current events and worldly facts). This "internal lexicon" is the buildup of information over the course of one's life (as part of crystallized intelligence).[22(p.352)] Semantic memory changes portray a complex picture in that elders have more word-finding problems (such as the tip-of-the-tongue phenomenon), but vocabulary may even improve into old age.[19,25]
- **Procedural memory**: Procedural memory is performance based, for example, remembering how to ride a bicycle or the motoric steps to completing a recipe or self-care task. Because daily performance tasks are often overlearned and have become automatic, this type of memory is often maintained into old age. This situation can be problematic at times, for example, when a person with dementia remembers the procedure of driving (e.g., inserting the key, turning the wheel, pushing on the gas pedal) but has forgotten how to manage the more cognitively challenging aspects of driving (e.g., problem solving in the midst of traffic or navigating in unfamiliar territory).

In summary, a great number of studies have been completed on memory and aging. Notable is that not all types of memory are affected equally by the typical aging process. Critical differences have been found among the various memory systems. Research in the area of episodic versus semantic memory has often demonstrated a more severe decline in memory for events (episodic memory tasks), whereas verbal memory such as vocabulary (semantic memory) tends to be better preserved.[26] Working memory tends to decline more sharply with age than immediate or primary memory. Most elderly people were able to retain 7-digit telephone numbers as well as their younger counterparts (primary memory task); however, when a 10-digit number was used (e.g., a long-distance telephone number), the older participants did not perform as well.[27] Studies showing a memory decline with age have often involved more complicated tasks.[19,22] Older people also seem to have more difficulty ignoring distractions during working memory tasks, and they are less able to ignore irrelevant thoughts.[28,29]

Compensatory techniques and adaptive measures may be necessary to maintain quality of life if memory skills start to diminish significantly. Self-help books on this subject are readily available. For the healthcare professional, several tactics may be helpful when working with people who tend to be forgetful:

- Make the material to be learned interesting (applicable to the client's life). A story, an anecdote, or even a song may more easily catch and hold the client's attention.
- Use multimodal sensory input (e.g., let the person hear and read the information, as well as use other senses to interact with the material as appropriate).

- Use repetition, but not to the point of boredom or becoming condescending as if you are testing the person.
- Use cuing, but only as needed.
- Have clients work with or manipulate the information if at all possible (e.g., have them write out or input their own schedule rather than just giving them the printed schedule).
- Information that the older person perceives to be important will more likely be able to find a place in memory storage banks.
- Immediately following an instruction session, have clients paraphrase what was just conveyed or show-and-tell the information they just encountered; both can be effective techniques to enhance the learning process, applying the adage that one learns best by teaching.

Following are some tips to stimulate remembering (or compensate for decreased memory), adapted from Lucci[30] and Strauss[31]:

- *Pay attention.* Information can be remembered only if it is initially acknowledged.
- *Repeat what you want to remember by rehearsing aloud.* If you meet someone and want to remember his or her name, be sure to use the name in conversation within the next few minutes.
- *Make lists or use a date book (or electronic calendar).* Write down what you want to remember (but then practice remembering without the list).
- *Establish habits.* For example, always put your keys on the hook beside the door, or always park in the same section of the parking lot at the mall. Make healthy habits of proper diet and exercise for physical and cognitive well-being.
- *Relax.* Relaxation may allow the mind to clear itself of problems, which may help to facilitate recall, whereas excess stress can hinder learning and memory.
- *Use self and environmental cues.* These cues can be invaluable for stimulating memory skills. Environmental cues can be as diverse as signs, kitchen timers, or alarm clocks. Use memory triggers; look over photos to provoke memories.

Problems with memory tasks, both subjective (memory complaints) and objective (actual losses), are probably the most commonly acknowledged types of age-related cognitive decline.[32] Displaying poor memory skills does not mean that a person has dementia. Mild forgetfulness, when it is an isolated cognitive impairment, is not cause for alarm and is experienced by young and old alike. Decreased memory, or **age-associated memory impairment** (AAMI), is widespread and refers to memory skills that are lower than average. AAMI is not as serious and may or may not relate to mild cognitive impairment.

Mild cognitive impairment (MCI) refers to lower than expected cognitive performance in memory or other cognitive tasks (usually defined as more than 1.5 standard deviations below the typical group mean during neuropsychological testing). MCI usually does not interfere with day-to-day activities.[33] There are four subtypes of MCI. Amnestic MCI (aMCI) is the most common, and generally has a more rapid progression. MCI affects approximately 16% of older adults who do not have dementia, and it impacts men more often than women.[34]

A meta-analysis of 41 cohort studies conducted by Mitchell and Shiri-Feshki[35] found an eventual 39.2% conversion rate from MCI to dementia, and a 5–10% conversion rate per year. Therefore, the majority of people with MCI do not develop more serious cognitive declines commensurate with dementia.[35]

Risk factors for MCI are much like those for dementia in general, and include diabetes, smoking, hypertension, sedentary lifestyle, lack of engagement in cognitively challenging tasks, high cholesterol levels, and depression.[33] Preserving cognition often can be facilitated by a healthy, engaging, and active lifestyle. Malek-Ahmadi et al. determined that four questions on the Alzheimer's questionnaire were most predictive of aMCI.[36] These are:

1. Does the patient have trouble remembering the date, year, and time? (most predictive)
2. Does the patient repeat questions/statements in the same day?
3. Does the patient have difficulty managing finances?
4. Does the patient have a decreased sense of direction?

Memory remediation may be possible for those who are motivated to improve their ability to remember. Compensating for, rather than trying to improve, decreased memory performance, however, seems to work best for most older people who sometimes get creative in their approaches to reminding themselves. For example, putting car keys in the refrigerator as a reminder to bring lunch with them or keeping pill boxes at the dinner table as a reminder to take medications can both be helpful.

One way to assess whether older people have memory impairments is simply to ask them. Yet it is worth noting that people, in general, do not have a good sense of how well they can remember. Although self-assessments are efficient and easy to use, their usefulness is questionable because the correlation between level of memory impairment per self-report and level determined through objective neuropsychological testing has typically been insignificant or low.[37-39] Keep in mind that we are asking those with less than perfect memory capabilities to make judgments about their ability to *remember*. A more objective measure would be observing functional memory performance, for example, noting whether the person has left the stove on, has had difficulty with medication routines, or has forgotten important appointments. Compensatory measures, including perhaps reminders from others, may be necessary.

Healthcare practitioners can use various screens to assess cognitive function. The results can influence the approach to rehabilitation, offer suggestions for caregivers, and provide strategies for managing cognitive decline. **Table 4-2** provides a brief list of possible tools.

CRYSTALLIZED AND FLUID INTELLIGENCE

Crystallized intelligence tends to remain strong in those who are aging typically and includes skills such as language comprehension, educational qualifications, and life and occupational skills. Baltes compared this type of intelligence with what we term wisdom,

TABLE 4-2 Tools for Assessing Cognition

Name	Tool Description
Montreal Assessment of Cognition (MoCA)[a]	Rapid screening tool for mild cognitive dysfunction that assesses attention and concentration, executive functions, memory, language, visuo-constructional skills, conceptual thinking, calculations, and orientation.
The Saint Louis University Mental Status (SLUMS)[b]	Examination with oral and written content for detecting mild cognitive impairment and dementia; results can help a doctor determine if further diagnostics are needed if dementia is suspected.
Mini Mental State Exam (MMSE)[c]	Common screening tool that provides quantitative measure of cognitive impairment.
Loewenstein Occupational Therapy Cognitive Assessment (LOTCA)[d]	Battery of assessments for adults with neurological impairments to assess cognitive function.
Short Blessed Test (SBT)[e]	Sensitive screen used to detect early cognitive changes associated with Alzheimer's disease.
Executive Function Performance Test (EFPT)[f]	Top-down functional assessment that assesses executive cognitive function in an environmental context by way of task initiation, execution, and completion.

Data from: [a] Nasreddine. http://www.mocatest.org; [b] St. Louis University. http://medschool.slu.edu/agingsuccessfully/pdfsurveys/slumsexam_05.pdf; [c] Folstein & Folstein. http://www4.parinc.com/Products/Product.aspx?ProductID=MMSE-2; [d] Itzkovich, Averbuch, Elazar, & Katz. http://www.therapro.com/The-Loewenstein-Occupational-Therapy-Cognitive-Assessment-LOTCA-2nd-Edition-P7732.aspx; [e] Washington University School of Medicine. http://alzheimer.wustl.edu/adrc2/Images/SBT.pdf; [f] Washington University School of Medicine. http://www.ot.wustl.edu/ot/otweb.nsf/5af541d3cfd036a986257260005bc07d/ecc9551f54901f1d8625791e0063d1a7!OpenDocument

or "an expert knowledge system in the fundamental pragmatics of life permitting excellent judgment and advice involving important and uncertain matters of life."[40] Older adults may be more skilled at making decisions, perhaps because of their ability to take life's ambiguities into account.[41]

Despite a strong perceived link between wisdom and aging, even highly intellectual older individuals in our society are not necessarily revered for their level of understanding of life's complexities. In certain cultures, especially ancient ones, elders are expected to share historical stories, songs, rituals, and traditions with future generations. They are considered the sages of the community. Yet, in our modern Western society, older people rarely have such important societal roles, and therefore the wisdom of aging may often get lost in favor of individualism, materialism, and the quest for eternal youth.[42] According to do Rozario, in our developed world we may have lost "our sense of history and real wisdom."[42(p.121)] Schachter-Shalomi and Miller, in their book *From Age-ing to Sage-ing: A Profound New Vision of Growing Older*, put forward the idea that older people who work on expanding their consciousness and promoting their spiritual growth may demonstrate wisdom in their actions, thereby attaining "the crowning achievement of life."[43(p.17)]

If we buy into their proposal, rather than the "inevitable" decline and disengagement expected by many—young and old alike—older people could (again) be considered the wise pillars of the community. Some might say that by honoring the wise and respecting their collective insight, these elders with superior judgment would be returning to their rightful place in society. At least we could be open to the hopeful possibilities.

Fluid intelligence includes the speed and accuracy of information processing, such as discrimination, comparison, and categorization. It has been deemed to be largely evolutionarily and genetically based. Baltes researched the two types of intelligences in young and old subjects and found that only fluid intelligence, or "biologically based mechanics," showed a significant decline in older adults. He proposed that when learning potential was no longer evident (i.e., when practice or memory training no longer had an additional effect), the participant could be starting the process of pathologic rather than typical aging.[40] However, even though this study and others[24,44] have shown that the human mind has its limitations in old age, Baltes and associates[45] also point out that these limits often are not apparent because the brain is generally not used to its full potential. Baltes draws an interesting analogy of a young and an old person strolling together. Walking together works out well until the couple approaches a hill; the steeper the hill, the more difficult it may be for the older person to keep up. This is true not only with physical performance, but also with mental functioning, especially processing speed.

Gerontological researchers have studied the cognitive changes of aging. Cross-sectional studies comparing the young to the old at one point in time tend to show definitive differences favoring the young in various aspects of thinking, with the declines more pronounced in the realm of fluid intelligence. Longitudinal studies, such as the Seattle Longitudinal Study (SLS),[24] examine individuals over time (since 1956 for the SLS). These studies generally have found less change over time within the individual than across individuals. Several factors are associated with worse or better performance over time. The genetic factors (e.g., race, gender, innate intelligence) cannot be changed, but people can influence many factors related to cognitive performance. For example, physical exercise, cognitive stimulation, nutrition, smoking, alcohol use, level of education, and employment type have all been shown to correlate to cognitive functioning.[46,47] In a recent article on training the brain, Curlik and Shors purport that aerobic physical exercise helps the brain produce new neurons in the hippocampus, while mental stimulation, such as learning novel tasks, helps those new neurons survive.[48] Making and sustaining positive lifestyle choices can have lasting effects well into old age.

LEARNING

The ability to learn new information can change as people age. Certainly, the old (and we hope outdated) adage that "an old dog can't learn new tricks" does not apply to older people who are aging well. Ongoing research, such as that cited by Curlik and Shors and taking place at the Salk Institute,[48] has unequivocally demonstrated that even older (middle-aged and beyond) brain cells can regenerate, an exciting finding with huge implications for stroke rehabilitation and medicine in general.[49] We have known for years that brain cells can develop new interneuronal connections and "add system capacity" to enhance learning.[50] Older individuals indeed may need more practice sessions than their younger counterparts to master a task. They also may need to have the instructions presented in a variety of ways (e.g., verbal, written, or demonstrated) and perhaps geared toward their sensory capacities (e.g., larger print) before learning can occur.

Neuropsychologist Dr. Paul Nussbaum, in his book *Brain Health and Wellness*, promotes the idea that learning should no longer be considered merely a means to an end, but that learning on its own ought to be seen as crucial to maintaining health, both physical and cognitive.[51] He expands on the adage "use it or lose it" by suggesting that we not only need to use our brains to maintain brain health, but also further stimulate our brains by engaging in activities both "novel and complex" on a regular basis.[51(p.162)] By challenging our brains through new learning, we can, throughout life, enhance the thinking process and potentially create brain reserve.[52] Additionally, energizing environments that engage participants in socialization, physical activity, and mental stimulation help to create a healthy brain—one that may be able to delay the onset of disease.[52,53] One example of brain health was discovered by den Dunnen and colleagues, who studied the brain donated to science by the oldest Dutch woman, who lived to be 115 and died in 2005.[54] Contrary to expectations, the woman's cognition was at a relatively high performance level until she died, and the autopsy revealed no significant pathology. This hopeful finding relates to the idea of brain preservation throughout life, even a very long life.

DEMENTIA

Normal aging does include a slowing down and a gradual wearing out of bodily systems. It does not include dementia, which is considered a pathologic aging process. **Dementia** is defined as progressive cognitive impairment that eventually interferes with daily functioning. The prevalence of dementia among 60-year-olds is only 1–2%, but dementia becomes increasingly more common with advancing age.[50] Now with a much higher proportion of the population of industrialized nations living into old age, the prevalence of dementia has been increasing. Worldwide, there were 26.6 million people with Alzheimer's disease in 2006, with an estimated 5.4 million people in the United States. A new case of Alzheimer's disease (AD) surfaces every 68 seconds.[4,55] AD is more common in women because they live longer. Therefore, two-thirds of those with AD in the United States are women.[4] The mean age of onset is 81 years of age.[56] AD is the most common form of dementia (comprising about two-thirds of all dementia types).[57] Due to its high prevalence, the discussion here focuses on AD specifically. Interested readers are encouraged to find out more information on other forms of dementia they encounter in clients or patients, such as Lewy body dementia, frontotemporal dementia, or dementias related to Parkinson's disease or stroke (cerebrovascular accidents).

Certain causes of dementia may be treatable, and given the appropriate treatment, cognitive functioning may be restored. Causes of dementia-type symptoms may include infections (such as urinary tract infections), metabolic and endocrine disturbances, malnutrition, alcohol and/or drug abuse, psychiatric disorders, deficiency states, trauma, Huntington's disease, Pick's disease, and Parkinson's disease.[58]

Dementia, specifically AD, encompasses multiple cognitive, psychological, and functional deficits, including memory impairment, which is always present (**Figure 4-2**). The following signs and symptoms may be present as well:

- Difficulties with understanding or communicating through language.
- Difficulty with problem solving and other high-level cognitive tasks, such as abstract reasoning. A common cognitive test used with people who are suspected of having dementia is the Mini Mental State Examination, which is a brief and readily available cognitive screening tool.[59]
- Impaired visual spatial skills, which can impair the ability to drive safely.[60]
- Behavioral disturbances such as depression, anxiety, wandering, and neglect of personal hygiene.[56]

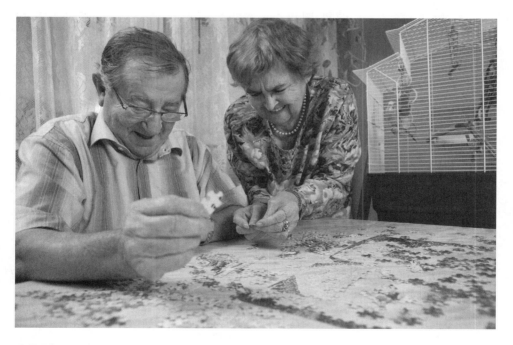

FIGURE 4-2
© iStockphoto/Thinkstock

During the early stages of AD (usually the first few years following onset), physical symptoms are not as common. The person is able to walk and displays normal movement patterns and posture. As the disease progresses, however, the impairments associated with AD worsen. People with AD usually regress developmentally until, when near death, they may display some behaviors similar to a newly born infant. **Table 4-3** describes some of the progression of features commonly seen in AD. It needs to be pointed out that each person displays an individual course of the disease and therefore may have only a few rather than all of these traits.

AD progresses through three stages: mild, moderate, and severe. Because there is no cure, the current emphasis of medical providers is to prolong the first two stages. Medications to maintain cognitive functioning and manage agitation are constantly being tested. The Cochrane Database of Systematic Reviews provides up-to-date overviews of different medications being proposed as treatment for AD.[61,62] Scientists try to ward off the third

TABLE 4-3 Alzheimer's Disease Symptom Progression

	Initial	End Stage
General behavior	Indifferent; may be delusional or depressed; may deny problems	Withdrawn, agitated, mood may change abruptly
Language	Normal or mild word finding difficulties	Severe impairment, words may be meaningless "word-salad"
Memory	Mild short-term deficits	Unable to test
Orientation	Fully oriented	Oriented to self only
Personal care/ADL skills[a]	Inattention to detail, but able to complete basic personal care	Dependency, may show fear of bathing
Instrumental ADLs[b]	Slight impairment, carelessness, decreased safety awareness, may need supervision	Unable to complete
Mobility	Normal	Abnormal, may not be able to walk or transfer independently
Posture	Normal	Flexed, often preferring a fetal position
Range of motion/ movement	Normal or within functional limits	Increased muscle tonus; contractures[c] common

[a]ADLs (activities of daily living) include bathing, dressing, self-feeding, grooming, and so forth.
[b]IADLs (instrumental activities of daily living) include home management, money management, care of others, and so forth.
[c]A contracture is defined as a decrease of 50% or more of normal passive range of motion. It is a painful condition affecting many in long-term care settings, including more than three-quarters of patients who can no longer walk (Souren, LE, Frensses, EH, Reisberg, B. Contractures and loss of function in patients with Alzheimer's disease. *Journal of the American Geriatrics Society*, 1995;43(6):650–655).
Data from: Ham, RJ. Making the diagnosis of Alzheimer's disease. *Patient Care*, June 15, 1995: 104–120; Morris, JC. The Clinical Dementia Rating (CDR): Current version and scoring rules. *Neurology*, November 1993: 2412–2414; and Cole, SA. Behavioral disturbances in Alzheimer's disease. *Patient Care*, June 15, 1995: 121–131.

stage because they believe that initially and into the middle stages for those with AD "most of the person is still there." Someone in the initial stages is still physically capable and can still find joy in living.[60] As healthcare professionals, we need to emphasize these beliefs with caregivers, who greatly need support when caring for someone with AD.

WORKING WITH THOSE WHO HAVE DEMENTIA

There are some general guidelines to follow when working with persons who have dementia. Again, remember that these are suggestions only; what works for one may have the opposite impact on another.

- Caring and respect are essential, even when the person cannot reciprocate.
- Healthcare professionals (or anyone) should never speak about persons with dementia in front of them as if they were not there.
- The behavior of those with AD may try your patience even as a professional, but controlling your emotions is crucial. Remember that the person is not intentionally trying to provoke you.
- Soothing music may defuse the intensity of an uncomfortable situation and foster relaxation.
- A sense of humor, so that you can laugh together, also can be extremely helpful, although it is important never to let the person think that you are laughing at him or her.
- Diversion may help to calm a stressful situation, including the following:
  - Involvement in simple (not childish) activities
  - Playing games, playing or enjoying music, and singing songs they have enjoyed formerly
  - Drawing, writing, or painting
  - Looking through old photograph albums; creating albums or scrapbooks for the future
  - Reminiscing ("Tell me about . . .")
  - Involving them in tasks or parts of tasks they enjoy, for example, helping with meal preparation or taking care of or just interacting with a pet

Several books are available for those who want to improve their ability to work with older people who have dementia. A few examples are *A Dignified Life: The Best Friends Approach to Alzheimer's Care* by Bell and Troxel,[63] *The Best Friends Book of Alzheimer's Activities* (Volumes I and II),[64] and *Talking to Alzheimer's* by Strauss and Khachaturian.[65] **Table 4-4** offers some more specific, though not prescriptive, suggestions as well.

RELATED DISORDERS

Sometimes what appears to be dementia is actually another medical disorder in disguise. Gaining a basic understanding of some of these common disorders may help you decide when to make referrals. Some of the more common ailments with signs and symptoms similar to dementia are briefly described here.

TABLE 4-4 Dementia: Problems and Potential Solutions

Functional Problem Area	Potential Solutions
Decreased self-care skills (ADLs)	• Offer supervision • Simplify clothing/environment • Gently encourage person to do as much as possible without nagging • Remove safety hazards • Obtain an occupational therapy referral
Decreased involvement in daily activities	• Encourage involvement in what person can still do well • Praise successes and have patience • Try safe, simple repetitive chores • Offer items of interest
Wandering	• Take walks together in safe areas • Purchase identification bracelet • Alert neighbors • Remove obstacles indoors • If balance is decreased, obtain physical therapy referral
Impaired communication	• Speak slowly and calmly; do not yell • Give simple directions, one step at a time • Use repetition as needed • Obtain speech therapy referral
Sleep disturbance	• Establish a bedtime routine • Make sure person gets enough exercise/activity during the day • Limit liquid before bedtime • Encourage toileting immediately before bedtime • Omit obstacles in bedroom to bathroom route or purchase bedside commode • A back rub may promote restful sleep
Problem Behavior	**Possible Solutions**
Inappropriate behavior	• Always treat person with dignity and respect • Divert person to another activity • Watch for signs of overstimulation and try to avoid these situations • Listen and respond to the feeling behind the words being said, rather than the words themselves • Ask for help (e.g., from team, doctors, support group, adult day care) • Use humor • Do not ignore requests for assistance
Anxiety and/or agitation	• Structure environment • Establish daily routine with lots of opportunity for structured activities • Promote the feeling of security

TABLE 4-4   Dementia: Problems and Potential Solutions (*continued*)

Problem Behavior	Possible Solutions
Anger	• Offer a drink, a snack, or a favorite item • Do not confront, tease, or argue with the person • Listen and divert to new topic if possible • Limit stimulation • Remove from disruptive environment • Take care of your own safety

Data from: Cole, SA. Behavioral disturbances in Alzheimer's disease. *Patient Care,* June 15, 1995: 121–131; Gwyther, LP. General guidelines for caregivers and tips for communicating with your relative. *Patient Care,* June 15, 1995: 132–134; and Colorado State University. *Guidelines for Working with People with Alzheimer's Disease* [class handout]. Fort Collins, CO: Alzheimer's Disease and Aging Research, Department of Psychology, 1989.

Malnutrition   Deficiencies of the B-complex vitamins, vitamin C, zinc, magnesium, folic acid, and protein, or **malnutrition**, can cause behavioral disturbances, including those implicated in the diagnosis of clinical depression.[66]

Cerebrovascular Accident (CVA) or Stroke   **Cerebrovascular accident** (CVA) or stroke, especially small infarcts with limited accompanying functional declines, may cause behavior disturbances much like those brought about by depression or AD. In fact, a rather common type of dementia (multi-infarct dementia) is caused by a series of small strokes.

Hypothyroidism   Hypothyroidism slows metabolic processes, which causes the affected person to respond slowly and to be lethargic.

Failure to Thrive   A related syndrome to ones previously described is **failure to thrive** (FTT). An insidious deterioration in functioning that is not related to a specific disease, FTT can be caused by depression, dementia, chronic conditions, or drug reactions. Social isolation, low socioeconomic status, and functional dependency all are predisposing factors of FTT. Case examples are common; perhaps we all know of someone who just seemed to wither away prior to dying. Common features of FTT include weight loss resulting from lack of appetite, social withdrawal, lack of concern about appearance, memory loss, impaired ambulation, and incontinence (common in nearly half the cases described).[67] Those with this syndrome simply seem to be giving up on life. A referral to a geriatrician is usually appropriate for those with (potential) FTT.

Lack of Oxygen   Certain disorders (e.g., lung disease, pneumonia) are associated with a lowered ability of the body to complete oxygen uptake. *Hypoxemia* refers to insufficient oxygen levels in the blood. Oxygen saturation levels (O_2Sat) for most people should be 95% or higher. The saturation level is measured by a pulse oximeter that is placed on the finger. Although a physician must determine what is abnormal for any one person, in general hypoxemia can lead to tissue damage as well as mental confusion, including impaired judgment and problem-solving ability. Therefore, someone with low blood oxygen levels may appear to have dementia. Fortunately, administering oxygen, often through a nasal cannula per physician's orders, may improve mental status quickly.

Learned Helplessness   Another complication that has received little attention as a problem of aging is **learned helplessness**, which is a condition that develops when living beings "learn that their responses are independent of desired outcomes."[68] Consequently, they learn to not respond to stimulation from their environment. For example, in experiments when dogs learned that they could not control the onset of electric shocks, they eventually gave up and became helpless and apathetic. Similar results can occur in human beings, perhaps especially older people who may receive (too much) care from others.

For example, Mr. M., who came in as a patient for rehabilitation in a skilled nursing unit after rather minor surgery, was unable to complete his self-care skills, even though he had no medical or physical reason not to (other than deconditioning). It turned out that his home health aides, provided by his well-intentioned family, had taken over doing everything for him, even the most basic self-care tasks such as dressing. He had *learned* to become compliant and helpless. Fortunately for Mr. M., he was able to unlearn his helplessness and was actually surprised about what he could accomplish for himself when given the chance. Caregivers, who may be overly caring, do more than necessary for their patients and therefore may inadvertently "help" them lose the ability to complete vital life tasks.

DEPRESSION IN OLDER ADULTS

At least 1 out of every 10 adults in the United States report having symptoms of depression.[69] The Centers for Disease Control and Prevention found **depression** to be most prevalent in persons 45–64 years of age, women, blacks, Hispanics, non-Hispanic persons of other races or multiple races, persons with less than a high school education, those previously married, individuals unable to work or unemployed, and persons without health insurance.[69] At least 1 out of 20 community-dwelling people older than age 65 have clinical depression. This number rises sharply in hospitals and long-term care facilities, where the prevalence of depression reaches at least 10% to over 30%.[70,71] Despite this high proportion of depression in older adults, depression as a clinical condition often goes unnoticed and therefore undiagnosed. This is an especially heart-wrenching fact considering that depression is often amenable to treatment.

Cognitive symptoms of depression may include decreases in episodic memory, language processing, working memory, executive function, and processing speed. Cognitive changes in older adults with symptoms of depression can be related to the biological function of the thyroid gland, hypothalamic-pituitary functions, hippocampal function, and vascular disease.[72]

The purpose of this section is to make healthcare professionals aware of the signs and symptoms of clinical depression and to offer guidelines for treatment and referral. The Geriatric Depression Scale (GDS), a brief, convenient self-report screening measure for depression among older adults, is shown in **Table 4-5**.

TABLE 4-5   Geriatric Depression Scale (Short Form)

Patient's Name: _____ Date: _____

Instructions: Choose the best answer for how you felt over the past week. Note: When asking the patient to complete the form, provide the self-rated form.

No.	Question	Answer	Score
1.	Are you basically satisfied with your life?	Yes / *No*	
2.	Have you dropped many of your activities and interests?	*Yes* / No	
3.	Do you feel that your life is empty?	*Yes* / No	
4.	Do you often get bored?	*Yes* / No	
5.	Are you in good spirits most of the time?	Yes / *No*	
6.	Are you afraid that something bad is going to happen to you?	*Yes* / No	
7.	Do you feel happy most of the time?	Yes / *No*	
8.	Do you often feel helpless?	*Yes* / No	
9.	Do you prefer to stay at home, rather than going out and doing new things?	*Yes* / No	
10.	Do you feel you have more problems with memory than most people?	*Yes* / No	
11.	Do you think it is wonderful to be alive?	Yes / *No*	
12.	Do you feel pretty worthless the way you are now?	*Yes* / No	
13.	Do you feel full of energy?	Yes / *No*	
14.	Do you feel that your situation is hopeless?	*Yes* / No	
15.	Do you think that most people are better off than you are?	*Yes* / No	
		TOTAL	

Scoring:

Answers indicating depression are in bold and italicized; score one point for each one selected. A score of 0 to 5 is normal. A score greater than 5 suggests depression.

*Apps are now available on the iPhone and Android for this screen.

Source: Reproduced from Sheikh JI, Yesavage JA: Geriatric Depression Scale (GDS): Recent evidence and development of a shorter version. *Clinical Gerontology: A Guide to Assessment and Intervention.* 1986;5(1/2):165–173, NY: The Haworth Press, 1986.

DSM-IV-TR CRITERIA FOR DEPRESSION

According to the *Diagnostic and Statistical Manual of Mental Disorders*, 4th edition (DSM-IV-TR),[73] the following are common signs and symptoms of depression:

- *Depressed mood "most of the day, nearly every day"*[73(p.356)]: The person may feel sad or appear tearful. The person may complain of feeling hopeless. (This may be the easiest symptom to recognize, but because we all have "off" days, it may go unnoticed.)
- *Anhedonia:* The person has difficulty experiencing pleasure doing formerly enjoyable activities.
- *Weight gain or loss:* More than 5% of body weight within 1 month.

- *Sleep disturbances:* Sleeping either more or less than usual.
- *Psychomotor disturbances:* Either slowness in movements or agitated/hyperactive movements.
- *Feelings of worthlessness or lowered self-esteem.*
- *Decreased energy nearly every day.*
- *Cognitive changes:* These changes may include inability to concentrate or to complete cognitive tasks that were formerly successfully completed.
- *Indecisiveness nearly every day.*
- *Recurrent thoughts of death and/or suicide.*
- *Guilt:* The DSM-IV-TR also lists guilt as a symptom of depression,[73] but others claim that the expression of guilt is not a common feature of depression in older adults.[74]

If several of these signs and symptoms, especially one of the first two, are present for two weeks or more, a referral to the person's physician is in order because he or she may have clinical depression, a serious but often treatable disorder.[73] As a healthcare professional, you may need to confer with the doctor and/or healthcare team to let them know of your concern, while being careful not to violate patient confidentiality. A crucial point to keep in mind is that older people do not tend to "fake" the signs and symptoms of depression.[75]

SUICIDE IN OLDER ADULTS

Despite societal beliefs to the contrary, feeling down and depressed is not a natural or normal consequence of the aging process. Unusual mood disturbance must be taken seriously. **Suicide** was ranked the tenth leading cause of death in the United States in 2009, accounting for over 38,000 deaths.[76] The suicide rate in the United States for men was the highest among those who were 75 and older, at 16.3 per 100,000.[76] Fixed risk factors for suicide in the United States include being male (currently 4 to 1 ratio),[77] single, older, and having a family history of suicide. Although suicide is not always a consequence of depression, death is the most definitive outcome of depression.

Other risk factors for suicide include psychiatric illness (schizophrenia, schizoaffective illness, and delusion disorder, as well as anxiety disorders and substance abuse); social disconnectedness of the older person from his or her family, friends, and community (caused by stress, loss of loved one, disruption of family ties, and/or employment changes); perceptions of burdensomeness on loved ones and/or society; feelings of not belonging to valued groups or relationships; chronic physical illness and pain; decreased functional capacity (for example, impairments in instrumental activities of daily living [IADLs]); and depression or poor cognition.[78,79]

Healthcare professionals need to be aware of the potential for suicide and give serious consideration to *any* indication that the person may be thinking about it. Older adults may be less likely to seek mental health services, but when they seek medical care, they may report somatic symptoms related to depression and suicidal ideation (e.g., insomnia, loss of appetite, or gastrointestinal symptoms).[80] Practitioners should listen with great care to the older person's stories and make a referral if there is *any* cause to think suicide may be a possibility.

The following are common indicators of possible impending suicide:

- Past history of suicidal attempts or current/past threats of suicide, especially direct threats
- Symptoms of depression, ongoing bodily complaints, or other psychiatric disorders[81]
- Discharge from a healthcare facility against medical advice or recommendation
- Spontaneous recovery from a depressed mood, including sudden euphoria
- Substance abuse or dependence
- Bereavement, severe losses in life, or identifying with a person who is deceased, especially a life partner
- Giving things away or putting one's affairs in order[82]

Although it is beyond the scope of this text to discuss the ethical issues raised by suicide undertaken to escape excruciating, irreversible pain and/or terminal illness, it suffices to reiterate that depression, which often precedes a suicide attempt, is generally amenable to treatment. Through medication management, psychotherapy, and/or electroconvulsive shock treatment there is good potential for restoring the quality of life for elderly people who are depressed. More than 80% of older adults with clinical depression who are properly diagnosed and treated can recover and return to their prior and usual level of functioning.[83] Depression can happen to anyone; no amount of education, money, or social status can guarantee it will not surface. According to Dr. Ira Katz, who was director of geriatric psychiatry at the Hospital of the University of Pennsylvania, as healthcare professionals our job is "to explain to patients that we think they may have an illness that is treatable, and with treatment they can feel better and function better."[84]

DEATH AND BEREAVEMENT

Dying and death are natural life events during old age. They are nonetheless events that are, at best, accepted but more often feared or dreaded for self and loved ones. Our society has done a good job of neatly tucking away the dying process into institutions, where the final event of death is sometimes forestalled for a very long time. In 2004 approximately 73% of deaths of those age 75 and over occurred in institutions (e.g., hospitals and nursing homes); less than 21% died at home,[85] whereas a century ago institutional deaths were rare.[86] Many ethical issues related to death and dying are particularly pertinent for older people. They or their family members are more likely to need to make a decision about the level of medical care desired for the eventual time when they would be unable to make a decision for themselves. Living wills and advance directives can outline one's wishes and everyone (of any adult age) is encouraged to have them. They can ease the sense of uncertainty when a loved one must make those life-or-death decisions.

Generally people experience an increased number of losses involving significant others as they age. Not only the death of spouses, but also the death of siblings and friends occur more frequently as a person reaches the end of his or her own life, especially if it is particularly long. However, just because one experiences these death events more often does not imply that **bereavement** gets any easier. The healthcare professional should keep in mind that grieving persons of all ages may need additional emotional support, and each grieving process is highly individualized with regard to duration and coping methods.

Several theorists have described the models and theories for stages of grief or the grieving process (see **Table 4-6**).

These stages are neither set to specific timelines nor completely distinct from one another. However, in our society, grieving is expected to last only a short while, and then those who are grieving are encouraged to "get on with things" or "snap out of it."[91] Unfortunately, the feelings of loss, isolation, and extreme sadness may persist for years— sometimes much longer than is socially expected or accepted.[92] Healthcare professionals often encounter older people who are in the midst of some stage of bereavement sometimes even many years after the loss occurred.

Caregivers of people who are dying are enmeshed in an extremely stressful situation. Healthcare professionals can ease the burden of caregiving at least a little by promoting wellness practices, setting limits, and providing "opportunities for distraction, humor and relaxation."[86] These caregivers already are grieving the impending loss of their loved one, even if they seem to be in denial about the upcoming death event. Caregiver stress is a real thing, and should be addressed for the safety and well-being of the caregiver and care recipient. Ways to manage caregiver stress include knowing about and utilizing local resources (e.g., adult day programs, visiting nurses, meal delivery, respite care), getting help

TABLE 4-6 Models and Theories for Stages of Grief

Model	Description
Parkes (1972)	Four stages: numbness, yearning/protest, disorganization, and developing a new identity.[87]
Kübler-Ross (1970)	Five stages: shock/denial, anger, bargaining, depression, and finally acceptance.[88]
Dual Process Model (Stroebe & Schut, 1999)	The individual confronts and avoids the task of grieving, which gives way to adaptive coping of loss.[89]
Tasks of Mourning (Milstein, Kovar, Kovar, & Paterniti, 2012)	Four steps to mourning are suggested: accept the reality of the loss, express the pain of grief, adjust to life without the deceased, and withdraw emotional energy from the deceased and reinvest it in other relationships.[90]

by talking with friends or family or attending support groups, using relaxation techniques, staying physically active and taking care of oneself, making time for personal activities, and attaining education about other healthy ways to cope.[5]

Several recommendations are offered for those working with bereaved individuals or families. Keep in mind that each person has his or her own way of handling grief, yet many have found the following suggestions helpful:

- As much as time allows, let the person talk about the loved one and the loss. Asking about the deceased person, even a spouse or child, is generally acceptable and may even be desired. You can assess quickly whether this is a subject the person would rather not broach. Shedding tears is a natural, healthy experience that can aid the healing process.
- Assure the bereaved person that his or her feelings are legitimate. Stating "I understand" is usually not helpful, unless you truly have been in a similar situation. Euphemistic comments such as "He was quite old" or "It's all for the best" are better left unspoken. Even if the person was old, the death of a loved one is never easy.[91] Clichés and sympathizing remarks are generally regarded as not helpful.
- It is okay not to have the right words or answers. Just being there and offering your compassion and support does often seem to help.[93]
- Allow the bereaved person to make decisions. According to Alty, well-meaning individuals often will take over decision making for grieving persons. However, just because a person is grieving does not mean that he or she cannot think rationally (or that the person wants to give up decision making).[94]
- Discuss counseling or contacting their spiritual adviser for those who need additional help. Behavior that is harmful to self or others is an example of pathologic bereavement. For the person talking about suicide, telling you that his or her life is now over, or communicating with the deceased person as if he or she were still alive, a referral is in order.[91] Social workers can be extremely helpful to the grieving individual because they can assist clients and their significant others "to cope with their feelings, . . . to recognize their choices, . . . to develop and maintain meaningful communication with one another, and to link up with people and services beyond themselves."[95]

Remember, older people may have had to contend with a number of losses in a short period of time. Not only are their loved ones and friends more apt to die or become ill, but they may be dealing with other personal losses as well. For example, older people may have physical losses related to abilities in life skills, or they may need to move out of their long-term homes. In addition, the older person may be demonstrating anticipatory grief of his or her own approaching death.[94] Sensitivity and knowing one's own limits as a healthcare professional are necessary ingredients for working with bereaved clients effectively.

PERSONALITY DEVELOPMENT

Personality is what makes a person a unique individual. Each of us has a set of character traits, attitudes, habits, and emotional tendencies that distinguish us from everyone else. These dispositions can be intimated by our appearance (e.g., tattoos, clothing styles, or level of care taken in grooming), but are essentially inner characteristics causing us to behave as we do. To a degree, one's personality also predicts life events, such as quality of relationships, ability to accept change, employment choices and successes, happiness, and health and mortality.[96] Many studies have explored the development of personality in youth and into young adulthood, whereas fewer studies have concentrated on personality evolvement during older adulthood. The question is whether significant personality change takes place during old age (in both healthy adults and those afflicted with disease).

There are many theories on personality, yet the well-known theorists (e.g., Maslow, Piaget, Freud) devoted little attention to the personality of older people. One theorist who may already be familiar to many readers is Erik Erikson, who initially proposed eight stages of psychosocial development.[97] Originally, the final stage was integrity versus despair. Erikson viewed those who were successful in this stage as being able to develop a sense of pride in their past accomplishments and present lives. They judge their own lives as having been worthwhile. Others, who do not successfully complete this stage, experience instead a feeling of despair, not only about the course of their lives thus far, but also because they do not believe that they have enough time left to improve the course of their life. Overall, Erikson proposed that this then-final stage of life was both a positive and integrating time for well older adults.[98] In an updated version of personality development, Erikson and Erikson include a ninth stage in their theory: **gerotranscendence**, which is associated with wisdom and a moving away from early and midlife materialism.[99] Ardelt describes this "transcendence of the self" as a move toward selflessness, compassion, and reflection, all characteristics of a truly wise person (**Figure 4-3**).[100]

Social scientists are beginning to show more interest in the final years of life with regard to personality development. The trait theory espoused by McCrae and Costa is perhaps the most well known.[101] Their five-factor model of personality is as follows:

1. *Neuroticism:* Associated with hostility, depression, anxiety, and impulsiveness
2. *Extraversion:* Associated with a high level of energy and being outgoing in social situations
3. *Openness to experience:* Associated with open-mindedness, curiosity, and adjustment to change
4. *Agreeableness:* Associated with affection, compassion, and being altruistic
5. *Conscientiousness:* Associated with a strong commitment to goals and being a principled person

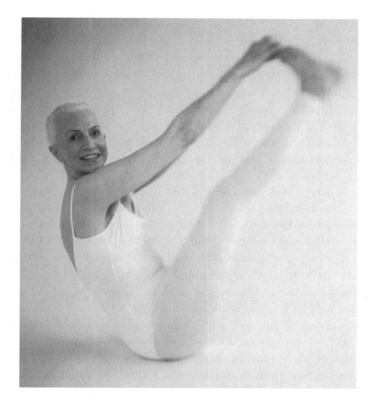

FIGURE 4-3   Both inner and outer stretching are beneficial at any age.
© Ryan McVay/Photodisc/Getty Images

Each of us falls on a continuum for each of these traits. Research conducted on these traits has determined they have the greatest instability between the ages of 17 and 35 years, and then they tend to become more fixed. When these traits were studied in older people over 3- and 6-year intervals, strong stability of all five traits was found using both self and spousal reports. Even when the intervals between testing increased to as much as 50 years, stability coefficients still remained statistically significant, indicating that overall personality traits, at least in these five realms, are relatively fixed, with life events exerting little overall influence for major change.[102] Weiss and colleagues also found few differences in the five traits based on age when looking at more than 1,000 Medicare patients from ages 65 to 100.[103] In the Weiss study, the older participants did show a higher level of agreeableness, which may be the result of a cohort effect or higher death rates for those with lower levels of this trait (those with an intense "type A" personality have proportionately more heart disease, which ultimately leads to an earlier death).

Other evidence also supports the relative permanence of personality traits in typically aging older adults. For example test-retest correlations of optimism scores have been found to be high (over 0.7) over a 10-year period even when considerable life change was occurring in the participants' lives, and when scores did vary, they tended to veer in the direction toward being more optimistic.[104] Hayflick, in citing the results of the Baltimore Longitudinal Study of Aging (BLSA), maintains that personality traits remain essentially the same throughout the life span in typically aging older adults, although most people older than age 50 do begin to prefer slower-paced activities.[105] This is a valuable piece of information for healthcare professionals who work with older people. Pacing healthcare intervention for the convenience of the client, rather than the provider, is essential for good care (and perhaps getting more difficult in these hectic times for health care).

Although overall they are stable, nonetheless personality changes can and do occur. Wood and Roberts suggest that personality traits are open systems that are plastic and can be influenced throughout life.[106] Research has shown that men, as they get older, may become more nurturing and open about their feelings, whereas women may become more assertive, confident, and comfortable with themselves. Social scientists believe these changes could be influenced by hormonal fluctuations perhaps causing a diminution of the character distinctions between the genders.[104] Levels of agreeableness and conscientiousness also tend to increase with age (at least until age 70) for both genders.[107]

Representations of the self, such as one's goals, values, coping styles, and control beliefs, are likely to change over the course of a lifetime. In a pivotal study done by Erikson and colleagues, older people described themselves as more tolerant, patient, open-minded, understanding, compassionate, and less critical than when they were younger.[97] However, many study participants viewed both themselves and the other older adults in the study as more set in their ways. This seeming contradiction was explained by the suggestion that as people age typically, they increasingly integrate their own personal style, but they also can gain a new understanding and tolerance of others' behavioral styles. Conceivably, people may be able to improve their character throughout life by simply doing what they would do if they were who they wanted to be ("acting as if");[108] for example, if a woman wants to be an altruistic person, she decides to take on the role of a volunteer.

Personalities come in many flavors, and not all are compatible with one another. As healthcare professionals, we need to make a concerted effort to provide excellent customer service to all our clients of any age. We now have substantial evidence that old age does not equate with any specific personality traits, especially those often heard on the street (e.g., grumpy [old men], doddering [old woman], stubborn, disagreeable, closed-minded, etc.). Some people were this way their whole lives, whereas others may become "better all the time."[108] Others may have personality disorders associated with disease, such as AD. In these cases, it is crucial to remember the people are not necessarily still "themselves" and may be acting out due to the disease process rather than the behavior being self-directed. One person diagnosed with AD described his experience as, "Sometimes I'm me, and sometimes I don't know who I am. I don't know, it comes and it goes; I never know."[109(p.115)] Even when working with people who have challenging personality types, compassion is the path of least resistance and the most fulfillment, when all things are considered at the end of the day.

Self-efficacy is a construct that was introduced by Bandura in the 1970s.[110] It relates to the beliefs that each person has about their own capacity to function based on their perceived locus of control.[111] Those who have strong self-efficacy, or internal locus of control, feel empowered to shape their own futures. On the other hand, those with low self-efficacy or external locus of control believe that the course of their lives is determined by the whims of the world and that they, personally, can have little influence over the course of their own future. The person's belief in intrinsic or extrinsic locus of control can stem from physical limitations (actual or perceived) and the ability for the person to adapt their thinking or learning in new situations.[111] People who can adapt as they age and who continue lifelong learning tend to have a higher level of self-efficacy and potentially a higher quality of life (and vice versa).[111]

The tendency has been to attribute a lower level of self-efficacy and to expect an external locus of control in older people. Because of various hardships (e.g., medical emergencies, living on fixed incomes) that usually occur more frequently as people age, it makes sense that older people would feel a diminished sense of control. Older people also may have fewer choices about their personal living arrangements and variety of physical pursuits. However, surprisingly, Rhee and Gatz drew a different conclusion.[112] Older adults in their study showed a higher level of self-perceived internal control when compared to college students. Additionally, the college students as a group actually had even a lower level of self-perceived locus of control than attributed to them by the older adults.

The strength of one's sense of self-efficacy may be variable across time and across different domains of life.[113] For example, people may feel empowered about financial matters, yet feel that their health is beyond their personal control. Other domains besides health and finances include work or productivity, transportation, family, friends, safety, and living arrangements. McAvay and her colleagues were interested in looking at older people's perceptions of self-efficacy in the different domains mentioned and the potentially influencing factors of these perceptions over time.[113] They found the trait of self-efficacy in any domain was quite stable over the course of 2 months. For each domain listed, a majority of older respondents (65% to 95%) reported a high degree of self-efficacy, indicating that at least *these* older people believed that they have a high level of control over many aspects of their lives. The only domain in which less than half of the respondents reported a high level of self-efficacy was finances. This finding is logical; many elderly people may feel a lack of control over finances because they are on fixed incomes.

A decline in health (as evidenced by an increase in number of medical conditions) was significantly correlated to decreased self-efficacy in the domains of productivity, family, friends, and living arrangements. Perhaps somewhat expectedly, prior depression was the one factor corresponding most closely with a low level of self-efficacy across all domains. Older people who feel depressed have a tendency to feel powerless about the course of their lives, which subsequently can lead to even further social isolation. The downward spiral of depressed mood and withdrawal emphasizes the need for a medical referral and intervention.

In a study of perceived self-efficacy, a high level of spiritual self-efficacy was most highly predictive of lower levels of psychological distress. Low levels of self-efficacy in other domains also predicted loneliness and distress.[114] A significant correlation has been found between a high level of self-perceived self-efficacy and positive health behaviors such as healthy diet, exercise, and nonsmoking.[115,116] On the other hand, chronic illnesses may lower the level of perceived control, and this in turn may decrease one's motivation to maintain a healthy lifestyle.[115] Both McAvay and colleagues and Blazer have stressed the importance of developing and maintaining social support systems and learning effective coping strategies to boost self-efficacy and deal effectively with daily problems.[113,116]

Healthcare providers can use the General Self-Efficacy Scale, provided in **Table 4-7**, with older adults to assess optimistic self-beliefs for coping with aging and life demands. It is available free online in 31 different languages. Based on the responses given, healthcare providers can address issues and concerns to facilitate gains in self-efficacy to improve quality of life in the aging population.

Overall, in the realm of personality, there are no definitive answers with regard to aging. People who go through typical life development adhere to their personhood throughout life: they remain unique individuals with distinct features. Disease processes, especially AD, absolutely can rob people of their essential personality, leaving someone quite different in their wake. Also, extreme diversity is found even within a set cohort of people, especially as the cohort grows older. Although we can use stereotypes to explain and explore the personality of older people in general, these theories will never adequately illuminate any one person.

TABLE 4-7   General Self-Efficacy Scale

Rate the following questions with this scale: 1 = Not at all true, 2 = Hardly true, 3 = Moderately true, 4 = Exactly true	
1	I can always manage to solve difficult problems if I try hard enough.
2	If someone opposes me, I can find the means and ways to get what I want.
3	It is easy for me to stick to my aims and accomplish my goals.
4	I am confident that I could deal efficiently with unexpected events.
5	Thanks to my resourcefulness, I know how to handle unforeseen situations.
6	I can solve most problems if I invest the necessary effort.
7	I can remain calm when facing difficulties because I can rely on my coping abilities.
8	When I am confronted with a problem, I can usually find several solutions.
9	If I am in trouble, I can usually think of a solution.
10	I can usually handle whatever comes my way.

Reproduced from Schwarzer, R., & Jerusalem, M. (1995). Generalized Self-Efficacy scale. In J. Weinman, S. Wright, & M. Johnston, *Measures in health psychology: A user's portfolio. Causal and control beliefs* (pp. 35–37). Windsor, England: NFER-NELSON.

QUALITY OF LIFE

Quality of life (QOL) is an elusive construct about which a profusion of documents have been written, but it can only truly be understood on a personal level. Each person has his or her own sense of what constitutes a high level of quality in life (**Figure 4-4**).

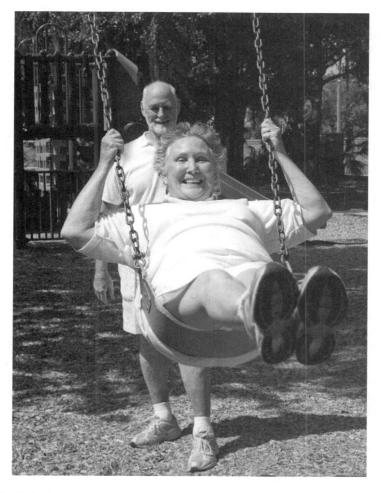

FIGURE 4-4   Enjoying time with loved ones can boost quality of life at any age.
© iStockphoto/Thinkstock

A study by Molzhan, Kalfoss, Makaroff, and Skevington compared QOL across different cultures. Researchers found that older adults in developed countries often citied general health and attributes of physical health such as sleep quality, energy, and being free of pain as of high importance for QOL. In contrast, older adults in less developed countries cited energy, happiness, and home environment as areas of QOL with high importance.[117] Healthcare professionals must keep in mind that stereotypical information, although helpful in understanding older people as a global population, again will not likely fit any one situation. Factors such as age, socioeconomic status, cultural beliefs, and self-reported health status will impact self-rated QOL.

According to Schalock, quality of life is an overarching, multidimensional concept made up of several core principles[118]:

- QOL is best understood from the perspective of the individual.
- QOL embodies feelings of well-being.
- A high QOL is experienced when a person's basic needs are met and he or she has opportunities to pursue and meet personal goals and challenges.
- QOL can be enhanced by giving people choices and encouraging them to make decisions that affect their own lives.
- A sense of community enhances QOL.
- QOL for all persons (including those with disabilities and older adults) may be composed of the same dimensions (although the level and priority of these dimensions will differ among individuals). These dimensions are as follows:
  - Basic material well-being (e.g., food and housing)
  - Emotional well-being, including safety and spirituality
  - Interpersonal relations
  - Engagement in meaningful activities (life occupations)
  - Personal development, including education, learning, and skills
  - Physical well-being (health and wellness)
  - Self-determination, including personal control and goals/values
  - Social inclusion, including roles and supports
  - Human rights, such as voting and accessible housing

Among the older population, it is assumed that the degree of health or illness can have a significant impact on the level of quality of life. In a study done on life satisfaction in older adults, lack of health was listed as the biggest threat to happiness five times more frequently than any other threat, even death.[119] Kehn concluded that health status was a strong predictor of happiness.[119]

Although increasing age was a relatively negative risk factor for attaining the status of robust aging, Garfein and Herzog found that many older people even over 80 years fit into the "robust aging" category.[120] Robust aging is defined by these authors as productive involvement, and positive affective status, functional status, and cognitive status.[120] Therefore, older age per se should no longer be considered a "phase of waning health and declining resources,"[120] but rather a time to learn to age well. In a qualitative study of eight people ages 85 to 100,

Ward-Baker determined that ongoing engagement in productive activities such as work, resilience in the face of hardships, and a high degree of self-efficacy were crucial to living a satisfying life among the oldest-old.[121] Close relationships, lifelong learning, being an optimist, and accepting one's circumstances also came out as important contributing factors, but not for everyone. In another study on robust or successful aging (which could also be viewed as aging with a comparatively high quality of life), four factors were determined to promote well-being in these "successful agers" (and distinguish them from those who were aging less well): social contact and support, *subjective* satisfaction with health, low vulnerability scores (on the personality scale), and fewer stressful life events in the past 3 years.[120]

From a different perspective, a research effort spearheaded by Ardelt explored the impact of wisdom on life satisfaction in old age.[122] She found objective life conditions, such as health, finances, social relationships, and physical environment, could explain only a small portion of the variation of life satisfaction scores in previous studies. Her contention is that a person's level of wisdom explains much of the variability of life satisfaction in older adults. She defines wisdom as "an integration of cognitive, reflective and affective elements" including an "awareness and acceptance of human limitations" allowing us to view the human condition with humor, compassion, and detachment. This is an interesting premise because it allows those with even poor *objective* life conditions to have a great amount of *subjective* life satisfaction.

One's existential sense of personal control, insight, and/or attitude may indeed affect personal quality of life more than anything else. There may even be reason to believe that the hardships of life could challenge a person in such a way as to stimulate increased wisdom and thereby improve satisfaction with life. When viewed in this light, we can more easily understand why there are many older people who, despite ongoing, daily concerns and frequent losses, continue to find their lives satisfying and fulfilling. So many older people report a high level of satisfaction with life (despite ongoing losses) that this finding has been termed "the paradox of aging."[123(p.346)]

Despite ongoing research, QOL remains a nebulous construct. We need to keep in mind that each older person is unique and deserving of respect for his or her own opinions. Exploring these important life concepts with clients can help promote an optimal level of life satisfaction. As healthcare professionals, our contributions to clients' life quality may be minimal, or by using keen listening skills, client-centered approaches, and creative problem solving, and/or by making referrals to others who may be able to provide direct assistance, our input may be invaluable and much appreciated.

SUMMARY

Although change is inevitable throughout life, the essential core of the human being is not likely to be altered by the aging process alone. As people age, if they experience typical aging, they *tend* to exhibit the following characteristics:

- Take longer to learn new tasks
- Become more forgetful, especially of short-term information

- Prefer somewhat slower-paced activities
- Retain essential personhood
- Continue to perceive level of life quality as satisfactory

However, many cognitive, psychological, and personality changes can and do occur over time. These changes can be positive, such as when someone makes an effort toward self-improvement by making significant adjustments in lifestyle patterns. Other times disease, misfortune, or injurious lifestyle choices impose detrimental influences on cognitive functioning, personality, and quality of life. Each age cohort becomes more diverse as their ages increase. Although, as a group, the members tend to show the signs of aging already mentioned, within each age group there are those who continue to perform essentially as well as they ever did (or even better) and those who have succumbed to the "ravages of old age."

Although no one is guaranteed a long life that includes success or happiness throughout the aging process, everyone can take steps to improve their odds of living *well* into old age. The value of close human connections, physical and mental exercise, and ongoing involvement in occupations (in the global sense of the term) and important life roles have been written about extensively.[124–126]

By listening, being supportive and considerate, promoting a personal level of independence, and making referrals as appropriate, we can help older persons live their best potential quality of life and remain as productive or engaged as they choose to be. Our goal, as a caring, highly developed society, should be to promote meaningful involvement in life endeavors at a level of challenge fitting the person right up until their final days of life.

Review Questions

1. The "paradox of aging" refers to
   A. A high quality of life despite the problems of aging
   B. Wisdom despite cognitive losses
   C. Lower levels of depression among older people
   D. Long life despite various medical conditions

2. Which personality trait tends to decrease in typically aging older people?
   A. Optimism
   B. Extraversion
   C. Neuroticism
   D. Agreeableness

3. Self-efficacy, or the sense that one has control over one's life
   A. Tends to remain stable over all domains over the course of adulthood
   B. Tends to be lowest in older adults for the domain of finances
   C. Increases significantly after one retires
   D. Was found to be at a lower level in older adults as compared to college students

4. Which of the following statements about attention and aging is true?
   A. Sustained attention declines significantly with age.
   B. Older people have more difficulty dividing attention between complex tasks.
   C. Attentional switching does not decline with age.
   D. Older people have difficulty paying attention for more than 5 to 10 minutes.

5. A&O × 2 means a person is alert and oriented to
   A. Self and others only
   B. Time and self only
   C. Situation and self only
   D. Self and place only

Learning Activities

1. Think of the role models you know who are at least 60 years old. What personality traits do you appreciate in these older people? How can you ensure that you will have some of these same traits when you are older? Do you think one can develop these traits? Why or why not?

2. It may be interesting to interview a few older people. Ask them how they think their personalities and thinking skills have changed over the course of years. How does this compare with the research data? How do you think you will change as you get older?

3. Discuss the concept of self-efficacy (having a sense of control over one's life). Do you think that for yourself your sense of self-efficacy will increase, decrease, or stay the same as you get older? In one or all domains? Explain your answer.

4. Generally the level of cognition declines as one gets older. How can you ensure that this decline will be minimal? List five things that you can do to improve your cognitive level.

5. Discuss wisdom. What is it, and what makes someone wise? Do you equate being wise with being older? Why or why not? How do we view wisdom compared to other world cultures?

6. Discuss quality of life, which means many things to different people. What aspects of your life give it a high level of quality? Share these with the group. Do you think these will change as you age? Why or why not?

7. Discuss depression in older adults. What are some of the reasons that older people become depressed? (Include life events and changes that tend to occur.)

8. Handling grief is a personal issue. Discuss with one other person what actions you think would be helpful if you were grieving for a significant other. What actions would cause you to feel worse? Do you think this will change as you get older? If so, how? Discuss the themes in a larger group. Afterward discuss how this knowledge will change how you might interact with a grieving person as a friend or as a professional.

CASE STUDY

Emma is an 85-year-old white female who was recently widowed. She lives independently in her small home in a large city. She is fairly active in her community; she likes to attend church, weekly exercise classes, and social outings with her friends. Recently, she has found little interest or joy with leaving her home; this began after a bout of the flu where she was hospitalized for 3 days. She was happy enough with her medical care, and was glad to be feeling well enough to return home. However, she finds she has little energy to manage her home, let alone socialize with friends. Her visiting nurse asks her often about her mood, appetite, and sleep patterns. Emma is vague with her responses and says she's "fine." The nurse requests a social worker to speak with Emma to see if any community services would help her recover and get back to her former routine. Additionally, home health–based occupational and physical therapists visit the client at home to address her self-care and mobility needs. After evaluations are completed, the team discusses Emma's care, and they are all concerned about possible depression and her self-perceived life satisfaction post-illness.

1. What are some assessments that can be completed with Emma to glean more information?
2. What factors are likely impacting her recovery?
3. Who should potentially be on Emma's healthcare team, and why?
4. What are some potential interventions the professionals can provide?

REFERENCES

1. Budd, K. New adventures, new risks, new you. *AARP Magazine,* 2012 June 7: 51–53. Copyright 2012 AARP. All rights reserved.
2. Perlmutter, M. Cognitive potential throughout life. In JE Birren, VL Bengston (Eds.), *Emergent Theories of Aging.* New York: Springer, 1988.
3. Levy, BR. Mind matters: Cognitive and physical effects of aging self-stereotypes. *Journals of Gerontology, Series B: Psychological Sciences and Social Sciences,* 2003;58B(4):P203–P211.
4. Bennett, T, Gaines, J. Believing what you hear: The impact of aging stereotypes upon the old. *Educational Gerontology,* 2010;36(5):435–445. doi: 10.1080/03601270903212336.
5. Alzheimer's Association. Facts and Figures. 2012. Retrieved May 13, 2013, from http://www.alz.org/downloads/facts_figures_2012.pdf

6. Terry, DF, Sebastiani, P, Andersen, SL, Perls, TT. Disentangling the roles of disability and morbidity in survival to exceptional old age. *Archives of Internal Medicine,* 2008;168(3):277–283.
7. Thomas, D. Do not go gentle into that good night. In D Jones (Ed.), *The Poems of Dylan Thomas.* New York: A New Directions Book, 1971.
8. Santayana, G. *The Philosophy of Travel.* 1964.
9. *Stedman's Concise Medical Dictionary for the Health Professions.* 3rd ed. Baltimore, MD: Williams & Wilkins, 1997.
10. Drag, LL, Bieliauskas, LA. Contemporary review 2009: Cognitive aging. *Journal of Geriatric Psychiatry and Neurology,* 2010;23(2): 75–93. doi: 10.1177/0891988709358590.
11. Zec, RF. The neuropsychology of aging. *Experimental Gerontology,* 1995;30:431–442.

12. Vasilevskis, EE, Jan, JH, Hughes, CG, Ely, EW. Epidemiology and risk factors for delirium across hospital settings. *Best Practice and Research in Clinical Anaesthesiology,* 2012;26:277–287. doi: 10.1016/j.bpa.2012.07.003.

13. Flinn, DR, Diehl, KM, Seyfried, LS, Malani, PN. Prevention, diagnosis, and management of postoperative delirium in older adults. *Journal of the American College of Surgeons,* 2009;209(2): 261–268. doi: 10.1016/j.jamcollsurg.2009.03.008.

14. Keyser, SE, Buchanan, D, Edge, D. Providing delirium education for family caregivers of older adults. *Journal of Gerontological Nursing,* 2012; 38(8):24–31.

15. Tun, PA, Wingfield, A. Does dividing attention become harder with age? Findings for the divided attention questionnaire. *Aging and Cognition,* 1995;2(1):39–66.

16. Verhaeghen, P, Cerella, J. Aging, executive control, and attention: A review of meta-analyses. *Neuroscience and Biobehavioral Reviews,* 2002;26(7):849–857.

17. Parkin, AJ, Java, RI. Determinants of age-related memory loss. In TJ Perfect, EA Maylor (Eds.), *Models of Cognitive Aging.* Oxford, UK: Oxford University Press, 2000: 188–203.

18. Connor, LT. Memory in old age: Patterns of decline and preservation. *Seminars in Speech and Language,* 2001;22(2):117–125.

19. Hoyer, WJ, Verhaeghen, P. Memory aging. In JE Birren, KW Schaie (Eds.), *Handbook of the Psychology of Aging.* Burlington, MA: Elsevier, 2006: 209–232.

20. Baddeley, AD. The psychology of memory. In AD Baddeley, BA Wilson, FN Watts (Eds.), *The Handbook of Memory Disorders.* Chichester, UK: John Wiley and Sons, 1995.

21. Birren, JE, Schroots, JJF. Autobiographical memory and the narrative self over the life span. In JE Birren, KW Schaie (Eds.), *Handbook of the Psychology of Aging.* Burlington, MA: Elsevier, 2006: 477–498.

22. Bäckman, L, Small, BJ, Wahlin, A. Aging and memory: Cognitive and biological perspectives. In JE Birren, KW Schaie (Eds.), *Handbook of the Psychology of Aging.* San Diego: Academic Press, 2001.

23. Hultsch, DF, Hertzog, C, Dixon, RA, Small, BJ. *Memory Change in the Aged.* Cambridge, UK: Cambridge University Press, 1998.

24. Prull, MW, Gabrieli, JDE, Bunge, SA. Age-related changes in memory: A cognitive neuroscience perspective. In FIM Craik, TA Salthouse (Eds.), *The Handbook of Aging and Cognition.* 2nd ed. Mahwah, NJ: Lawrence Erlbaum Associates, 2000.

25. Schaie, KW. *Intellectual Development in Adulthood: The Seattle Longitudinal Study.* New York: Cambridge University Press, 1996.

26. Hultsch, DF, Dixon, RA. Learning and memory in aging. In JE Birren, KW Schaie (Eds.), *Handbook of the Psychology of Aging.* 3rd ed. San Diego, CA: Academic Press, 1990: 258–274.

27. Gorman, WF, Campbell, CD. Mental acuity of the normal elderly. *Journal of the Oklahoma State Medical Association,* 1995;88:119–123.

28. Hasher, L, Zacks, RT. Working memory, comprehension, and aging: A review and a new view. In GH Bower (Ed.), *The Psychology of Learning and Motivation.* New York: Academic Press, 1988: 193–225.

29. Gazzaley, A, Sheridan, MA, Cooney, JW. Age-related deficits in component processes of working memory. *Neuropsychology,* 2007;21(5): 532–539.

30. Rosenthal, HF. Spring cleaning turns up some leftover news tidbits. *Portland Press Herald* (Portland, ME), March 26, 1997.

31. Straus, C. (2009). Strategies for Improving Memory. Retrieved June 18, 2013, from http://psychcentral.com/lib/2009/strategies-for-improving-memory/

32. Bartrés-Faz, D, et al. Neuropsychological and genetic differences between age-associated memory impairment and mild cognitive impairment entities. *Journal of the American Geriatrics Society,* 2001;49(7):985–990.

33. Mayo Clinic. Mild Cognitive Impairment. 2013. Retrieved February 13, 2013, from http://www.mayoclinic.com/health/mild-cognitive-impairment/DS00553

34. Petersen, RC, et al. Prevalence of mild cognitive impairment is higher in men. The Mayo Clinic Study of Aging. *Neurology,* 2010;75(10): 889–897.

35. Mitchell, AJ, Shiri-Feshki, M. Rate of progression of mild cognitive impairment to dementia—meta-analysis of 41 robust inception

cohort studies. *Acta Psychiatrica Scandinavica,* 2009;119(4):252-265. doi: 10.1111/j.1600-0447.2008.01326.x.

36. Malek-Ahmadi, M, Davis, K, Belden, CM, Jacobson, S, Sabbagh, MN. Informant-reported cognitive symptoms that predict amnestic mild cognitive impairment. *BMC Geriatrics,* 2012; 12:3. doi:10.1186/1471-2318-12-3.

37. Knight, RG, Godfrey, HPD. Behavioral and self-report methods. In AD Baddeley, BA Wilson, FN Watts (Eds.), *The Handbook of Memory Disorders.* Chichester, UK: John Wiley and Sons, 1995.

38. Craik, FIM, Anderson, ND, Kerr, SA, Li, KZH. Memory changes in normal aging. In AD Baddeley, BA Wilson, FN Watts (Eds.), *Handbook of Memory Disorders.* Chichester, UK: John Wiley and Sons, 1995. (pp. 211-241).

39. Ryan, EB. Beliefs about memory changes across the adult lifespan. *Journal of Gerontology: Psychological Sciences,* 1992;47:41–46.

40. Baltes, PB. The aging mind: Potential and limits. *Gerontologist,* 1993;33:580–594.

41. Kim, S, Hasher, L. The attraction effect in decision making: Superior performance by older adults. *Quarterly Journal of Experimental Psychology,* 2005;58A(1):120–133.

42. do Rozario, L. From ageing to sageing: Eldering and the art of being as occupation. *Journal of Occupational Science,* 1998;5(3):119–126.

43. Schachter-Shalomi, Z, Miller, R. *From Age-ing to Sage-ing: A Profound New Vision of Growing Older.* New York: Warner, 1995.

44. Schaie, KW, Hofer, SM. Longitudinal studies in aging research. In JE Birren, KW Schaie (Eds.), *Handbook of the Psychology of Aging.* San Diego: Academic Press, 2001.

45. Baltes, PB, et al. People nominated as wise: A comparative study of wisdom-related knowledge. *Psychology of Aging,* 1995;10:155–166.

46. Robnett, RH, Porell, FW, Turner, BF, Tun, PA. The correlates of cognitive and metacognitive stability and change in the first five waves of the Health and Retirement Study (1992–2000). Unpublished dissertation. Boston, University of Massachusetts, 2007.

47. Yu, F, Ryan, LH, Schaie, KW, Willis, SL, Kolanowski, A. Factors associated with cognition in adults: The Seattle Longitudinal Study. *Research in Nursing and Health,* 2009;32(5):540–550.

48. Curlik, DM, Shors, TJ. Training your brain: Do mental and physical (MAP) training enhance cognition through the process of neurogenesis in the hippocampus? *Neuropharmacology,* 2012;64:506–514.

49. Dana Alliance for Brain Initiatives. Stem Cells and Neurogenesis, Progress Report 2006. Retrieved July 5, 2008, from http://www.dana.org/news/publications/detail.aspx?id=4234

50. Hotz, RL. Probing the workings of hearts and minds. Research. *Los Angeles Times,* April 3, 1997.

51. Nussbaum, PD. *Brain Health and Wellness.* Tarentum, PA: Word Association, 2003.

52. Nussbaum, PD. Brain health: Bridging neuroscience to consumer application. *Generations,* 2011;35(2):6–12.

53. Metz, AE, Robnett, R. Engaging in mentally challenging occupations promotes cognitive health throughout life. *Gerontology Special Interest Section Quarterly,* 2011;34(2):1–4.

54. den Dunnen, WFA, et al. No disease in the brain of a 115-year-old woman. *Neurobiology of Aging,* 2008;29(8):1127–1132.

55. Rocca, WA, et al. Trends in the incidence and prevalence of Alzheimer's disease, dementia, and cognitive impairment in the United States. *Alzheimer's and Dementia,* 2011;7(1):80–93. doi: 10.1016/j.jalz.2010.11.002.

56. Cole, SA. Behavioral disturbances in Alzheimer's disease. *Patient Care,* June 15, 1995:121–131.

57. Ebly, EM, et al. Prevalence and types of dementia in the very old: Results from the Canadian Study of Health and Aging. *Neurology,* 1994; 44:1593–1600.

58. Cummings, JL, et al. Dementia. In CK Cassell et al. (Eds.), *Geriatric Medicine,* 3rd ed. New York: Springer-Verlag, 1997: 897–913.

59. Folstein, MF, Folstein, SE, McHugh, PR. "Mini-Mental State": A practical method for grading the cognitive state of patients for the clinician. *Journal of Psychiatric Research,* 1975;12(3):189–198.

60. Ham, RJ. Making the diagnosis of Alzheimer's disease. *Patient Care,* June 15, 1995: 104–120.

61. Birks, J, Grimley-Evans, J, Iakovidou, V, Tsolaki, M. Rivastigmine for people with

Alzheimer's disease. *Cochrane Database of Systematic Reviews,* 2009;2(CD001191). doi: 10.1002/14651858.CD001191.pub2.

62. Birks, J. Cholinesterase inhibitors for Alzheimer's disease. *Cochrane Database of Systematic Reviews,* 2006;1(CD005593), doi: 10.1002/14651858.CD005593.

63. Bell, V, Troxel, D. *A Dignified Life: The Best Friends Approach to Alzheimer's Care.* Deerfield Beach, FL: Health Communications, 2002.

64. Bell, V, Troxel, D, Cox, TM, Hamon, R. *The Best Friends Book of Alzheimer's Activities* (Vol. I and II). Baltimore, MD: Health Professions Press, 2008.

65. Strauss, CJ, Khachaturian, ZS. *Talking to Alzheimer's.* Oakland, CA: New Harbinger, 2002.

66. Patenaude, J. Nutrient deficiency-related depression and mental changes in elderly persons. *Home Health Care Management and Practice,* 1996;9(1): 29–39.

67. Palmer, RM. "Failure to thrive" in the elderly: Diagnosis and management. *Geriatrics,* 1990; 45(9):47–55.

68. Fincham, FD, Cain, CM. Learned helplessness in humans: A developmental analysis. *Developmental Review,* 1986;6:301–333.

69. Centers for Disease Control and Prevention (CDC). An Estimated 1 in 10 U.S. Adults Report Depression. 2011. Retrieved from http://www.cdc.gov/features/dsdepression/

70. Johnson, JC. Depression and dementia in the elderly: A primary care perspective. *Comprehensive Therapy,* 1996;22:280–285.

71. National Institute of Mental Health. Older Adults: Depression and Suicide Facts. Retrieved July 7, 2008, from http://www.nimh.nih.gov/health/publications/older-adults-depression-and-suicide-facts.shtml#role

72. Thomas, AJ, O'Brien, JT. Depression and cognition in older adults. *Current Opinion in Psychiatry,* 2008;21(1):8–13.

73. American Psychiatric Association. *Diagnostic and Statistical Manual of Mental Disorders.* 4th ed. (text revision). Washington, DC: American Psychiatric Association, 2001.

74. McIntyre, LG, et al. Depression and suicide: Assessment and intervention. *Home Health Care Management and Practice,* 1996;9(1):8–17.

75. Juratovac, E. The Ohio Nurses Association presents "Anxiety and depression in older adults": An independent study. *Ohio Nurses Review,* March 1996:4–13.

76. Centers for Disease Control and Prevention (CDC). Suicide: Facts at a Glance. 2012. Retrieved June 18, 2013, from http://www.cdc.gov/violenceprevention/pdf/suicide-datasheet-a.PDF

77. Centers for Disease Control and Prevention. Web-based Injury Statistics Query and Reporting System (WISQARS). Retrieved June 13, 2013, from http://www.cdc.gov/injury/wisqars/index.html

78. Conwell, Y, Van Orden, K, Caine, ED. Suicide and older adults. *Psychiatric Clinics of North America,* 2011;34(2):451–468. doi:10.1016/j.psc.2011.02.002.

79. Cukrowicz, K, Cheavens, JS, Van Orden, KA, Ragain, RM, Cook, RL. Perceived burdensomeness and suicide ideation in older adults. *Psychology and Aging,* 2011;26(2):331–338. doi: 10.1037/a0021836.

80. Neufeld, E, O'Rourke, N. Impulsivity and hopelessness as predictors of suicide-related ideation among older adults. *Canadian Journal of Psychiatry,* 2009;54(10):684–692.

81. Welton, RS. The management of suicidality: Assessment and intervention. *Psychiatry,* May 2007:2–12.

82. Hemphill, BJ. Depression among suicidal elderly: A life-threatening illness. *Occupational Therapy Practice,* 1992;4(1):61–66.

83. National Institute of Health. Retrieved July 11, 2013 from http://www.nimh.nih.gov/health/publications/older-adults-depression-and-suicide-facts.shtml#role

84. Adams, RC. Geriatric rehab treats depression to improve function. *Advance for Occupational Therapists,* December 9, 1996:19.

85. Centers for Disease Control and Prevention (CDC). Worktable 309. Deaths by Place of Death, Age, Race, and Sex: United States, 2004. Retrieved May 15, 2013, from http://www.cdc.gov/nchs/data/dvs/MortFinal2004_Worktable309.pdf

86. McCue, JD. The naturalness of dying. *Journal of the American Medical Association,* 1995; 273:1039–1043.

87. Parkes, CM. *Bereavement*. London: Penguin, 1972.

88. Kübler-Ross, E. *On Death and Dying*. New York: Macmillan, 1970.

89. Stroebe, M, Schut, H. The dual process model of coping with bereavement: Rationale and description. *Death Studies*, 2009;23(3):197–224.

90. Milstein, JM, Kovar, LB, Kovar, LJ, Paterniti, DA. A path to wholeness. *Journal of the American Medical Association*, 2012;308(10):985–986.

91. Waltman, RE. When a spouse dies. *Nursing*, 1992;92:48–52.

92. Goleman, D. Grief may not follow a predictable pattern. In W Dudley (Ed.), *Death and Dying: Opposing Viewpoints*. San Diego, CA: Greenhaven Press, 1992: 139–144.

93. Chessler, BR. Friends can help the grieving cope with death. In W Dudley (Ed.), *Death and Dying: Opposing Viewpoints*. San Diego, CA: Greenhaven Press, 1992: 155–160.

94. Alty, A. Adjustment to bereavement and loss in older people. *Nursing Times*, 1995;91(12): 35–36.

95. Davidson, KW, Foster, Z. Social work with dying and bereaved clients: Helping the workers. *Social Work in Health Care*, 1995;21(4):3.

96. McAdams, DP, Olson, BD. Personality development: Continuity and change over the life course. *Annual Review of Psychology*, 2012;61:517–542. doi: 10.1146/annurev.psych.093008.100507.

97. Erikson, EH, et al. *Vital Involvement in Old Age*. New York: W. W. Norton; 1989: 36.

98. Erikson, EH. *Childhood and Society*. 2nd ed. New York: W. W. Norton; 1963.

99. Erikson, EH, Erikson, JM. *The Life Cycle Completed: Extended Version with New Chapters on the Ninth Stage of Development*. New York: W. W. Norton, 1998.

100. Ardelt, M. Self-development through selflessness: The paradoxical process of growing wiser. In HA Wayment, JJ Bauer (Eds.), *Transcending Self-Interest: Psychological Explorations of the Quiet Ego*. Washington, DC: American Psychological Association, 2008: 221–223.

101. McCrae, RR, Costa, PT. *Personality in Adulthood*. New York: Guilford Press, 1990.

102. Costa, PT, Herbst, JH, McCrae, RR, Siegler, IC. Personality at midlife: Stability, intrinsic maturation, and response to life events. *Assessment*, 2000;7(4):365–378.

103. Weiss, A, Costa, PT, Karuza, J, Duberstein, PR, Friedman, B, McCrae, RR. Cross sectional age differences in personality among Medicare patients aged 65 to 100. *Psychology and Aging*, 2005;20(1):182–185.

104. Carver, CS, Scheier, MF, Segerstrom, SC. Optimism. *Clinical Psychology Review* 2010; 30:879–889.

105. Hayflick, L. *How and Why We Age*. New York: Ballantine; 1994: 145.

106. Wood, D, Roberts, BW. The effect of age and role information on expectations for big five personality traits. *Personality and Social Psychology Bulletin*, 2006;32(11):1482–1496.

107. *Harvard Mental Health Letter*. As a man (or woman) grows older. May 2006.

108. Sohn, E. Better all the time. *Health*, 2004;18(1). Retrieved June 28, 2008, from http://O-web .ebscohost.com.lilac.une.edu/ehost/detail? vid+11& hid+8&sid+063f0b6a-4740

109. Harris, PB. The sense of self in Alzheimer's disease: The person's perspective. In BM Oberg, E Nasman, E Olsson (Eds.), *Changing Worlds and the Ageing Subject: Dimensions in the Study of Ageing and Later Life*. Hants, UK: Ashgate, 2004: 115–132.

110. Bandura, A. Self-efficacy: Toward a unifying theory of behavioral change. *Psychology Review*, 1977;84:191–215.

111. Leung. DSY, Liu, BCP. Lifelong education, quality of life and self-efficacy of Chinese older adults. *Educational Gerontology*, 2011;37(11): 967–981.

112. Rhee, C, Gatz, M. Cross-generational attributions concerning locus of control beliefs. *International Journal of Aging and Human Development*, 1993;37:153–161.

113. McAvay, GJ, et al. A longitudinal study of change in domain-specific self-efficacy among older adults. *Journals of Gerontology Series B: Psychological Sciences and Social Sciences*, 1996;51B:P243–P253.

114. Fry, PS, Debats, DL. Self-efficacy beliefs as predictors of loneliness and psychological distress in older adults. *International Journal of Aging and Human Development*, 2002;55(3):233–269.

115. Deeg, DJH, et al. Health behavior and aging. In JE Birren, KW Schaie (Eds.), *Handbook of the Psychology of Aging*. 4th ed. San Diego, CA: Academic Press, 1996: 129–149.

116. Blazer, DG. Self-efficacy and depression in late life: A primary prevention proposal. *Aging and Mental Health*, 2002;6(4):315–324.

117. Molzhan, AE, Kalfoss, M, Makaroff, KS, Skevington, SM. Comparing the importance of different aspects of quality of life to older adults across diverse cultures. *Age and Ageing*, 2011;40(2): 192–199. doi: 10.1093/ageing/afq156.

118. Schalock, RL. Reconsidering the conceptualization and measurement of quality of life. In *Quality of Life*. Washington, DC: American Association on Mental Retardation, 1995: 123–138.

119. Kehn, DJ. Predictors of elderly happiness. *Activities, Adaptation and Aging*, 1995;19(3): 11–30.

120. Garfein, AJ, Herzog, AR. Robust aging among the young-old, old-old, and oldest-old. *Journals of Gerontology Series B: Psychological Sciences and Social Sciences*, 1995;50B:S77–S87.

121. Ward-Baker, PD. The remarkable oldest old: A new vision of aging. *Dissertation Abstracts International Section A: Humanities and Social Sciences*, 2007;67(8-A):3115.

122. Ardelt, M. Wisdom and life satisfaction in old age. *Journals of Gerontology Series B: Psychological Sciences and Social Sciences*, 1997;52B(1): P15–P27.

123. Carstensen, LL, Mikels, JA, Mather, M. Aging and the intersection of cognition, motivation, and emotion. In JE Birren, KW Schaie (Eds.), *Handbook of the Psychology of Aging*. Burlington, MA: Elsevier, 2006: 343–362.

124. Adelmann, PK. Multiple roles and psychological well-being in a national sample of older adults. *Journals of Gerontology Series B: Psychological Sciences and Social Sciences*, 1994;49:S277–S285.

125. Ruuskanen, JM, Ruoppila, I. Physical activity and psychological well-being among people aged 65 to 84 years. *Age and Ageing*, 1995; 24:292–296.

126. Netuveli, G, Wiggins, RD, Hildon, Z, Montgomery, SM, Blane, D. Quality of life at older ages. *Journal of Epidemiology and Community Health*, 2006;60(4):357–363.

FUNCTIONAL PERFORMANCE IN LATER LIFE: BASIC SENSORY, PERCEPTUAL, AND PHYSICAL CHANGES ASSOCIATED WITH AGING

REGULA H. ROBNETT, PhD, OTR/L,
JESSICA J. BOLDUC, DrOT, MS, OTR/L, and
JOHN MURRAY, MPH, RPSGT, RRT

Old age is not an illness—it is a stage of life.

—Sr. Marie Antoinette de la Trinité, L.S.P.*

Chapter Outline

Behavioral Objectives

Upon completion of this chapter, the reader will be able to:

1. List at least four recommendations for healthcare professionals who work with people who have diminished visual skills.
2. Define perception and describe how perceptual skills may change as one ages.
3. Describe compensatory measures related to decreased perceptual functioning.
4. Describe how sensory systems tend to change over the course of aging, including the impact on life functioning.
5. List compensatory measures for each of the sensory changes related to aging.

*With permission from Little Sisters of the Poor, Publications Office, 601 Maiden Choice Lane, Baltimore, MD 21228.

6. List at least four recommendations for healthcare professionals who work with people who are hard of hearing.
7. Describe the basic physical changes of aging related to range of motion, strength, motor control, and endurance.
8. Discuss how physical changes affect performance in various life skills including self-care and work.
9. Describe how sleep patterns change with age.
10. Describe the components of cognitive behavioral therapy for sleep disorders.

Key Terms

Agnosia	Perception
Anosmia	Praxis
Apraxia	Presbycusis
Cognitive behavioral therapy (CBT)	Range of motion
Contracture	Reaction time
Dyspraxia	Restless leg syndrome (RLS)
Endurance	Scotoma
Hyposmia	Senescence
Insomnia	Sleep hygiene
Motor coordination	Sleep restriction
Maximum Muscle strength	Stimulus control
Obstructive sleep apnea (OSA)	Vision
Olfaction	

Ironically, change may be the only constant in our lives. This chapter explores the sensory, perceptual, and physical changes associated with the aging process. The intent of the chapter is to provide a brief overview of these potential changes and to provide suggestions that may help the healthcare professional in assisting older people who have experienced these age-related changes. The chapter is not intended as a fully developed source book of interventions in these realms. It merely offers a springboard of ideas and information. The charts and lists of potential interventions are starting points only and not all inclusive.

Healthcare professionals who are rehabilitation specialists, such as occupational and physical therapists and speech-language pathologists, are the experts in the realm of sensory, perceptual, and physical changes, including how to remediate these problems or compensate for the problems not amenable to restoration. They are skilled at in-depth interventions to improve functional performance based on extensive professional theories and evidence-based research and practice. Although intended to be helpful to those who are rehabilitation specialists and those who are not, as well as students and other healthcare professionals, this chapter is not a comprehensive guidebook or a cookbook for intervention. Each of the mentioned professions has textbooks (often several hundred pages long) focusing precisely on the topics in this chapter. The interested reader can view this chapter as a mere appetizer; those with the skill and motivation can go for the "main course" through additional reading and education.

In this chapter the focus is on the typical physical, sensory, and perceptual changes taking place within the aging body, especially as these changes relate to function. **Senescence**, or the process of physical decline, does occur, but often at a slower and more variable rate than is customarily believed.

An important aspect to consider, along with these physical and sensory changes, is associated performance levels. Even though the described changes related to aging are rarely outwardly encouraging, nonetheless daily functioning throughout life can remain adequate or even good given enough drive, good fortune, the right genes, and the absence of disease. Seventy-five percent of adults aged 65 or older have at least one chronic illness.[1] In 2005, one out of every two Americans had a chronic condition, with arthritis being the most common cause of disability.[2] Yet most of those who do have chronic conditions are still able to live well and would be able to improve their functioning with a little assistance or a bit of education to promote small changes. The chapter starts with an overview of sensation including vision, perception, hearing, olfaction, taste, and touch and then provides a review of physical changes. The emphasis is always on what the healthcare professional needs to know when working with older people in various capacities.

SENSATION AND PERCEPTION

VISION

Sensory changes occur with aging. Some of these changes are quite familiar and arrive almost expectedly after a half century of life. For example, visual skills are known to decrease with age, beginning already in the third decade of life. The good news is, generally, older people are able to maintain an acuity level close to unimpaired (20/20) with corrective lenses at least until age 88 (see **Table 5-1**).[3(p.138)]

Other visual skills known to show a decline with advancing age are the following:

- Visual processing speed
- Sensitivity to light
- Ability to see well in dim light
- Near **vision**, especially problematic for reading small print
- Upward gaze without moving head
- Contrast sensitivity, separate from visual acuity
- Color sensitivity, especially along the blue–yellow axis of color
- Dynamic vision, which includes
  - Smooth visual pursuits of a moving target (such as watching the movement of a tennis ball), especially with distractions or with increased velocity of targets
  - Visual tracking or saccades, the small ballistic eye movements needed for reading (although decline with age is less than for pursuits)[3]

TABLE 5-1   Common Visual Diagnoses and Functional Implications in Old Age

Disease of the Eye	Prevalence by Age		Functional Implications
Cataracts	50–54[a]	5%	World appears dull, as if seeing through dusty or cloudy lens; readily amenable to treatment, usually on an outpatient basis.
	80+[a]	68%	
Age-related macular degeneration (AMD)	50–54[a]	<0.05%	Central field vision is impaired, affecting reading and other fine detail work.
	80+[a]	<12%	
Glaucoma	50–54[a]	<1%	Loss of peripheral vision, usually gradually; may lead to tunnel vision or total blindness.
	80+[a]	<8%	
Diabetic retinopathy (DR)[b]	40–49	7–31%	The person with diabetes and DR has blind spots or **scotomas**; visual skills may fluctuate; may be associated with depressed mood.
	>75	12–23%	
Retinal detachment	10 to 12.5 of 100,000 population annually (approximately 0.001%), typically between ages 40 and 70[c]		Tearing or separation of retina from underlying tissue that can be caused by trauma or illness.[d]
Dry eyes	48–91	14%[e]	Poor lubrication of the eye due to poor tear production.[d]

[a] Schieber, F. Vision and aging. In JE Birren, KW Schaie (Eds.), *Handbook of the Psychology of Aging*. Burlington, MA: Elsevier, 2006: 129–161.
[b] Eye Diseases Prevalence Research Group, Diabetic Retinopathy Subsection. The prevalence of diabetic retinopathy among adults in the United States. *Archives of Ophthalmology*, 2004;122:552–563.
[c] Larkin, GL. Retinal Detachment. 2009. Retrieved from http://emedicine.medscape.com/article/798501-overview.
[d] American Optometric Association. Adult Vision: Over 60 Years of Age. 2013. Retrieved from http://www.aoa.org /x9454.xml
[e] Gayton JL. Etiology, prevalence, and treatment of dry eye disease. *Clinical Journal of Opthamalogy*, 2009;3:405–412.

Visual skills that tend to be preserved include basic color vision and the ability to maintain fixation on a target.[4] The healthcare professional working with older persons may offer several simple compensatory measures to mitigate the effects of decreased eyesight. **Table 5-2** outlines some of these measures. Although these can be helpful, general suggestions, they cannot be expected to be comprehensive or work for everyone. If the older person is having difficulty with daily tasks because of impaired visual skills, a certified low vision therapist (CLVT; who works exclusively with blind persons and persons with visual impairment), another low vision specialist such as a behavioral optometrist, or an occupational therapist may be of assistance.

TABLE 5-2   Selected Compensatory Measures Related to Specific Visual Impairments

Visual Impairment	Compensatory Measures
Decreased visual acuity	• Corrective lenses (clean and in good repair) • Larger print—font size 10–12 points • Larger images/signs • Magnifiers • Closed-circuit television (a device to magnify objects or written material) • Tactile cues for phone, oven, or microwave dials/buttons
Central vision loss	• Visual scanning training and eccentric viewing
Increased sensitivity to light	• Use nonreflective materials on walls, floors, and ceilings (environmental modifications) • Use yellow film to reduce glare • Wear protective lenses • Shield eyes from bright lightbulbs • Provide overhangs on windows
Decreased ability to see in dim light	• Use task lighting directed at work area (environmental modification) • Use nightlights • Avoid driving at night, dawn, or dusk
Decreased ability to see contrasts	• Use black with white or yellow contrasts • Highlight obstacles or changes in floor surface levels (environmental modification) • Avoid difficult color discriminations, such as blue/green when safety is a concern (otherwise, a safety pin on the waistband of a blue pair of pants can distinguish them from a green pair)

Source: Data from Charness, N, Bosman, EA. Human factors design for the older adult. In JE Birren, KW Schaie, M Gatz, TA Salthouse, C Schooler (Eds.), *Handbook of the Psychology of Aging*, 3rd ed. San Diego, CA: Academic Press, 1990: 452–453; Zoltan, B. *Vision, Perception and Cognition.* Thorofare, NJ: Slack, 1996; and Pizzimenti, JJ, Roberts, E. The low vision rehabilitation service: Part two. Putting the program into practice. *Internet Journal of Allied Health Sciences and Practice*, 2005;3(3):1–11.

VISUAL PERCEPTION

Perception is the ability to make sense of incoming sensory information. Usually this refers to being able to interpret visual data, but it can also refer to auditory, olfactory, and gustatory sensation as well. One must have the foundation of adequate acuity for visual perception to be intact. Surprisingly, visual perceptual skills do not show a uniform decline with aging. For example, Lindfield and colleagues researched the ability of people of varying ages to complete visual closure tasks (in which one must identify a given object when shown only fragments of the object).[5] In this study, the older adults were actually able to identify the fragmented pictures more accurately than their younger counterparts, perhaps because of their experience perceiving the world. Because of decreased sensory functioning, older people may become more proficient at inferring meanings from less sensory input.[4] However, they tend to be slower at processing the information and take in less information per unit of time.

Decreases in perceptual skills, such as not understanding what common objects are used for (**agnosia**), loss of spatial awareness (e.g., right/left, back/front), and impaired visual constructional abilities (e.g., completing puzzles, assembling common objects), are not usually associated with typical aging to any notable degree. When perception is awry, the problems are usually related to disease processes such as dementia, stroke (cerebrovascular accident), or psychiatric disorders. Because intact perceptual skills are generally necessary for typical or normal everyday living, deficits need to be addressed. Rehabilitation specialists such as occupational therapists can work with those who have perceptual difficulties in adapting the environment and adapting daily tasks to promote function.

AGE-RELATED HEARING LOSS: PRESBYCUSIS

Hearing is another sensory modality with a tendency to decline with age. **Presbycusis** occurs in both genders, but men, especially, tend to lose the ability to hear higher frequencies. Older people have more difficulty distinguishing higher pitched consonant sounds; understanding of lower pitched vowel sounds tends to remain intact. Also, older people in general cannot recall as much of the previous conversation if the number of words spoken per minute is increased. Both younger and older subjects were able to recall more verbal information if the words were spoken in the context of normal sentences rather than in random word strings. However, older adults' accuracy decreased more dramatically than did the younger participants' with unrelated words.[4]

Older women are more likely to report hearing loss and compensate by searching for nonverbal cues during conversation, and are also more likely to seek treatment. In contrast, older men, who are more likely to have hearing loss, also are more likely to deny a problem and not seek treatment.[6] Older people also tend to have more difficulty tuning out background noise, which often leads to discomfort or frustration during noisy social gatherings as the person struggles to attend to what is going on. Thus a hearing impairment easily may lead to social isolation. In a large-scale population-based study, Kramer, Kapteyn, Kuik, and Deeg found that older people with hearing impairments reported feeling more symptoms of depression (including loneliness) and had lower self-efficacy scores than older people with intact hearing.[7] Not surprisingly, those with hearing loss also had fewer people in their social network. Additionally, being socially isolated (i.e., lonely) can lead to mental decline due to lack of cognitive stimulation. One idea is that during conversations, people with hearing loss tend to use more of their cognitive reserve to compensate for hearing loss and/or perceptual processing, leading to decline in other areas of cognition (e.g., memory).[8]

These studies and past experiences lead to the following recommendations for working with older adults:

- Speak in a *tone* that can be heard. Although some older people do need you to increase your volume or decibel level, do not assume this is the case. More likely, the person who has difficulty hearing will need you to lower the pitch of your words. It is always all right to ask the person what is best for him or her.
- If possible, face the person so they can see you speak. You may want to start by saying their name to get their *attention*. Make and keep eye contact, and keep your hands away from your face and mouth to enable lip reading. (Speak in a natural way.)[9]
- Make sure that your *rate* of speech is not too fast, but also not so slow as to sound condescending. Rephrase rather then repeat when necessary.
- Avoid *elderspeak*, which is described as baby talk for older adults (e.g., use of more diminutives, slower speech, more repetition, and simpler words with fewer syllables).[10] Even though older people may have difficulty hearing, this does not imply that they need to be talked to as if they have lost their cognitive capacity.
- Whenever possible, keep background noise to a minimum.
- Do not verbally jump from one idea to the next too quickly because older people are more likely to use the context of what is being said to understand the conversation.

SMELL AND TASTE

Other sensory perceptions that change over time include smell (**olfaction**) and taste. These closely related declines have psychological implications. The ability to detect smells in general and correctly identify differing odors decreases with age. The majority of people older than age 80 have impaired olfaction.[11] Studies have shown a high prevalence of **hyposmia** (decreased smell sensation) and **anosmia** (complete loss of smell) in participants age 65 and older. Additionally, in a study by Nordin, Monsch, and Murphy, 77% of the older participants with smell loss (but no other apparent disease diagnoses) reported that they had a normal sense of smell.[12] This loss tends to be insidious and therefore may go unnoticed. This sensory loss, with its associated lack of awareness, can constitute a serious safety issue for those wishing to remain independent in their own homes. Compensatory measures, such as natural gas/smoke detectors and having someone else with a normal sense of smell check for spoilage of food, are recommended.

Because olfaction provides a backdrop for taste sensation, decreased smell sensation can contribute to decreased pleasure in eating, with a subsequent increased potential for malnutrition. Olfaction impairments, common in those who are 70 and over, are associated with depressive symptoms and poorer quality of life, which can also impact enjoyment of food, drink, and socialization.[13] As people age, their ability to detect salty, bitter, and sour tastes decreases as the threshold needed for detection increases.[14] The ability to taste sweets does not appear to change with age.[14] This may contribute to an overreliance on sweets and an oversalting of food. Thirst sensation also declines, which increases the probability of dehydration in older persons.[15] Booth and colleagues suggest that inadequate dietary intake may actually cause a loss of taste perception, rather than the reverse being true.[16] This implication points to the extreme importance of maintaining an adequate diet, especially as we age.

PHYSICAL CHANGES AND PERFORMANCE

RANGE OF MOTION

Range of motion (ROM) refers to the ability of a joint to move through its natural pattern of movement. For example, the shoulder of a typical healthy person can flex up (toward the sky) nearly straight (about 170°).[17] This amount of movement is considered normal for that joint. Every joint in the body has a typical range. Older age does relate to a decline in joint range of motion in areas including the shoulder,[18] hip, and wrist.[19] That being said, chronological age alone may affect range of motion less than several age-related conditions, which can definitely have a negative effect on smooth movements and maximum range. For example, arthritis; muscle disuse, misuse, or overuse; injuries; stroke; Parkinson's disease; and dementia have all been associated with less than optimal movement patterns. Various forms of arthritis are the most common cause of disability in the United States, with more than 50 million people (50% of adults over age 65) currently living with the associated functional losses.[2]

Nonresistive, repetitive range of motion exercises may be able to maintain or improve current range, or may slow down the progression of disease processes such as osteoarthritis.[20] Physicians and other professionals who are experts in movement (e.g., physical therapists) can help older persons develop optimal movement programs for their needs, working toward their best possible performance, staving off loss of motion secondary to disease, maintaining current range, increasing range of motion, and increasing strength. No matter what the person's life situation is, regular movement (especially by engaging in meaningful life tasks) is important if the person is at all able. People who tend to be sedentary or immobile, such as those who are bedridden for a prolonged period in the hospital or in long-term care facilities, are especially at high risk of sustaining joint **contractures**.

Contractures are generally caused by joint immobilization and result in decreased range of motion, stiffening and subsequent structural changes, and pain on movement at one or more joints. Joints typically affected are hips, shoulders, and knees. The best treatment is actually to prevent contractures from occurring through regular movement and exercise/stretching. However, in treatment the approach is to increase joint mobility if at all possible through a passive, active-assisted, or (best) active range of motion program established by a rehabilitation specialist. If contractures are not resolved, occasionally surgical intervention is required due to pain or immobility preventing the completion of basic daily tasks, such as bathing, dressing, and grooming.

STRENGTH

Maximum muscle strength tends to occur in early adulthood; middle age is generally a time of only slight decline. By age 65, a 20% reduction in strength is common, with losses tending to occur even more rapidly thereafter. An additional 30% reduction is common after age 70.[21] However, this potential consequence of aging is based on average losses in the population. This trend does not necessarily link specifically to individuals, who may *not* get progressively weaker with age. Older people, if physically capable, can still be involved in and even improve in sports requiring practice and skill such as tennis, golf, skiing, boating, and bowling (**Figure 5-1**). Studies have shown that older adults who exercise can reduce the pain caused by arthritis, restore balance to reduce fall potential, strengthen bones, maintain weight, improve glucose control for diabetes management, and improve heart health.[22] Also, by adding a prescribed exercise routine, people can improve their muscle strength and may even get strong enough to participate in the Senior Olympics and win competitions. Encouraging physical activity is almost always appropriate, although the level of exertion and duration of activity need to be determined by the person's primary healthcare provider(s).

ENDURANCE

Endurance is usually defined as the ability to sustain involvement in a physical activity. Although not the same as strength, the two are closely related. Several studies have noted that the decrease in muscular endurance during one's lifetime is proportionately less than the decrease in muscle strength.[23] Endurance training has been found to have a positive impact on heart and pulmonary function along with improving cognition.[24,25]

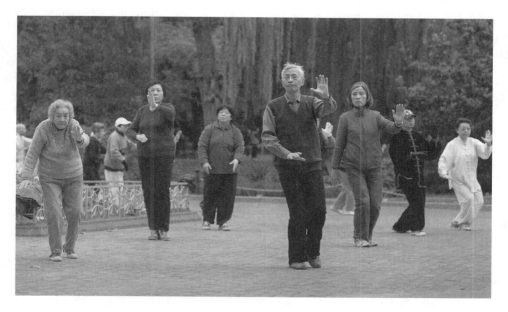

Figure 5-1 Exercise can boost both physical and mental functioning.
Source: © jacus/iStockphoto.com

EXERCISE

A meta-analysis of 13 aerobic exercise training programs for older people demonstrated that long-term programs (more than 30 weeks in duration) were associated with improved endurance.[26] On a hopeful and health-related note, an active lifestyle involving stretching, aerobic activity, and strength building can improve range of motion, strength, and endurance, and in so doing may actually slow the course of physiologic aging (**Figure 5-2**). In a recent review of both physical and mental training, Curlik and Shors found that both types of exercise were important for maintaining brain health, at least in animal studies.[27] Although aerobic activity fosters the production of new neurons in the hippocampus, mental activity, especially learning new skills, helps the newly formed neurons survive over the long term.

PRAXIS

Praxis is defined as the ability to carry out purposeful motor actions. **Dyspraxia** refers to a decreased ability to plan and/or execute purposeful movements, whereas **apraxia** refers to the complete inability to carry out these motor plans. During most common everyday routines, most people do not need to think consciously about their performance; simple tasks (such as eating or dressing) are completed automatically. Repetition of these routines over time allows the conversion of initially novel actions into established habits. Goal-directed actions occur throughout the day during self-care, work, leisure, and home management tasks. If the level of motor (or cognitive) performance significantly decreases for any reason (e.g., injury, aging, or disease), one's ability to live independently can be threatened.

Also worth noting is the fact that people do not lose functional performance rapidly from one day to the next because of the aging process; however, they can have sudden physical losses caused by accidents or medical issues. Often, rehabilitation with the overall goal of helping one to regain lost skills and learning to work with the remaining abilities is warranted.

When reviewing studies that have explored the physical performance of older people, we find cross-sectional differences between age groups, for example, when 20-year-olds are compared to 80-year-olds, as well as longitudinal changes within the same person over time (for example, from age 60 to age 80). The changes are not always in the expected direction of deterioration. Age-related performance has been measured in several domains: gross motor coordination (including balance and mobility), reaction time, strength, endurance, and work-related performance.

Reaction Time Perhaps the most straightforward trend when examining performance is the slowing of **reaction time** as people head into old age. An example of needing to take action quickly with a specific response is in driving a car: Brake lights directly ahead indicate an immediate need to step on the brake. As people age, in general, they are not

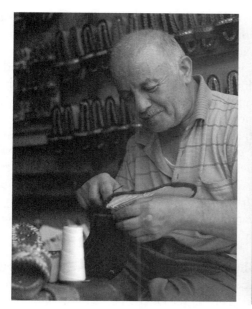

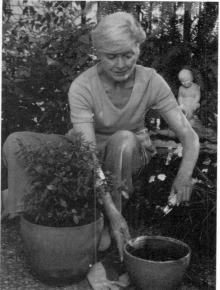

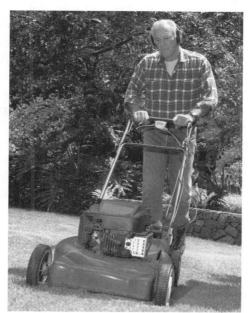

Figure 5-2   The diligent older worker makes a substantial contribution to society.
(top left) © asliuzunogu/ShutterStock, Inc.
(top right) © Photodisc
(bottom) © LiquidLibrary

able to react as quickly. In the Baltimore Longitudinal Study of Aging (BLSA), researchers determined that the slowing of behavior was a continuous process over the course of a lifetime, and that increasing the complexity of task demands further increased the response time needed.[28] (In the case of driving, worse traffic conditions than usual would be an example of this.) Stimulus–response time tends to become about 20% slower between the ages of 20 and 60, and the responses in later life are less likely to be accurate.[29] However, the BLSA study and others note that the variability within any one age group (cohort) also significantly increases with age. Therefore, at age 80, for instance, a man still can be nearly as fast in responding as he ever was and still have perfectly adequate reaction time to be successful in independent living skills such as driving. (A masculine example is used purposefully because studies have tended to show that slowed reaction time is more pronounced in older women.[28]) It is also interesting to note that when only verbal (instead of psychomotor) responses were required, the slowing has not been nearly as pronounced and may not be evident at all.[23]

Motor Coordination   Gross **motor coordination** is another crucial prerequisite to completing daily tasks without assistance. Specifically, mobility, or ambulation, seems to be an extremely valued skill. Falls are more prevalent in the elderly population; one out of every three adults age 65 and older has one fall yearly. Of these 2.3 million falls, more than 600,000 resulted in hospitalization.[30] Unfortunately, falling once increases the risk of the older person falling again.[31] Twenty to thirty percent of people who fall sustain injuries such as lacerations, hip fractures, or head traumas. These injuries can make it hard to get around or live independently, and increase the risk of early death.[30] In 2009, over 20,000 older adults died from unintentional falls.[30] Repeated falls generally are associated with declines in balance, coordination, and/or strength. All these areas have been studied and have generally shown age-correlated declines. Again, it is worth pointing out the increasing variability among older cohorts, and the fact that the vast majority of elderly people still have adequate amounts of strength and coordination to do the tasks that they want or need to do, including walking, as part of their daily routines.

Impaired ambulation may be cause for a referral to a physical therapist, who can help remediate physical skills or possibly recommend assistive devices for safe ambulation. Local Area Agencies on Aging may be able to recommend local programs designed for older people who want to improve their sense of balance, for example, the Matter of Balance program started by rehabilitation specialists at Boston University.[32] There are several ways to improve postural control (for example, exercises, sports, and yoga or tai chi).[33] Also, for those with a decreased sense of balance, it is vital to make sure the home or environment is clutter-free and that obstacles (such as loose rugs, cords, and pets) do not present hazards. Rehabilitation specialists such as occupational or physical therapists are good resources to contact for additional balance-related treatment strategies.

Fine motor coordination refers to hand-based skills such as writing, self-feeding, buttoning, and working with tools. Considering age alone, we see little change in a person's ability to complete fine motor tasks. Older people who are aging in a typical fashion (i.e., without disease) are just as capable as their younger counterparts are in tasks such as typing, cooking, and card playing. This maintenance of skill could be based on two potential explanations: (1) ongoing practice over the years has improved skill level over time, or (2) with ongoing repetition these tasks become more automatic and therefore require less skill for completion. Salthouse, a well-known researcher in the field of aging, has yet another explanation for the continued good performance of professionals using these types of skills (such as typing), which is explained in the following subsection. When fine motor skills are impaired, as they often are in old age, the culprit is more than likely arthritis, stroke, or another skill-robbing disease, rather than *typical* aging.

Any significant decreases in level of functioning, occurring either suddenly or over the course of a few weeks or months, are not generally consistent with the typical aging process. Of course, emergency situations necessitate immediate action, but even relatively rapidly declining physical and/or cognitive performance also requires prompt medical attention. Abrupt behavioral changes should send up warning flags to the older person, family, and friends warranting a call and probably a visit to the person's physician. The physician can then make referrals for further medical care or for rehabilitation.

WORK PERFORMANCE

With the alleged age-related deterioration of functional component skills, such as aspects of cognition, balance, reaction time, and muscle strength, you might surmise that the work performance of older workers would be inferior to that of their younger counterparts. However, as a group, older workers do very well. The following empirical evidence is offered to debunk ageist myths with regard to older workers:

- Based on actual attendance records, older workers have less absenteeism than younger workers do.[34,35]
- Age is not linked to job performance by empirical research, even on the established platform of slowed cognitive functioning in old age.[34,36]
- Older workers have proportionately fewer workplace injuries.[34,35]
- Older workers demonstrate less workplace aggression and substance abuse, and are more dependable.[34]

One employer praised older workers' stronger work ethic[37]; others lauded the older employees' experience and sense of leadership.[38] Salthouse, who completed a series of studies on the performance of older workers, found past relevant work experience to be a more important factor than specifically tested cognitive abilities in predicting work performance.[36] After studying older architects, engineers, and secretaries, Salthouse proposed that occupation-specific experience, although it did not seem to moderate the inverse relationship between age and basic cognitive processes, did, however, contribute to successful job performance. The older secretaries, for example, had slower reaction times, but they still were able to type as proficiently as their younger counterparts through the use of a phenomenon Salthouse named "anticipatory processing."[36] This developed job skill allows the older secretaries to more effectively scan ahead and maintain their speed.

Overall, although there do seem to be age-related declines in cognition, sensation, perception, and physical performance, for most typically aging older people these changes do not make a substantial impact on either their comprehensive work performance or essential daily living skills. Rather, being productive in a work environment can help keep older adults active and connected with their communities, and foster a sense of well-being and self-esteem. Employers will be faced (if they are not already) with retaining an older workforce due to economic and population changes. Older adults can do very well in the workplace with minimal modifications (e.g., workstation setup, lighting) for their health and safety (which benefits everyone).[39]

SLEEP AND AGING

Sleep is considered an activity of daily living (ADL) because it is an essential part of everyday life. This daily task is completely different from other daily activities, but we cannot live without doing it regularly. Sleep has become an increasingly important and studied factor in older adults because of its central role in promoting a high quality of life. Lack of sleep can cause dramatic changes in how one feels (and acts) during the day. The National Sleep Foundation reports that 65% of people over the age of 55 have reported sleep problems at least a few times per week. Also, according to a 2003 survey by the Foundation, 26% of those ages 55–64 reported that their sleep was either fair or poor, while 21% of those ages 65–84 reported fair or poor sleeping habits.[40] Nationally, over 50 million Americans of all ages and socioeconomic statuses report sleep-related problems.[41]

NORMAL SLEEP

To discuss sleep disorders we must first have an understanding of normal sleep and the typical sleep cycle. People have a sleep–wake cycle that is known as the circadian rhythm: the 24-hour clock responsible for keeping most people awake during the day and allowing them to feel sleepy and go to sleep at night. The stimulating effects of light through the retinohypothalamic tract control this rhythm in the hypothalamus. The light causes alerting signals to help maintain wakefulness. As the day progresses the sleep load increases and the alerting signals must get stronger for continued feelings of alertness. When darkness falls, evening/nighttime routines such as dinner and relaxation are associated with the decrease of alerting signals. Melatonin is released, causing further reduction in the alerting signals until the sleep load overtakes wakefulness and sleep ensues. For many, this often happens between 9 and 11 p.m.

Once asleep, we also have a rhythm to our sleep. Sleep is broken into two states, nonrapid eye movement (NREM) and rapid eye movement (REM) sleep. Non-REM sleep consists of three stages: N1, N2, and N3. N1 is the link between consciousness and unconsciousness. In this stage of sleep we may have some awareness of surroundings and are easily aroused. We spend about 5% of our time asleep in stage N1. In stage N2, we lose consciousness, but we are still in a light stage of sleep and can be aroused easily. Approximately 50% of our sleep time is spent in stage N2. Stage N3 is considered deep sleep. When we are in deep sleep, arousal is difficult. If aroused during deep sleep, we are usually somewhat disoriented. During this stage, growth hormone is released, which continues to be needed for tissue repair as we age. The N3 stage of sleep is when we experience the most restorative sleep so essential to functional performance and feeling refreshed during the day. Unfortunately, as we age, this stage of sleep decreases and is replaced by the lighter stage N2 (**Figure 5-3**).

Stage R, or rapid eye movement (REM), sleep is when we dream. During this stage of sleep, the brain is more active than when we are awake. REM sleep is thought to be responsible for reorganization of our thoughts similar to rebooting a computer. During stage R, we experience muscle atonia, preventing us from acting out our dreams. We also lose a degree of autonomic control, which leads to heart rate variability, irregular respiration, and fluctuations in blood pressure. Stage R comprises about 25% of our sleep.

The sleep cycle consists of four to five periods of non-REM and REM sleep, each lasting about 90 minutes. The first part of the night consists of more deep sleep and shorter REM sleep, and the latter part of the night consists of longer REM periods and shorter deep sleep (N3) periods.

THE AGING PROCESS AND ITS IMPACT ON SLEEP

Sleep requirements change over the life course; infants need approximately 16 hours per day and adults need about 8 hours per day. One longstanding misconception is that

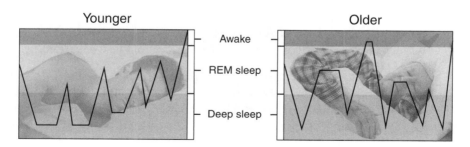

Figure 5-3 REM cycles of younger and older people.
(left) Photo © George Doyle/Stockbyte/Thinkstock
(right) Photo © Wavebreak Media/Thinkstock

older people need less sleep. They actually need the same amount of sleep as they get older, but getting enough of the refreshing type of sleep may become more difficult. The major reasons are related to the decrease in time spent in deep sleep and more time spent in lighter stages. While in these lighter stages of sleep we are more able to be aroused and therefore are more susceptible to the sleep disruptions caused by pain or discomfort that may come with aging. Older people take more medications than any other age group, and many of these medications have a negative effect on sleep, including exhaustion,[42] hypotension, morning sedation, central nervous system overstimulation and depression, daytime drowsiness, and somnolence.[43] This leads to a more disruptive and fragmented sleep for many older people. Although their sleep requirements stay the same throughout adulthood, their sleep efficiency (time asleep to time in bed) is reduced over time, requiring older people to spend more time in bed to get the required amount of sleep.[44]

The circadian rhythm also changes as we age. The rhythm becomes phase advanced, which results in melatonin being released earlier in the evening. This may lead to moving bedtime up and early morning awakenings. Instead of getting sleepy between 9 and 11 p.m., sleepiness may occur as early as 7 p.m. This then leads to earlier wake-up times (usually between 4 and 5 a.m.). Although this change is considered normal, it can have a negative impact on one's life, for example, one's social life in the evening. The easiest way to delay the hour of sleep is exposure to bright light (either natural sunlight or artificial light) later in the day. Artificial light of at least 2,500 lux (five times brighter than house lights) is recommended.[44]

SLEEP DISORDERS

Sleep problems/disorders include the following:

- Difficulty falling asleep (sleep-onset **insomnia**)
- Waking up often during the night (sleep maintenance insomnia)
- Waking up too early and not being able to get back to sleep (terminal insomnia)
- Waking up not feeling refreshed
- Snoring, which may be related to pauses in breathing (sleep apnea)
- Unpleasant feelings in the legs (restless leg syndrome)

Overall, about two-thirds of older adults report experiencing one or more of these symptoms at least a few nights a week, with 55- to 64-year-olds (71%) being most likely to report problems sleeping, compared to adults 65–74 years old (65%) and 75–84 years old (64%).[40]

Insomnia   Insomnia is the most common symptom of more than 30 different sleep disorders.[45] Acute insomnia is fewer than 30 days in duration whereas chronic insomnia lasts longer than a month. The onset of insomnia may begin with some type of emotional event such as the loss of a loved one or a recent stay in the hospital. During the event, the normal rhythm of sleep is disrupted and an abnormal sleep cycle ensues. The new cycle may then become the norm; many people have difficulty resuming their previous sleep routine.

Although many believe the most effective treatment for insomnia is in the form of a sleeping pill, this may only rarely be true. Sleeping pills are perhaps a good short-term solution, especially for those who have had a traumatic or emotional event that is interfering with sleep (e.g., death of a spouse or a forced move). However, in the long run, other techniques such as sleep restriction, stimulus control, sleep hygiene, and cognitive behavioral therapy can offer a more sustainable positive impact on the older person's overall quality of life. Underlying health issues such as stress, illness, medication side effects, environmental causes (light or noise), depression, and/or pain should be addressed prior to considering sleep medications.[46]

Obstructive Sleep Apnea Signs and symptoms of **obstructive sleep apnea** (OSA) include snoring and witnessed apnea during sleep and/or complaints of excessive sleepiness during the day. OSA occurs because the trachea is either totally or partially obstructed, causing the body's oxygen level to drop. This in turn signals the brain to get in gear (i.e., wake up), which increases muscle tone and subsequently raises the oxygen level back to normal. This disruption of the sleep pattern can occur up to 60 times an hour, so a person may need 10–12 hours of sleep to attain just enough restorative sleep per night. Prior to the time of menopause, twice as many men as women are afflicted with OSA, but after people reach their 50s the gender numbers even out. Approximately 5–8% of older adults in the United States have some level of OSA.[47]

Loss of oxygen to the brain obviously can be life threatening, and this condition can have serious consequences, including heart arrhythmias and mood and memory problems.[47] Whereas repositioning to side-lying may help (lying on one's back seems to exacerbate the problem), the use of a continuous positive airway pressure (CPAP) device is considered the leading therapy for OSA, and has helped millions to overcome the negative impact of sleep apnea. The CPAP is often prescribed after a sleep study has been completed to determine the diagnosis after studying sleep state, eye movement, muscle activity, heart rate, respiratory effort, airflow, and blood oxygen levels.[47] The CPAP machine does not involve oxygen transmission; it simply keeps the airway path unobstructed through air pressure.[48] The CPAP hoses and masks require regular maintenance and cleaning. If not maintained, the buildup of bacteria can cause additional harm just by using the machine.

Restless Leg Syndrome/ Periodic Leg Movements of Sleep **Restless leg syndrome** (RLS) is a neurologic disorder including "creepy crawly feelings" or other unpleasant sensations in the legs, usually while in bed. These symptoms lead to periodic leg movements during sleep (PLMS), and thus hinder people from getting a good night's sleep. According to the National Institute of Neurological Disorders and Stroke, PLMS may occur every 10 to

60 seconds and may last the entire night.[49] This need to move almost constantly also causes the brain to wake up, disrupting the sleep cycle akin to sleep apnea. Parkinsonian-type medications (Levodopa), along with anticonvulsants, benzodiazepines, and narcotics, have been able to afford some relief to PLMS sufferers.[49,50] Additionally, avoidance of caffeine, chocolate, tea, and soft drinks may lessen the symptoms.[50]

TREATMENT OF SLEEP DISORDERS

There are four primary types of treatments for sleep disorders:

- Sleep restriction
- Stimulus control
- Sleep hygiene
- Cognitive behavioral therapy

Although the typical healthcare professional is not expected to help an older person overcome serious sleep disorders, there are nonetheless some relatively simple helpful hints that could benefit older people in their quest for regular restful nights of sleep.

Sleep restriction does not refer to actually restricting sleep, but rather to restricting one's time in bed. The goal is to be asleep 90% of the time that one spends in bed. Often those who have insomnia will spend many hours in bed but not sleeping. This leads to poor sleep habits whereby one learns (subconsciously) that a bed is not for sleeping. If people aim for the 90% rule, they can determine how long they would need to be in bed to get the desired number of hours of sleep. Whether or not they have slept enough, they get out of bed at the allotted time. The person forces himself or herself to stay awake (and out of bed) until it's time to go to sleep again. Later, time spent in bed can be gradually added back in.

Stimulus control also refers to the amount of time spent in bed, in this case attempting to get to sleep or back to sleep. If someone cannot fall asleep within a half hour, it's best to get out of bed and do something relaxing. When the person is sleepy, she or he can go back to bed and try again to go to sleep. Rather than tossing and turning, consumed with worry that one will not get enough sleep, one gets out of the bedroom and does an activity. This ritual should be individualized because some find reading or puzzles relaxing, whereas others may have differing interests.

Sleep hygiene involves those activities and habits that are conducive to sleeping soundly. To some degree these factors are also individualized, although most find that a quiet, cool, dark room is helpful for inducing sleep, whereas eating, exercising, or a blaring television are more likely to keep one awake. Exercise should take place at least 2 to 3 hours before bedtime, and taking a hot bath can be helpful an hour or more before heading to bed. Some find it helpful to write down a to-do list for the next day to put the next day's demands into perspective. It can certainly be helpful for those having sleep disturbances to spend time devising their own personal sleep hygiene "dos and don'ts" list so that they can work on promoting healthy, restful sleep patterns for themselves.

Finally, **cognitive behavior therapy** (CBT) has been found to be helpful for those having difficulty sleeping. A therapist who specializes in sleep disorders can teach the client about sleep and work with the person to understand that it is not necessarily catastrophic if one occasionally does not get enough sleep. Worrying about a lack of sleep only exacerbates the situation. CBT puts the daily activity of sleep into perspective, and the therapist attempts to get those with sleep disorders to relax more about their sleep patterns. This attitude adjustment along with the other techniques mentioned may be all that is needed for a person to regain sound sleeping habits. For example, Edinger, Wohlgemuth, Radke, Marsh, and Quillian completed a randomized controlled trial comparing CBT to relaxation therapy and a placebo treatment for 75 adults.[51] They not only determined that CBT led to better sleep outcomes over the 6-week study period, but also found that these gains were sustained over a 6-month period.

With regard to sleep, overall people need adequate amounts of varying durations, typically around 8 hours per night. As people age, various diagnoses, medication side effects, general aches and pains, or the need to get up for toileting in the middle of the night can interfere with healthy sleep patterns. Fortunately, sleep disorders are usually treatable. The importance of normal sleep was emphasized in a large study by Ancoli-Israel, who found that those with fewer sleep disturbances were more likely to be "successful agers."[52]

SUMMARY

This chapter reviews some of the sensory and physical changes that tend to accompany the aging process, especially as these changes relate to day-to-day functioning. It also covers work performance and sleep because these are two functional areas relevant to older people. The fact is that the vast majority of older people manage their daily routines just fine. Those who are afflicted with one of the diseases associated with aging or the consequences of poor lifestyle choices may not do as well as the typically aging population, but people, even those with chronic conditions or physical decline secondary to ill health, can sometimes be surprisingly resilient and outperform the expectations placed upon them. As healthcare professionals, it is at least part of our job to instill hope for the future. We can almost always make small but significant positive changes to any life situation.

Highlights of the changes addressed in this chapter are as follows:

- Common visual diagnoses include decreased acuity, cataracts, macular degeneration, glaucoma, and diabetic retinopathy, yet the majority of older people are able to maintain adequate visual skills for the completion of daily tasks.
- Visual perceptual skills, or the ability to interpret incoming visual information, is more affected by disease processes (such as stroke) than by the aging process alone.
- Physical skills such as joint range of motion, strength, endurance, reaction time, and motor coordination do change over the course of time, with older adults generally not performing as well as their younger counterparts. However, several measures can be taken to improve performance even among the oldest members of the population.

- Perhaps surprisingly, for various reasons older workers tend to perform as well as or better than their younger counterparts.
- Sleep disorders are common among older adults, and several treatment techniques for improving quality and quantity of sleep are available for those needing help in this area.

CASE STUDY

Cecil is an 85-year-old married male who lives in Naples, Florida. He is in good physical shape; he swims daily and continues to play golf on the weekends with his former work buddies. Prior to retirement (5 years ago), Cecil was a car salesman for antique cars, and also worked as the town clerk. He reports he enjoys being social, reading, and putting together model antique cars. Cecil had a right hip replacement a few years ago (after retirement) that he states gave him a new lease on life. Generally, Cecil has no complaints regarding aging, except for his diminishing eyesight. Cecil was diagnosed with macular degeneration a few years ago, but most recently he has noted difficulties with some of his favorite hobbies. Cecil now finds that even with his newest pair of glasses he is not able to read the paper as easily, has difficulty putting together the small parts of his model cars, and even has occasional trouble putting his golf ball on the tee. He has stopped driving, but luckily his friends or wife drive him to the beach to swim or to the golf course.

One day his wife read an article in the *New York Times* talking about various tools available to enhance reading or fine motor tasks for individuals with macular degeneration. Cecil was intrigued and soon spoke with his doctor, who referred him to a low vision specialist. A functional assessment was completed to assess Cecil's visual acuity, visual fields, and contrast sensitivity. A clinical exam was completed not too long ago by his ophthalmologist who prescribed his current corrective lenses. The low vision specialist also discussed what activities Cecil would like to resume and which activities are the most troublesome.

Can you come up with a few recommendations before reading further?
What types of healthcare professionals might be able to help Cecil maintain or enhance his quality of life?

The specialist makes a few recommendations. You can discuss these and look up anything you do not understand to enhance your learning:
For reading:

- Additional magnifiers that can be handheld or worn around the neck for a hands-free approach. This will make the font size of the reading material appear larger, permitting Cecil to adjust his central vision for reading.
- Additional lighting through the use of task lights that simulate daylight.
- Practice/training with scanning and eccentric viewing through the use of a reading guide. Eccentric viewing training requires practice to change seeing from central vision to peripheral vision.

For golfing or being outdoors:

- Use contrasting colors for the ball and tee (e.g., white and black) and use eccentric viewing when possible.
- Consider wearing tinted glasses to control for glare and enhance contrast.

Cecil is eager to try some new strategies so he is able to resume the hobbies that he finds meaningful. He plans to continue working with his low vision specialist for continued follow-up and training as his vision changes and new tasks become more challenging.

Review Questions

1. Perceptual skills in older adults
   A. Decrease dramatically with age
   B. Are more likely to be affected by disease than by the typical aging process
   C. Are more accurate and show decreased response time than for younger people
   D. Do not change with the aging process

2. Choose the *false* statement about sensation and aging:
   A. Men, more than women, lose the ability to hear high frequencies as they age.
   B. The ability to taste sweet and sour is maintained.
   C. Thirst sensation declines with age.
   D. Most older people who have hyposmia are aware of their impairment.

3. Older workers tend to
   A. Be slower and therefore less efficient
   B. Have less of a work ethic driving them
   C. Use past experience to work efficiently
   D. Withdraw from leadership roles

4. The most common visual condition (and the one most directly related to the aging process) is
   A. Cataracts
   B. Diabetic retinopathy
   C. Macular degeneration
   D. Glaucoma

5. Generally, the best way to compensate for presbycusis is by
   A. Yelling in the person's ear
   B. Speaking very slowly and simply
   C. Decreasing background noise
   D. Raising the pitch of your voice

Learning Activities

1. (Do the first part of this learning activity before reading the chapter.) On the left side of a piece of paper, make a list of the following: vision, visual perception, hearing, smell, taste, range of motion, strength, endurance, work performance, and sleep. For each category, write down what you expect to happen with this factor as you get older. Then, read the chapter and compare what you expected with what you learned in the chapter. Were you surprised about any of the results?

2. Based on what you learned in the chapter, why does driving become more difficult with advancing age? What other life tasks may be more difficult for older adults, and why?

3. Two, three, or four people should choose a card game they all know how to play. One player will wear glasses smeared with petroleum jelly; another player should wear earplugs and heavy leather gloves. The third player must keep his or her hands in a fist and wear dark sunglasses. If there is a fourth player, he or she will cover one eye and can move her arms only by sliding them across the table due to arm weakness (although she can still move her fingers). Any time a player cheats, he or she will lose a point toward the total score. After the game, discuss how the simulated age-related changes affected your ability to play the game.

4. Review the activity in item 3. How could you make it easier for the players to enjoy their game of cards? Come up with several suggestions.

5. Make a personal list of sleep hygiene "dos and don'ts" for yourself. Discuss with the group.

REFERENCES

1. Agency for Healthcare Research and Quality. (2002). Preventing Disability in the Elderly with Chronic Disease. Retrieved June 24, 2013, from http://www.ahrq.gov/research/elderdis.htm

2. Centers for Disease Control and Prevention. (2012). Arthritis-Related Statistics. Retrieved June 24, 2013, from http://www.cdc.gov/arthritis/data_statistics/arthritis_related_stats.htm

3. Schieber, F. Vision and aging. In JE Birren, KW Schaie (Eds.), *Handbook of the Psychology of Aging.* Burlington, MA: Elsevier, 2006: 129–161.

4. Fozard, JL. Vision and hearing in aging. In JE Birren, KW Schaie, M Gatz, TA Salthouse, C Schooler (Eds.), *Handbook of the Psychology of Aging.* 3rd ed. San Diego, CA: Academic Press, 1990: 150–170.

5. Lindfield, KC, et al. Identification of fragmented pictures under ascending versus fixed presentation in young and elderly adults: Evidence for the inhibition-deficit hypothesis. *Aging and Cognition,* 1994;1:282–291.

6. Gordon-Salant, S. (2005). Hearing loss and aging: New research findings and clinical implications. *Journal of Rehabilitation Research and Development,* 42(4):9–24. doi: 10.1682/JRRD.2005.01.0006.

7. Kramer, SE, Kapteyn, TS, Kuik, DJ, Deeg, DJH. The association of hearing impairment and chronic diseases with psychosocial health status in older age. *Journal of Aging and Health,* 2002;14(1):122–137.

8. Lin, FR, Metter, EJ, O'Brien, RJ, Resnick, SM, Zonderman, AB, Ferrucci, L. (2011). Hearing loss and incident of dementia. *Archives of Neurology,* 68(2):214–220.

9. Cleveland Clinic Foundation. (2012). Tips to Improve Communication When Talking with Someone with Hearing Loss. Retrieved June 24,

2013, from http://my.clevelandclinic.org /disorders/hearing_loss/hic-tips-improve-communication-when-talking-someone-hearing-loss.aspx

10. Thornton, R, Light, LL. Language comprehension and production in normal aging. In JE Birren, KW Schaie (Eds.), *Handbook of the Psychology of Aging*. Burlington, MA: Elsevier, 2006: 262–288.

11. Murphy, C, Schubert, CR, Cruickshanks, KJ, Klein, BEK, Klein, R, Nondahl, DM. Prevalence of olfactory impairment in older adults. *Journal of the American Medical Association*, 2002;288(18): 2307–2312.

12. Nordin, S, Monsch, AU, Murphy, C. Unawareness of smell loss in normal aging and Alzheimer's disease: Discrepancy between self-reported and diagnosed smell sensitivity. *Journals of Gerontology Series B: Psychological Sciences and Social Sciences*, 1995;50B:P187–P192.

13. Gopinath, B, Kaarin, A, Sue, CM, Kifley, A, Mitchell, P. Olfactory impairment in older adults is associated with depressive symptoms and poorer quality of life scores. *American Journal of Geriatric Psychiatry*, 2011;19(9):830–834.

14. Methven, L, Allen, VJ, Withers, CA, Gosney, MA. Aging and taste. *Proceedings of the Nutrition Society*, 2012;71(4):556–565. doi: 10.1017/S0029665112000742.

15. Smolowe, J. Older, longer. *Time*, Fall 1996;148(14): 76–80.

16. Booth, DA, et al. Measurement of food perception, food preference and nutrient selection. *Annals of the New York Academy of Sciences*, 1989;561:226–242.

17. Soucie, JM, et al. Range of motion measurements: Reference values and a database for comparison studies. *Haemophilia*, 2011;17(3):500–507. doi: 10.1111/j.1365-2516.2010.02399.x.

18. McIntosh, L, McKenna, K, Gustafsson, L. Active and passive range of motion in healthy older people. *British Journal of Occupational Therapy*, 2003;66(7):318–324.

19. Beal, MF, Lang, AE, Ludolph, A. Clinical aspects of normal aging. In *Neurodegenerative Diseases*. Cambridge, UK: Cambridge University Press, 2005.

20. King, OS, Halpern, BC. An exercise plan for older patients with arthritis: Keeping joints moving can stabilize or slow the degenerative process. *Journal of Musculoskeletal Medicine*, 2002;19(4):147–149.

21. American College of Sports Medicine. Position stand of exercise and physical activity for older adults. *Medicine and Science in Sports and Exercise*, 1998;30:992–1008.

22. Centers for Disease Control and Prevention. (2011). Why Strength Training? Retrieved June 24, 2013, from http://www.cdc.gov/physical activity/growingstronger/why/index.html

23. Spirduso, WW, MacRae, PG. Motor performance and aging. In JE Birren, KW Schaie (Eds.), *Handbook of the Psychology of Aging*. 3rd ed. San Diego, CA: Academic Press 1990: 183–200.

24. Muscari, A, et al. Chronic endurance exercise training prevents aging-related cognitive decline in healthy older adults: A randomized controlled trial. *International Journal of Geriatric Psychiatry*, 2010;25(10):1055–1064. doi: 10.1002/gps.2462.

25. National Institutes of Health. (2012). Exercise: Exercises to Try. Retrieved June 24, 2013, from http://nihseniorhealth.gov/exerciseandphysical activityexercisestotry/enduranceexercises/01.html

26. Huang, G, Shi, X, Davis-Brezette, JA, Osness, WH. Resting heart rate changes after endurance training in older adults: A meta-analysis. *Medicine and Science in Sports and Medicine*, 2005;37:1381–1386.

27. Curlik, DM, Shors, TJ. Training your brain: Do mental and physical (MAP) training enhance cognition through the process of neurogenesis in the hippocampus? *Neuropharmacology*, 2013;64:506–514.

28. Fozard, JL, et al. Age differences and changes in reaction time: The Baltimore Longitudinal Study of Aging. *Journals of Gerontology Series B: Psychological Sciences and Social Sciences*, 1994;49: P179–P189.

29. Hayflick, L. *How and Why We Age*. New York: Ballantine Books, 1994: 145.

30. Centers for Disease Control and Prevention. Falls Among Older Adults: An Overview. 2012. Retrieved June 24, 2013, from http://www.cdc.gov /homeandrecreationalsafety/falls/adultfalls.html

31. Ganz, DA, Bao, Y, Shekelle, PG, Rubenstein, LZ. Will my patient fall? *Journal of the American Medical Association*, 2007;297(1):77–86.

32. Maine Health. What Is a Matter of Balance? Retrieved January 20, 2009, from http://www .mmc.org/mh_body.cfm?id=432

33. Gillespie, LD, Gillespie, WJ, Robertson, MC, Lamb, SE, Cumming, RG, Rowe, BH. Interventions for

preventing falls in elderly people. *The Cochrane Library*, 2006;(1):CD000340.

34. Prenda, KM, Stahl, SM. The truth about older workers. *Business and Health*, May 2001: 30–38.

35. Ng, TWH, Feldman, DC. The relationship of age to ten dimensions of job performance. *Journal of Applied Psychology*, 2008;93(2):392–423.

36. Salthouse, TA. Age-related differences in basic cognitive processes: Implications for work. *Experimental Aging Research*, 1994;20:249–255.

37. Gunn, EP. Retire today, find a new job tomorrow. *Fortune*, July 24, 1995;132(2):102–106.

38. Lieberman, S, McCray, J. The coming of age(ism): Newsrooms should be wary of the generation gap. *The Quill*, April 1994;82(3):33–34.

39. Kenny, GP, Yardley, JE, Martineau, L, Jay, O. Physical work capacity in older adults: Implications for the aging worker. *American Journal of Industrial Medicine,* 2008;51(8):610–625.

40. National Sleep Foundation. Sleep in America Poll. Retrieved August 3, 2008, from http://www .kintera.org/atf/cf/%7BF6BF2668-A1B4-4FE8-8D1A-A5D39340D9CB%7D/2003SleepPoll ExecSumm.pdf

41. National Sleep Awareness Roundtable. Why Sleep Awareness Is Important. 2013. Retrieved June 24, 2013, from http://www.nsart.org/why-sleep-awareness-is-important

42. National Institutes of Health. Unexplained Fatigue in the Elderly [workshop]. June 25–26, 2007. Retrieved September 22, 2008, from http:// www.nia.nih.gov/ResearchInformation /ConferencesAndMeetings/Unexplained Fatigue.htm#summary

43. Ringdahl, DM, Snively, CG, Carney, PR. Pharmacological treatments. In PR Carney, RB Berry, JD Geyer (Eds.), *Clinical Sleep Disorders*. Philadelphia: Lippincott Williams & Wilkins, 2005: 485–486.

44. Phillips, B. Sleepiness. In PR Carney, RB Berry, JD Geyer (Eds.), *Clinical Sleep Disorders*. Philadelphia: Lippincott Williams & Wilkins, 2005: 101–112.

45. Nau, SD, Lichstein, KL. Insomnia: Causes and treatment. In PR Carney, RB Berry, JD Geyer (Eds.), *Clinical Sleep Disorders*. Philadelphia: Lippincott Williams & Wilkins, 2005: 157–190.

46. Cleveland Clinic. Insomnia. 2012. Retrieved June 24, 2013, from http://my.clevelandclinic.org /disorders/insomnia/hic_insomnia.aspx

47. National Sleep Foundation. Sleep Apnea and Sleep. 2011. Retrieved June 24, 2013, from http:// www.sleepfoundation.org/article/sleep-related-problems/obstructive-sleep-apnea-and-sleep

48. Berry, RB, Sanders, MH. Positive airway pressure treatment for sleep apnea. In PR Carney, RB Berry, JD Geyer (Eds.), *Clinical Sleep Disorders*. Philadelphia: Lippincott Williams & Wilkins, 2005: 290–310.

49. National Institute of Neurological Disorders and Stroke. Restless Legs Syndrome Fact Sheet. Retrieved September 22, 2008, from http://www .ninds.nih.gov/disorders/restless_legs/detail_ restless_legs.htm#106073237

50. Cleveland Clinic. Periodic Limb Movement Disorder. 2012. Retrieved June 24, 2013, from http:// my.clevelandclinic.org/disorders/periodic_limb_ movement_disorder/hic_periodic_limb_ movement_disorder.aspx

51. Edinger, JD, Wohlgemuth, WK, Radke, RA, Marsh, GR, Quillian, RE. Cognitive behavioral therapy for treatment of primary chronic insomnia. *Journal of the American Medical Association*, 2001;285(14):1856–1864.

52. Ancoli-Israel, S. Normal sleep linked to successful aging. *Science Daily*. 2008, June 11. Retrieved September 29, 2008, from http://www .sciencedaily.com/releases/2008/06 /080611071051.htm

GERIATRIC PHARMACOTHERAPY

CHRISTINE M. RUBY, PharmD, BCPS, and
THOMAS D. NOLIN, PharmD, PhD

Medicine sometimes snatches away health, sometimes gives it.

—Ovid, Roman poet

Chapter Outline

Behavioral Objectives

Upon completion of this chapter, the reader will be able to:

1. List the four pharmacokinetic parameters, all of which change in older persons.
2. Describe the primary alterations occurring with each of the pharmacokinetic parameters.
3. List at least five drugs/drug classes that require dosage adjustment in older persons.
4. Contrast pharmacokinetic and pharmacodynamic changes.
5. Describe factors contributing to polypharmacy and explain why polypharmacy is not desirable.

6. Define the term *medication-related problem*, and describe three common types.
7. Define the term *adverse drug reaction*, and differentiate it from side effect.
8. Describe the Beers and STOPP criteria and how these guidelines can be helpful to improve prescribing for older adults.
9. Identify the drug most likely to be abused by older persons.
10. Define the term *medication adherence*, describe barriers to it, and suggest possible strategies for maintenance of adherence.
11. Discuss an effective means of medication management in older persons.

Key Terms

Adherence	Medication-related problems
Adverse drug reaction	Pharmacodynamics
Beers criteria	Pharmacokinetics
Health literacy	Polypharmacy
Hydrophilicity	Screening Tool of Older Persons' Potentially
Lipophilicity	Inappropriate Prescriptions (STOPP)

The continued increase in life expectancy has translated to a growing number of older people worldwide. The percentage of the world's population over the age of 60 years doubled during the 20th century, and is projected to double or triple during the current century.[1] Moreover, older adults, especially those over 85 years, have become the fastest growing segment of the U.S. population. Individuals over age 65 currently represent 13.7% of the U.S. population and are expected to double in number to 70 million by 2030.[1,2] The majority of older people have at least one chronic disease and consequently use more medications than younger people do. A recent study found the prevalence of chronic conditions for seniors is 70.4%, and the medical expenditures for seniors with chronic conditions accounts for 92.7% of the total medical expenditures for seniors.[3] In addition, 25% of the medical expenditures in the United States are spent on the 8.2% of seniors who have five or more chronic conditions.[3] Seniors consume approximately 25% of the prescribed medications and spend nearly $3 billion per year in the United States alone.[3,4]

Older persons undergo well-documented age-related physiologic changes that directly influence drug disposition and response, a phenomenon that makes them susceptible to often preventable drug-related problems, particularly adverse drug reactions (ADRs).[5] An increased number of chronic illnesses contributes to polypharmacy, which may in turn lead to the development of ADRs and poor **adherence** to prescribed medication regimens.[1,4] An understanding of each of these issues is important in ensuring safe and effective pharmacotherapy. Clinicians familiar with them are better prepared to evaluate and individualize drug therapy in older adults.

PHARMACOKINETIC CHANGES

Pharmacokinetics is the study of what happens to a drug in the body. It takes into account all aspects of drug disposition in the body, including *absorption* from the administration site, *distribution* into various body compartments, and *clearance* from the body. Drug clearance is composed primarily of *metabolism* to active and inactive metabolites (by-products of drug metabolism) and renal *excretion* of parent drug and metabolites.

In short, the practice of clinical pharmacokinetics strives to reduce drug toxicity without compromising efficacy and/or to increase efficacy while avoiding toxicity. This is accomplished by maintaining blood concentrations of drugs within a proven therapeutic range. Age-related physiologic, and hence pharmacokinetic, changes affect the manner in which the body responds to medications (**Table 6-1**).[6,7] Careful consideration of these changes, combined with knowledge of which drugs are affected and how those drugs are influenced, allows a healthcare professional to determine the most appropriate dosing regimen.

ABSORPTION

Drugs are administered most frequently via the oral route, so changes in the gastrointestinal tract may translate into altered drug absorption and response. Age-related changes in the gastrointestinal tract include increased gastric pH, delayed gastric emptying time, and decreases in both intestinal motility and blood flow.[6] An increase in gastric pH can

TABLE 6-1   Physiologic Changes Affecting Drug Disposition in Older Adults

Physiologic Change	Pharmacokinetic Parameter Affected
↑ Gastric pH	Absorption
↓ Gastric emptying time	
↓ Gastrointestinal motility	
↓ Gastrointestinal blood flow	
↓ Lean muscle mass	Distribution
↑ Total body fat	
↓ Total body water	
↓ Serum albumin	
↓ Cardiac output	
↓ Liver mass	Clearance (metabolism)
↓ Hepatic blood flow	
↓ Enzyme activity	
↓ Renal blood flow	Clearance (excretion)
↓ Glomerular filtration rate	
↓ Renal tubular function	

interfere with the dissolution or breakdown and subsequent pharmacologic response of some drugs. For example, the antifungal agent ketoconazole requires a low gastric pH to be broken down and subsequently available for systemic absorption.[1] When used in the setting of an increased gastric pH, the drug exhibits lowered therapeutic responses because of incomplete dissolution.

The delay in gastric emptying allows more contact time between drugs and the stomach. This can be problematic with potentially ulcer-causing drugs such as the non-steroidal anti-inflammatory agents (e.g., ibuprofen, naproxen). Increased drug–drug inter-actions are also possible, as is the case with antacids and other compounds containing a cation or positively charged element (e.g., calcium carbonate, magnesium hydroxide, aluminum hydroxide, iron, ferrous sulfate), as a result of increased binding (chelation) of the cation to other medications, such as tetracycline and quinolone antibiotics. Generally, this can be avoided by administering them at least 2 hours apart from one another.

Decreased cardiac output and blood flow may slightly affect the rate of absorption of drugs administered orally, as well as those administered topically, intramuscularly, and subcutaneously, as a result of reduced regional blood perfusion.[8] In general, however, despite the preceding changes, the *extent* of absorption and resulting bioavailability of most drugs are not significantly affected in older adults.[4,8] Because of the delay in gastric emptying and decreased motility, the *rate* of absorption may potentially be reduced, but any reduction is usually minor.

DISTRIBUTION

Various changes in the composition of the aging body influence the distribution of drugs. The *volume of distribution* is a term that refers to the extent to which a drug distributes throughout bodily tissues. It does not represent a specific body fluid or volume per se, but a virtual volume in which a given amount of drug would have to distribute to gener-ate the measured concentration.[5] Drug distribution is dependent on several factors, including the extent of water solubility (**hydrophilicity**), fat solubility (**lipophilicity**), and plasma protein binding. Body composition changes with age, affecting each of these factors, so the volume of distribution of many drugs also changes.

The ratio of lean body mass to total body fat changes with age. Total body fat increases up to 45% as we grow older.[1,8] As a result, lipophilic drugs, which distribute extensively into fat tissue, may exhibit increased volumes of distribution. This is the case with the tranquilizing agent diazepam and the cardiovascular drugs amiodarone and verapamil. Consequently, lipophilic drugs often accumulate over time, resulting in a prolonged dura-tion of action and longer elimination half-lives as a result of delayed release from fat tissues.

Other drugs are hydrophilic (i.e., distribute primarily into water), and their volumes of distribution are proportional to lean body weight. Lean body weight reflects primarily skeletal muscle mass and total body water, which falls up to 15% by the age of 80 years compared to young healthy adults.[1,8] The decrease in both of these as we age reduces the volume of distribution of water-soluble compounds, resulting in higher plasma concentrations and more frequent toxicity than in younger people given the same dose.[8] Examples of hydrophilic drugs include ethanol, the antibiotics gentamicin and tobramycin, the antiulcer drug cimetidine, and lithium, a common mood-stabilizing medication.

As one ages, decreases in serum albumin concentrations may occur secondary to chronic disease states, malnutrition, and/or severe debilitation.[9] Because only the free, non-protein-bound fraction of a drug is active, a reduction in serum albumin concentrations may result in higher free drug concentrations and intensified pharmacologic effects. Acidic compounds, including oral antidiabetic agents, the antiepileptic agents phenytoin and phenobarbital, and the anticoagulant warfarin, bind primarily to albumin and should be used cautiously in patients with hypoalbuminemia.[9] Generally speaking, however, age-related changes in protein binding do not affect and are not clinically relevant for many drugs.[8,9]

METABOLISM

Enzymatic metabolism or biotransformation by organs such as the liver and intestine is a crucial step in the elimination of drugs from the body. It serves to convert drugs through various metabolic pathways to more hydrophilic metabolites, which can then be excreted by the kidneys.[5] Hepatic metabolism of drugs is dependent on the organ's mass, microsomal enzyme activity, and blood flow. Hepatic mass decreases by approximately 1% per year after the age of 40, and blood flow to the liver may be reduced by up to 40% in older individuals.[1] This reduction in blood flow results in less of the drug being presented to the liver and decreased drug metabolism.

In addition to changes in blood flow, age influences the hepatic clearance of drugs by causing alterations in the intrinsic activity of selected microsomal enzymes. Drug metabolism occurs primarily via two enzyme pathways: phase I functional reactions (e.g., oxidation, reduction, hydrolysis) and phase II conjugation reactions (e.g., glucuronidation, acetylation, sulfation).[5] The cytochrome P450 superfamily of enzymes is responsible for the overwhelming majority of phase I metabolism. Phase I reactions are typically reduced in older adults, whereas phase II pathways generally remain unaffected.[4] As depicted in **Table 6-2**, the clearance of numerous drug substrates of phase I and II metabolic enzymes is affected by age. For example, the benzodiazepine anxiolytic and hypnotic agents chlordiazepoxide, diazepam, and alprazolam all undergo phase I metabolism and have prolonged elimination half-lives in older adults.[5] Conversely, oxazepam, lorazepam, and temazepam undergo phase II conjugation because the metabolism of these agents is not affected by age. Therefore they are preferred for use in older adults.[5]

EXCRETION

Kidney function is the most predictable and quantifiable determinant of drug clearance from the body. Reduction in kidney mass, the number of functioning nephrons, renal

TABLE 6-2 Selected Drugs with Reduced Clearance in Older Adults

Clearance Pathway	Drugs	
Phase I metabolism	Alprazolam	Propranolol
	Amiodarone	Midazolam
	Amitriptyline	Theophylline
	Chlordiazepoxide	Verapamil
	Cyclosporine	
	Diazepam	
	Diltiazem	
	Imipramine	
Phase II metabolism	Acetaminophen	
	Isoniazid	
	Lorazepam	
	Morphine	
	Oxazepam	
	Temazepam	
Renal excretion	Acyclovir	Penicillins
	Atenolol	Ranitidine
	Ciprofloxacin	Sotalol
	Digoxin	Vancomycin
	Fluconazole	
	Gentamicin	
	Glyburide	
	Imipenem	
	Lithium	
	Nitrofurantoin	

blood flow, glomerular filtration rate (GFR), and the rate of tubular secretion account for the decreased renal excretory capacity observed with aging.[1] Between the ages of 30 and 80 years, kidney mass decreases by about 25% and renal blood flow and GFR decline approximately 1% per year after the age of 40 years.[1,8] An otherwise healthy 70-year-old person may have a 50% decrease in renal function, even in the absence of kidney disease.

Many drugs are renally excreted and require dosage adjustments in older adults to avoid toxicity (Table 6-2). Drug dosage adjustments are typically based on an individual's kidney GFR, which is easily estimated based on age, sex, race, and serum creatinine concentration.[10] This assessment must be done with caution in older adults, however. Serum creatinine is a by-product of muscle that is almost completely excreted by the kidneys, so it is an excellent endogenous marker of kidney function. In normal young individuals, a decline in kidney function results in a predictable rise in serum creatinine concentration. However, because muscle mass decreases with aging, creatinine production and presence in the serum also decrease so that the serum creatinine value may not accurately reflect the true level of renal function in older adults. It is not uncommon for older adults with markedly reduced kidney function to have seemingly normal serum creatinine concentrations.

Renally excreted drugs requiring dosage adjustments in older adults include numerous antimicrobials, the cardiovascular drug digoxin, lithium, and several antiulcer medications such as cimetidine, famotidine, and ranitidine (Table 6-2). Many drugs also require dose adjustment because of the production of active metabolites that are renally eliminated. These include the narcotic agents morphine and meperidine, the antiarrhythmics procainamide and disopyramide, and allopurinol, a drug used to prevent gout.

PHARMACODYNAMIC CHANGES

Pharmacodynamics refers to the biological effects resulting from the interaction between a drug and its receptor site, and generally describes the relationship between plasma drug concentrations and an observed effect or response.[11] Most age-related changes in drug response are a result of pharmacokinetic changes that alter the concentration of drug reaching the site of action or receptor site rather than changes at the site of action itself. In the setting of altered pharmacokinetics, target drug concentrations remain the same, and the dose or dosing interval is adjusted to compensate for the alteration to achieve the desired plasma concentration. However, despite these dosage adjustments and attainment of the desired drug concentrations, altered drug responses may still occur because of age-related pharmacodynamic changes.[11] The interrelationship between pharmacokinetics and pharmacodynamics is depicted in **Figure 6-1**.

Equal concentrations of drug at the site of action produce different effects in the young and the old. Although relatively understudied, age-related pharmacodynamic changes in older adults can greatly influence drug response, usually leading to increased sensitivity or an exaggerated pharmacologic response to a given drug.[11] This is seen with

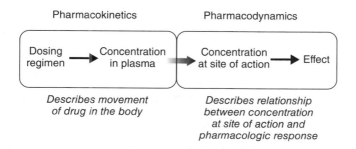

Figure 6-1   The interrelationship between pharmacokinetics and pharmacodynamics.

benzodiazepines (e.g., alprazolam, lorazepam, midazolam), narcotic analgesics (e.g., morphine), anticoagulants (e.g., warfarin), and many antihypertensive agents.[8,11] Diminished pharmacologic responses may also be seen with certain cardiovascular drugs including beta-blocking (e.g., propranolol), beta-adrenergic (e.g., isoproterenol), and calcium channel blocking agents (e.g., verapamil).[1,8,11] Altered responses may be the result of depletion of neurotransmitters and changes at the receptor site, including a decreased number of receptors and a decreased affinity or sensitivity of receptors overall. Changes in the sensitivity of older adults to drug therapy often require new target drug concentrations and more aggressive or alternative means of monitoring drug response to achieve the desired effects. In an effort to minimize adverse outcomes, it is always best to "start low and go slow" when initiating treatment with new drugs—that is, start new drug therapy with low doses and slowly titrate doses upward until the desired effects are achieved.

POLYPHARMACY

Polypharmacy, in simple terms, refers to the use of multiple medications in one individual.[12,13] In older adults, the use of multiple medications is often the rule rather than the exception.[14] Although the use of multiple medications often may be appropriate, the term *polypharmacy* usually connotes the use of more drugs than are clinically indicated or the excessive and unnecessary use of drugs, which in turn may lead to increased patient morbidity.[15] Indeed, as the number of medications taken increases, the likelihood of adverse drug reactions and drug–drug interactions also increases.[14,16] Furthermore, as the complexity of the drug regimen increases, the ability of older adults to adhere to the prescribed regimen diminishes.[17]

There are many possible reasons for polypharmacy. These include an increased number of chronic illnesses or physical ailments, a lack of one primary healthcare provider to coordinate medical care and drug use, subsequent use of multiple physicians (i.e., specialists), use of multiple pharmacies, and self-treatment, primarily with over-the-counter drugs, herbal remedies, or supplements.[13,18,19] A 2008 study by Qato and colleagues found 81% of 3,500 community-dwelling adults aged 57 to 85 years used at least one prescription medication, 42% used at least one over-the-counter medication, and 49% used a dietary supplement. Twenty-nine percent used at least five prescription medications concurrently.[19] It is not surprising that polypharmacy increases with advancing age.[20] In any age category, 50% of patients expect their physician to prescribe a drug at each office visit, and simultaneously, physicians often think that patients desire a prescription because it is seen as acknowledging the patient's ailment.[21] Ultimately, the final prescribing decision may result from the interaction of the patient, prescriber, and in some cases the family or caregiver.[22]

Studies have focused on establishing and quantifying the use of inappropriate medications in older persons and on discouraging their use.[12,15,23,24] One strategy to minimize polypharmacy requires shifting attention from specific inappropriate medications and refocusing on the appropriate use of medications.[16,22,25] It is important to distinguish between excessive and unnecessary drug use and a well-controlled drug regimen that appropriately and justifiably contains several agents. There is no magic number of drugs that equates to polypharmacy. We must resist the temptation simply to count the number of drugs a patient is receiving, determine it to be polypharmacy, and pass judgment on providers or the patient.

Strategies for reducing polypharmacy have been suggested.[14–16,21,26,27] A pharmacotherapeutic plan should be devised for every patient for whom drugs are prescribed.[16,22] Initially, nondrug therapies should be considered. Medications should only be prescribed with clear therapeutic goals in mind. Those with minimal side effects, the simplest dosing schedules, and the lowest cost should be selected whenever possible. Patients need to be educated regarding their drug regimens, and these should be routinely reevaluated at each healthcare visit. The use of several medications simultaneously can be managed if the prescriber assesses each patient's drug regimen every time the patient is seen.[16,28] It is entirely possible for a drug that was appropriately prescribed initially to subsequently become inappropriate for various reasons, including the development of adverse effects or therapeutic failure.[16] If these situations are identified and corrected, older patients will receive maximal benefits from the fewest number of medications.

MEDICATION-RELATED PROBLEMS

Drugs, if used inappropriately, may cause more harm than good.[29] It has been estimated that up to 200,000 people may die in the United States each year from **medication-related problems** (MRPs), which are defined as "events or circumstances involving a patient's drug treatment that actually, or potentially, interfere with the achievement of an optimal outcome."[30] If adverse drug reactions, one type of MRP, were classified as a distinct disease, it would rank as the fifth leading cause of death in the United States.[31] Moreover, MRPs also have a significant financial impact in this country. Overall, the cost of drug-related morbidity and mortality exceeded $177.4 billion in 2000.[29] Half of the morbidity and mortality caused by MRPs may be preventable.[32] By identifying, resolving, and preventing medication-related problems, a patient's medications are more likely to be appropriate, the most effective available, and correctly used. Common types of MRPs include untreated indications, drug use without indications, improper drug selection, incorrect dose, adverse drug reactions, drug interactions, and nonadherence. Each of these is described in the following subsections.

UNTREATED INDICATIONS

Untreated indications occur when the patient does not receive the therapy indicated for some medical condition or prophylactic need, such as immunizations.[33] Underuse of potentially beneficial medications is an increasingly recognized problem in older patients,[15,25,33] with some concluding that undertreatment of older persons is a problem equivalent to or of greater magnitude than medication overuse.[25,33,34] One example is the undertreatment of osteoporosis, a common condition resulting in significant adverse outcomes and an enormous economic burden.[27]

DRUG USE WITHOUT INDICATIONS

One of the primary goals of medication management in older adults is to eliminate medications being used without appropriate indications.[16] These include prescription and over-the-counter products for which there is currently no valid medical indication, the use of multiple drugs for a condition for which single-drug therapy is indicated, and drug therapy to treat an avoidable adverse effect caused by another medication. Use of unnecessary antihypertensive agents is a frequent example of this problem.[27] Frequent medication reassessment and cautious withdrawal of agents that do not have clearly defined indications improve the quality of pharmacotherapy in older adults.[35,36]

IMPROPER DRUG SELECTION

Improper drug selection occurs when the patient has a medical indication for which the prescribed drug is ineffective or less effective than alternatives, or if the patient has risk factors for which the medication is contraindicated, that is, prescribing a medication to which a patient is allergic.[27]

The American Geriatrics Society recently published updated **Beers criteria** for potentially inappropriate medication (PIM) use in older adults.[37] An interdisciplinary panel used a comprehensive, systematic review and grading of evidence for drug-related problems and adverse drug events in older adults to incorporate new evidence not considered in the last update published in 2003.[38] The new update categorized PIMs into three groups:

- Medications to avoid in older adults
- Medications considered potentially inappropriate when used in older adults with certain diseases or syndromes
- Medications to be used with caution (potential for misuse or harm, but evidence is still emerging)

Avoiding the use of inappropriate, high-risk drugs is an effective strategy for reducing medication-related problems. Selected examples from the 2012 Beers criteria are included in **Table 6-3**. Another, similar screening tool is called **STOPP (Screening Tool of Older Persons' Potentially Inappropriate Prescriptions)**. STOPP comprises 65 common potentially inappropriate prescribing practices including drug–drug and drug–disease interactions, drugs that adversely affect older persons at risk for falls, and duplicate drug class prescriptions.[39] Each criterion includes an explanation as to why the medication is potentially inappropriate.

TABLE 6-3   Selected Examples from Beers Criteria[37]

Drug Class	Examples
Antihistamines, 1st generation	Diphenhydramine, hydroxyzine
Cardiovascular	Alpha blockers, amiodarone, digoxin > 0.125 mg/d, dipyridamole IR, disopyramide, nifedipine IR, ticlopidine
Endocrine	Androgens, chlorpropamide, glyburide
GI agents	Antispasmodics, mineral oil, trimethobenzamide, metoclopramide
Musculoskeletal	Meperidine, chronic non-COX2-selective NSAIDs (unless receiving gastro-protection), pentazocine, cyclobenzaprine

Data from: American Geriatrics Society. Updated Beers Criteria for Potentially Inappropriate Medication Use in Older Adults. Retrieved January 15, 2013, from http://www.americangeriatrics.org/files/documents/beers/2012BeersCriteria_JAGS.pdf

INCORRECT DOSE

The interindividual variability of drug response increases with age, so finding the optimal dose is not always straightforward for older individuals.[6] Adjusting doses to match appropriate physical attributes and organ function is essential; however, it is often overlooked. The "start low and go slow" drug dosing strategy is typically recommended. That said, whereas clinicians are usually concerned about excessive medication dosing, occasionally an inadequate dosage of medication may be prescribed.[16] For instance, antidepressant therapy is typically initiated at a low dose and titrated upward to response. Failure to titrate upward in the event that a favorable response is not achieved (i.e., an inadequate dosage) may lead to therapeutic failure.[27] Documenting response to therapy provides a rational basis for the modification, continuation, or discontinuation of a drug.

ADVERSE DRUG REACTIONS

An **adverse drug reaction** (ADR) is defined as an "undesirable response associated with use of a drug that either compromises therapeutic efficacy, enhances toxicity, or both."[40] The U.S. Food and Drug Administration approves drugs on the basis that their benefits outweigh their risks. All drugs have the ability to cause problems, from minor side effects to permanent disability and even death.[41–43] It is important to differentiate ADRs from side effects of drugs, which are extensions of the known pharmacologic activity of the drug in question and are therefore expected and predictable. The clinical picture can often be so complex that this differentiation may be extremely difficult to determine. ADRs typically have the following characteristics[42]:

- Require a modification in drug therapy (e.g., drug discontinuation or dosage change)
- Cause or prolong admission to the hospital

- Require supportive treatment
- Negatively affect prognosis
- May result in disability or death

ADRs may go undetected because the presenting symptoms may mimic problems commonly associated with older age, such as forgetfulness, weakness, or tremor.[2] Common geriatric syndromes such as cognitive impairment, falls, and urinary incontinence may be caused or exacerbated by medications. ADRs also can be misinterpreted as a new medical condition and lead to drug use without indication.[2] A 2-year study of nursing home residents found that 74% had an ADR during their stay, and at least 61% of the ADRs were preventable.[44] Common drug categories implicated in ADRs in older patients include cardiovascular drugs, antibiotics, diuretics, anticoagulants, hypoglycemic drugs, steroids, opioids, anticholinergics, benzodiazepines, and nonsteroidal anti-inflammatory drugs.[32,45,46] In fact, adverse events stemming from use of only three drugs—warfarin, insulin, and digoxin—have been shown to be responsible for up to one-third of emergency department and outpatient care visits in people at least 65 years of age.[47]

DRUG INTERACTIONS

Older patients are at high risk of drug interactions. This risk may be because of patient factors (e.g., concurrent use of many drugs, numerous comorbidities), prescriber factors, or difficulties within the healthcare system such as inefficient communication between healthcare professionals and patients.[48] Several types of interactions exist, including drug–drug interactions, drug–disease interactions, drug–food interactions, and drug–alcohol interactions.[48–53] Drug–drug interactions can be pharmacokinetic or pharmacodynamic in nature. The understanding and management of these varied types of interactions can be challenging. Common drug interactions are often detected by commercial drug interaction software systems; however, the detection of complex interactions is often difficult. The individual choice of drugs for each disorder is usually appropriate, but when combined with several other agents in the same patient, this can yield unwanted results.[48] An expert panel identified 25 clinically important drug–drug interactions that are likely to occur in the community and ambulatory pharmacy settings.[54] Pharmacists and other healthcare professionals should take steps to prevent patients from receiving these interacting medications. Further, those developing computer software programs should focus interaction alerts on these and similarly important drug–drug interactions. Older patients have been shown to benefit by having their care managed by interdisciplinary teams that practice the principles of geriatric care focused on individualized pharmacotherapy.

NONADHERENCE

Nonadherence with prescribed drug regimens is a prevalent medication-related problem. In people age 60 years or older, rates of adherence to medication regimens range from

41% to 74%.[55] The term *adherence* more accurately reflects a therapeutic alliance or agreement between the patient and prescriber and is currently preferred over the now outdated term *compliance*, which suggests the passive following of the prescriber's orders.[56] Adherence also reflects the persistence, or length of time, with which regimen compliance has occurred.[57] Numerous potential barriers to adherence need to be considered when devising strategies for improvement.[58] These take into account factors under the patient's control, as well as interactions between the patient and the healthcare provider and between the patient and the healthcare system.[55]

Medication adherence and health outcomes are affected by **health literacy**, defined as "the degree to which people have the capacity to obtain, process, and understand basic health information and services needed to make appropriate health decisions."[59] Health literacy has been found to be significantly lower among older persons, even after adjusting for various types of cognitive impairments.[60] Knowledge of the patient's health literacy and efforts to enhance it may improve adherence rates and subsequent health outcomes. Methods to improve health literacy, and thus adherence, have been grouped into four general categories[58]:

- Providing patient education
- Improving dosing schedules
- Increasing access to clinic or office visits, such as providing longer open hours
- Improving communication between patients and healthcare providers

Despite use of these methods, low adherence is generally not "cured." So, efforts to improve adherence must be maintained for as long as the treatment is needed.[61]

DRUG ABUSE

Drug abuse among older adults may not be as prevalent as in younger age groups, but it does exist. Of the drugs abused by older adults, alcohol is the most common.[62] With age-related physiologic changes, older adults may experience unfavorable health effects even from relatively low levels of alcohol consumption.[63] Older patients are more likely to use multiple alcohol-interactive medications, as well as have interactive medical conditions and diminishing functional status.[53] Screening for alcohol use is essential to minimize adverse reactions, as is the provision of warnings to patients regarding potential detrimental effects.[53,54,63]

MEDICATION MANAGEMENT

Medication management generally involves periodic review of a patient's medications (prescription, nonprescription, vitamin supplements, herbal remedies, and nutritional products) to assess whether they are medically necessary, tailor prescriptions accordingly, and consult with patients to ensure that they understand the purpose and use of their medications.[64] Before initiating new drug therapy, nondrug treatments such as lifestyle modifications (e.g., diet and exercise programs), occupational and/or physical therapy, and psychotherapy should be employed, if possible. When medically justified, drugs should be prescribed with clear therapeutic goals in mind for each agent, including dosing schedule, monitoring parameters, duration of therapy, and desired outcome or endpoint. Medications should be discontinued when desired goals or outcomes are not met. Individual patients should be evaluated for issues that may contribute to poor adherence. Factors to consider when initiating new drug treatment include the drug's efficacy and side effect profile, cost, perceived and actual affordability, dosing schedule, and ease of administration. The effect of pharmacokinetic and pharmacodynamic changes and the likelihood of developing medication-related problems should be considered.

The lowest possible effective dose should be the starting point. Patients should be well informed regarding their new medications and provided with opportunities to express concerns or questions. The indications, benefits, potential adverse effects, and directions for use should be clearly explained. Well-written (i.e., clear and direct) instructions should also be provided. During subsequent visits, monitoring parameters should be reviewed and endpoints or outcomes desired initially should be assessed to determine whether they have been met.

Communicating the pharmaceutical care plan across all settings is essential to prevent medication-related problems as old prescriptions are discontinued and new drugs are initiated. This is vitally important during transitions of care; for example, when an older adult is admitted or discharged from the hospital. Effective communication with family members and caregivers is especially important to prevent hospitalizations or rehospitalizations because of side effects from unintended drug combinations.

PORTABLE PERSONAL MEDICATION RECORDS

An up-to-date medication list that is readily accessible to the patient and all caregivers is a critical component of medication management. This list should include all prescription medications, over-the-counter medications, herbal remedies, and dietary supplements. This comprehensive medication list allows efficient and ongoing drug regimen review and evaluation. A majority of patients do self-medicate with nonprescription alternatives, making it essential for these to be included in any medication list.

MEDICATION THERAPY MANAGEMENT SERVICES

The prevention and resolution of medication-related problems can be addressed through medication therapy management (MTM) services. This is a recognized covered service in the Medicare Part D drug benefit, some state Medicaid programs, and other private pay plans. MTM services are usually provided directly to the patient by licensed pharmacists, but may also be performed by other qualified healthcare providers. Comprehensive medication therapy management is considered the standard of care in the patient-centered medical home model, part of the Patient Protection and Affordable Care Act (ACA).

Taking into account the individual needs of the patient, MTM services include, but are not limited to, the following[65]:

- Performing or obtaining necessary assessments of the patient's health status
- Formulating a medication treatment plan
- Selecting, initiating, modifying, or administering medication therapy
- Monitoring and evaluating the patient's response to therapy, including safety and effectiveness
- Performing a comprehensive medication review to identify, resolve, and prevent medication-related problems, including adverse drug events
- Documenting the care delivered and communicating essential information to the patient's other primary care providers
- Providing verbal education and training designed to enhance patient understanding and appropriate use of his or her medications
- Providing information, support services, and resources designed to enhance patient adherence with his or her therapeutic regimens
- Coordinating and integrating medication therapy management services within the broader healthcare management services being provided to the patient

Further information regarding MTM services may be viewed at the website of the American Pharmacists Association (www.pharmacist.com/mtm).

SUMMARY

Drug therapy offers tremendous benefits to older people when used appropriately. However, inherent risks associated with suboptimal drug use in the vulnerable older population create challenges for professionals working with them. The effective management of medication regimens in older adults requires knowledge of the relevant issues. Pharmacokinetic and pharmacodynamic changes necessitate unique dosing and the careful selection of medications to minimize polypharmacy, minimize adverse effects, and improve adherence. We must become attuned to reviewing medication regimens with these issues in mind and develop a high index of suspicion for medication-related problems. In doing so, we will ensure that older patients receive maximal benefits from drug therapy while minimizing potential adverse outcomes.

Review Questions

1. Despite numerous pharmacokinetic changes in older adults, the extent of _____ is not significantly affected in older adults.
   A. Drug absorption
   B. Drug distribution
   C. Hepatic metabolism
   D. Renal excretion

2. Which of the following is the most predictable pharmacokinetic change in older adults?
    A. Absorption
    B. Distribution
    C. Hepatic metabolism
    D. Renal excretion

3. *Pharmacodynamics* refers to the
    A. Movement of drugs through the body
    B. Inability of drugs to move through the body
    C. Biological effects of drugs on the body
    D. Constantly changing pharmacokinetic parameters

4. Pharmacodynamic changes in older adults usually result in _____ pharmacologic responses.
    A. Diminished
    B. Unchanged
    C. Exaggerated
    D. Absent

5. Possible reasons for polypharmacy include which of the following?
    A. Lack of chronic illnesses
    B. Self-medication
    C. Use of a primary care physician
    D. Financial wealth

Learning Activities

1. Role-playing; two individuals required. One person plays an older adult patient with several chronic diseases, including arthritis and visual impairment, and limited income. Another plays a healthcare provider counseling the patient on how to take the medications. Generally speaking, what are the problems encountered by each individual and how can they be minimized?
2. Design a pharmacotherapeutic plan for the patient in activity 1. What strategies can be used by the healthcare provider to improve adherence?
3. Assume each of the following scenarios occurs in an older adult patient. Describe what the primary problem is and how it may be avoided or corrected.
    a. A patient taking an expensive medication every other day versus daily as prescribed so that it will "last longer."
    b. A patient started on a new H_2 antagonist for a peptic ulcer at normal dosing develops confusion a few days later.
    c. A patient receiving multiple medications, all of which are taken at different times of the day. When asked, he or she has no idea what each medication is, what it is used for, or when to take it.

REFERENCES

1. McLean, AJ, Le Couteur, DG. Aging biology and geriatric clinical pharmacology. *Pharmacological Reviews*, 2004;56(2):163–184.
2. U.S. Census Bureau. USA Quick Facts. Retrieved July 31, 2013, from http://quickfacts.census.gov /qfd/states/00000.html
3. Chi, MJ, Lee, CY, Wu, SC. The prevalence of chronic conditions and medical expenditures of the elderly by chronic condition indicator (CCI). *Archives of Gerontology and Geriatrics,* 2011;52(3):284–289.
4. Schwartz, JB. The current state of knowledge on age, sex, and their interactions on clinical pharmacology. *Clinical Pharmacology and Therapeutics*, 2007;82(1):87–96.
5. Bressler R, Bahl, JJ. Principles of drug therapy for the elderly patient. *Mayo Clinic Proceedings*, 2003;78(12):1564–1577.
6. Mangoni, AA, Jackson, SH. Age-related changes in pharmacokinetics and pharmacodynamics: Basic principles and practical applications. *British Journal of Clinical Pharmacology*, 2004;57(1): 6–14.
7. Cusack, BJ. Pharmacokinetics in older persons. *American Journal of Geriatric Pharmacotherapy*, 2004;2(4):274–302.
8. Turnheim, K. When drug therapy gets old: Pharmacokinetics and pharmacodynamics in the elderly. *Experimental Gerontology*, 2003;38(8): 843–853.
9. Grandison, MK, Boudinot, FD. Age-related changes in protein binding of drugs: Implications for therapy. *Clinical Pharmacokinetics*, 2000; 38(3):271–290.
10. Levey, AS, Bosch, JP, Lewis, JB, Greene, T, Rogers, N, Roth, D. A more accurate method to estimate glomerular filtration rate from serum creatinine: A new prediction equation. Modification of Diet in Renal Disease Study Group. *Annals of Internal Medicine*, 1999;130(6): 461–470.
11. Bowie, MW, Slattum, PW. Pharmacodynamics in older adults: A review. *American Journal of Geriatric Pharmacotherapy*, 2007;5(3):263–303.
12. Chutka, DS, Takahashi, PY, Hoel, RW. Inappropriate medications for elderly patients. *Mayo Clinic Proceedings*, 2004;79(1):122–139.
13. Stewart, RB. Polypharmacy in the elderly: A fait accompli? *Drug Intelligence and Clinical Pharmacy*, 1990;24(3):321–323.
14. Hayes, BD, Klein-Schwartz, W, Barrueto, F Jr. Polypharmacy and the geriatric patient. *Clinics in Geriatric Medicine*, 2007;23(2):371–390.
15. Hanlon, JT, Schmader, KE, Ruby, CM, Weinberger, M. Suboptimal prescribing in older inpatients and outpatients. *Journal of the American Geriatrics Society*, 2001;49(2):200–209.
16. Shrank, WH, Polinski, JM, Avorn J. Quality indicators for medication use in vulnerable elders. *Journal of the American Geriatrics Society*, 2007;55(Suppl 2):S373–S382.
17. Eisen, SA, Miller, DK, Woodward, RS, Spitznagel, E, Przybeck, TR. The effect of prescribed daily dose frequency on patient medication compliance. *Archives of Internal Medicine*, 1990; 150(9):1881–1884.
18. Anderson, GF. Medicare and chronic conditions. *New England Journal of Medicine*, 2005;353(3): 305–309.
19. Qato, DM, Alexander, GC, Conti, RM, Johnson, M, Schumm, P, Lindau, ST. *Journal of the American Medical Association*, 2008;300(24): 2867–2878.
20. Jyrkka, J, Vartiainen, L, Hartikainen, S, Sulkava, R, Enlund, H. Increasing use of medicines in elderly persons: A five-year follow-up of the Kuopio 75-plus Study. *European Journal of Clinical Pharmacology*, 2006;62(2):151–158.
21. Rollason, V, Vogt, N. Reduction of polypharmacy in the elderly: A systematic review of the role of the pharmacist. *Drugs and Aging*, 2003;20(11):817–832.
22. Spinewine, A, Schmader, KE, Barber, N, et al. Appropriate prescribing in elderly people: How well can it be measured and optimised? *Lancet*, 2007;370(9582):173–184.
23. Buetow, SA, Sibbald, B, Cantrill, JA, Halliwell, S. Appropriateness in health care: Application to prescribing. *Social Science and Medicine*, 1997;45(2):261–271.
24. Fick, DM, Cooper, JW, Wade, WE, Waller, JL, Maclean, JR, Beers, MH. Updating the Beers criteria for potentially inappropriate medication use in older adults: Results of a U.S. consensus

panel of experts. *Archives of Internal Medicine*, 2003;163(22):2716–2724.

25. Higashi, T, et al. The quality of pharmacologic care for vulnerable older patients. *Annals of Internal Medicine*, 2004;140(9):714–720.

26. Montamat, SC, Cusack, B. Overcoming problems with polypharmacy and drug misuse in the elderly. *Clinics in Geriatric Medicine*, 1992;8(1): 143–158.

27. Simonson, W, Feinberg, JL. Medication-related problems in the elderly: Defining the issues and identifying solutions. *Drugs and Aging*, 2005; 22(7):559–569.

28. Sherman, FT. Medication nonadherence: A national epidemic among America's seniors. *Geriatrics*, 2007;62(4):5–6.

29. Ernst, FR, Grizzle, AJ. Drug-related morbidity and mortality: updating the cost-of-illness model. *Journal of the American Pharmaceutical Association*, 2001;41(2):192–199.

30. Hepler, CD, Strand, LM. Opportunities and responsibilities in pharmaceutical care. *American Journal of Health-System Pharmacy*, 1990;47(3): 533–543.

31. Lazarou, J, Pomeranz, BH, Corey, PN. Incidence of adverse drug reactions in hospitalized patients: A meta-analysis of prospective studies. *Journal of the American Medical Association*, 1998;279(15): 1200–1205.

32. Gurwitz, JH, et al. Incidence and preventability of adverse drug events among older persons in the ambulatory setting. *Journal of the American Medical Association*, 2003;289(9):1107–1116.

33. Sloane, PD, et al. Medication undertreatment in assisted living settings. *Archives of Internal Medicine*, 2004;164(18):2031–2037.

34. Bain, K. Prevalence and predictors of medication-related problems. *Medicare Patient Management*, 2006:14–27.

35. Monane, M, Matthias, DM, Nagle, BA, Kelly, MA. Improving prescribing patterns for the elderly through an online drug utilization review intervention: A system linking the physician, pharmacist, and computer. *Journal of the American Medical Association*, 1998;280(14):1249–1252.

36. Tamblyn, R, et al. The medical office of the 21st century (MOXXI): Effectiveness of computerized decision-making support in reducing inappropri-ate prescribing in primary care. *Canadian Medical Association Journal*, 2003;169(6):549–556.

37. American Geriatrics Society 2012 Beers Criteria Update Expert Panel. American Geriatrics Society Updated Beers Criteria for Potentially Inappropriate Medication Use in Older Adults. Retrieved January 15, 2013, from http://www.americangeriatrics.org /files/documents/beers/2012BeersCriteria_JAGS .pdf

38. Fick DM, et al. Updating the Beers criteria for potentially inappropriate medication use in older adults: Results of a US consensus panel of experts. *Archives of Internal Medicine*, 2003;163: 2716–2724.

39. Gallagher, P, O'Mahony, D. STOPP (Screening Tool of Older Persons' Potentially Inappropriate Prescriptions): Application to acutely ill elderly patients and comparison with Beers criteria. *Age and Ageing*, 2008;37:673–679.

40. Joint Commission. Sentinel Event Glossary of Terms. 2007. Retrieved July 31, 2013, from http://www.e-moh.com/vb/t149271/

41. Kelly, WN. Potential risks and prevention, Part 2: Drug-induced permanent disabilities. *American Journal of Health-System Pharmacy*, 2001; 58(14):1325–1329.

42. Kelly, WN. Potential risks and prevention, Part 1: Fatal adverse drug events. *American Journal of Health-System Pharmacy*, 2001;58(14):1317–1324.

43. Marcellino K, Kelly, WN. Potential risks and prevention, Part 3: Drug-induced threats to life. *American Journal of Health-System Pharmacy*, 2001;58(15):1399–1405.

44. Cooper, JW. Adverse drug reaction-related hospitalizations of nursing facility patients: A 4-year study. *Southern Medical Journal*, 1999;92(5): 485–490.

45. Hajjar, ER, et al. Adverse drug reaction risk factors in older outpatients. *American Journal of Geriatric Pharmacotherapy*, 2003;1(2):82–89.

46. Routledge, PA, O'Mahony, MS, Woodhouse, KW. Adverse drug reactions in elderly patients. *British Journal of Clinical Pharmacology*, 2004; 57(2):121–126.

47. Budnitz, DS, Shehab, N, Kegler, SR, Richards, CL. Medication use leading to emergency department visits for adverse drug events in older adults. *Annals of Internal Medicine*, 2007;147(11):755–765.

48. Mallet, L, Spinewine, A, Huang, A. The challenge of managing drug interactions in elderly people. *Lancet*, 2007;370(9582):185–191.

49. Charrois, TL, et al. Community identification of natural health product–drug interactions. *Annals of Pharmacotherapy*, 2007;41(7):1124–1129.

50. Elmer, GW, Lafferty, WE, Tyree, PT, Lind, BK. Potential interactions between complementary/alternative products and conventional medicines in a Medicare population. *Annals of Pharmacotherapy*, 2007;41(10):1617–1624.

51. Fugh-Berman, A. Herb–drug interactions. *Lancet*, 2000;355(9198):134–138.

52. Juurlink, DN, Mamdani, M, Kopp, A, Laupacis, A, Redelmeier, DA. Drug–drug interactions among elderly patients hospitalized for drug toxicity. *Journal of the American Medical Association*, 2003;289(13):1652–1658.

53. Pringle, KE, Ahern, FM, Heller, DA, Gold, CH, Brown, TV. Potential for alcohol and prescription drug interactions in older people. *Journal of the American Geriatrics Society*, 2005;53(11):1930–1936.

54. Malone DC, et al. Identification of serious drug–drug interactions: Results of the Partnership to Prevent Drug–Drug Interactions. *Journal of the American Pharmacists Association*, 2004;44:142–151.

55. van Eijken, M, Tsang, S, Wensing, M, de Smet, PA, Grol, RP. Interventions to improve medication compliance in older patients living in the community: A systematic review of the literature. *Drugs and Aging*, 2003;20(3):229–240.

56. Steiner, JF, Earnest, MA. The language of medication-taking. *Annals of Internal Medicine*, 2000;132(11):926–930.

57. Gold, DT. Medication adherence: A challenge for patients with postmenopausal osteoporosis and other chronic illnesses. *Journal of Managed Care Pharmacy*, 2006;12(6 Suppl A):S20–S25.

58. Osterberg, L, Blaschke, T. Adherence to medication. *New England Journal of Medicine*, 2005;353(5):487–497.

59. Parker, RM, Ratzan, SC, Lurie, N. Health literacy: A policy challenge for advancing high-quality health care. *Health Affairs (Millwood)*, 2003;22(4):147–153.

60. Baker, DW, Gazmararian, JA, Sudano, J, Patterson, M. The association between age and health literacy among elderly persons. *Journal of Gerontology Series B: Psychological Sciences and Social Sciences*, 2000;55(6):S368–S374.

61. Haynes, RB, Yao, X, Degani, A, Kripalani, S, Garg, A, McDonald, HP. Interventions to enhance medication adherence. *Cochrane Database of Systematic Reviews*, 2005(4):CD000011.

62. Office of Applied Studies, Substance Abuse and Mental Health Services Administration. Substance Use Among Older Adults: 2002 and 2003 Update. 2005. Retrieved March 10, 2008, from http://www.oas.samhsa.gov/2k5/olderadults/olderadults.cfm

63. Fink, A, Elliott, MN, Tsai, M, Beck, JC. An evaluation of an intervention to assist primary care physicians in screening and educating older patients who use alcohol. *Journal of the American Geriatrics Society*, 2005;53(11):1937–1943.

64. Alkema, GE, Frey, D. Implications of translating research into practice: A medication management intervention. *Home Health Care Services Quarterly*, 2006;25(1–2):33–54.

65. Academy of Managed Care Pharmacy. In *Sound Medication Therapy Management Programs*: Version 2.0, 7–8. Retrieved July 31, 2013, from http://www.amcp.org/sound_mtm_program/

NUTRITION AND AGING

KATHRYN H. THOMPSON, PhD, RD

It's good food and not fine words that keep me alive.

—J. B. P. Moliere*

Chapter Outline

Behavioral Objectives

Upon completion of this chapter, the reader will be able to:

1. Demonstrate knowledge of current research on the impact of aging on nutrition status for healthy individuals and individuals with chronic diseases.
2. Describe the importance of early screening and intervention for nutritional risk in older adults.
3. Identify screening tools for the assessment of nutritional risk in the older adult.
4. Recognize the multiple factors that affect nutrition status in older adults (physiologic, social, psychological, economic, and environmental).
5. Describe the physiologic impact of aging on dietary intake and absorption.
6. Use MyPlate to advise the older adult about the implementation of the 2010 Dietary Guidelines for Americans.

---

*From WEBSTER'S NEW WORLD DICTIONARY OF QUOTATIONS. Copyright © 2005 by Houghton Mifflin Harcourt Publishing Company. Reprinted by permission of Houghton Mifflin Harcourt Publishing Company. All rights reserved.

7. Describe the basics of the Mediterranean diet and the DASH diet for the treatment of common chronic diseases in the older adult.
8. Recognize the impact of polypharmacy on nutritional status and drug–nutrient interactions in older adults.
9. Describe the appropriate use of nutritional supplements for the older adult.

Key Terms

Anorexia
Cachexia
Calcium
Carbohydrate
Cardiovascular disease
Celiac disease
Cholesterol
DASH (Dietary Approach to Stop Hypertension) diet
Dehydration
Diabetes
Dietary fiber
Dietary Guidelines for Americans
Dysphagia

Gluten
Hypertension
Lactose intolerance
Malabsorption
Malnutrition
Mediterranean diet
Nutritional supplements
Overnutrition
Protein
Sarcopenia
Vitamin B_{12}
Vitamin D
Weight loss

The importance of good nutrition throughout the life span and its contribution to health and quality of life cannot be overestimated. The average life span of individuals has increased dramatically over the past few decades. In 1940, only 7% of Americans aged 65 years were expected to live to age 90. Now, more than 27% are expected to become nonagenarians, and by 2050, given life circumstances similar to today, nearly 50% of 65-year-olds will reach this milestone.[1] In the next 20 years, the older population is predicted to reach 71 million, which will account for nearly 20% of the total U.S. population.

The aging population is a heterogeneous population ranging from healthy high functioning older adults living in the community to those who must depend on others for their care. Approximately 15% of older community-dwelling adults and 50% of hospitalized older adults are malnourished.[2] The incidence of chronic disease in this population is high, with 80% of older adults having at least one chronic disease and 50% having at least two.[3] Many of these chronic diseases can be managed successfully with nutrition intervention to improve both quality and quantity of life for aging individuals.

For many, the late-life years are a time of great change socially, economically, psychologically, and physically. With the death of a spouse and/or friends, many older adults find themselves living alone and eating meals alone. Changes in income as a result of retirement can mean fewer resources are available for food purchases. Older adults may also experience more limited mobility related to various joint, muscular, and other health problems. Individually or in combination, these factors interact and influence nutritional status in older adults.

The Older Americans Act of 2006 places special emphasis on integrated health promotion and disease prevention through nutrition education for older adults to improve the health of this population.[4,5] To realize these goals, all older adults should receive early nutrition screening and intervention for the problems of weight loss, nutrient deficiencies, and overnutrition. Nutritional recommendations and treatment plans should include a consideration of the effects of individual variations in physiological, environmental, and social changes associated with aging, as discussed in this chapter.

SCREENING

THE NUTRITION SCREENING INITIATIVE

One of the best ways to achieve high-quality nutrition care for older adults is to promote early screening and intervention. Since 1989, the American Dietetic Association, the National Council on Aging, and the American Academy of Family Physicians have collaborated in an effort called the Nutrition Screening Initiative (NSI) to encourage early and routine screening and intervention for nutrition risk in older adults.[6] The premise of the initiative is that nutrition status is a *vital sign* just as important in evaluating a person's health and well-being as the traditional vital signs of blood pressure and pulse.

The result of the Nutrition Screening Initiative is a self-assessment checklist that can be used in a variety of settings to help identify whether an individual is at risk for compromised nutritional well-being. In addition, the acronym DETERMINE is an educational device that can be used along with the checklist to help identify the warning signs of poor nutritional status in older adults. The self-assessment checklist and meaning of DETERMINE are presented in **Boxes 7-1** and **7-2**.

Three other screening instruments also might be helpful in assessing the nutritional status of your patient or client. They are the Subjective Global Assessment (SGA), the Mini Nutrition Assessment (MNA), and the Malnutrition Screening Tool (MST).

The SGA (available at www.hospitalmedicine.org/geriresource/toolbox/pdfs /subjective_global_assessmen.pdf) and MNA (available at www.mna-elderly.com/mna_ forms.html) are similar to the NSI and have been deemed valid and reliable tools to determine nutritional risk and the presence of **malnutrition**. The Malnutrition Screening Tool (MST) consists of two simple questions:

- Have you been eating poorly because of decreased appetite?
- Have you lost weight recently without trying?

In a study published in 2012 comparing nutrition screening tools, the MST and the MNA scored in the highest quartile for both sensitivity and specificity.[7] Both the SGA

BOX 7-1 Nutrition Screening Initiative Self-Assessment Checklist

Answer the following questions as carefully as you can. Add up the points for all yes answers and compare with the point evaluation scale. This checklist will help you determine if you are nutritionally at risk.

Question	Yes
I have an illness or condition that has recently made me change the kind and/or amount of food I eat.	2 pts
I eat fewer than two meals per day.	3
I rarely eat fruits, vegetables, and milk products.	2
I have three or more glasses of beer, liquor, or wine almost every day.	2
I have tooth or mouth problems that make it hard for me to eat.	2
I don't always have enough money to buy the food I need.	4
I eat alone most of the time.	1
I take three or more different prescription or over-the-counter drugs a day.	1
Without wanting to, I have lost or gained 10 pounds in the past 6 months.	2
I am not always physically able to shop, cook, and/or feed myself.	2

Total Score:

Point Evaluation Scale

0–2   Good! Recheck your score in 6 months.

3–5   You are at a moderate nutritional risk. See what can be done to improve your eating habits and lifestyle. The Area Agencies on Aging, senior nutrition programs, senior citizen centers, or health departments may be able to help. Recheck your score in 3 months.

6+   You are at nutritional risk. Bring this checklist the next time you see your doctor, dietitian, or other qualified healthcare provider. Ask for nutrition counseling.

Adapted from: The Nutrition Screening Initiative, a project of the American Academy of Family Physicians, the American Dietetic Association, and the National Council on Aging; 1989.

BOX 7-2   DETERMINE

Use this to help you remember the warning signs of nutrition risk.

D   *Disease:* The presence of any disease causing a change in eating habits may make it harder to eat right and will increase risk. Four of five adults have chronic diseases affected by diet. Confusion and memory loss may make it harder to plan healthy diets and even to remember what and when you last ate. Depression and loneliness can cause changes in appetite, digestion, energy level, weight, and well-being.

E   *Eating poorly:* Both eating too little and eating too much can cause a decline in health status. Lack of variety, poor quality foods, and poor balance of food types all lead to poor nutritional health. Many older adults skip meals and eat fewer than the recommended five servings daily of fruits and vegetables. Alcohol consumption is a concern, with one in four adults drinking too much.

T   *Tooth loss or mouth pain:* Healthy mouth, gums, and teeth are essential to good nutrition. When dental health is compromised, so is nutritional well-being.

E   *Economic hardship:* Although Social Security and Medicare have made great progress in combating poverty among older adults (approximately 35% were below the poverty level in 1959, whereas in 2003 only 10.2% fell below the poverty level; U.S. Department of Commerce, Bureau of the Census, 2003), financial struggles may make it harder to eat right and stay healthy.

R   *Reduced social contact:* Approximately one-third of all older people live alone. For a variety of reasons, aging brings with it fewer meaningful social contacts. This, too, can affect nutritional well-being.

M   *Multiple medicines:* Polypharmacy, the use of multiple drugs, can also compromise nutritional well-being. Almost half of older Americans take multiple medicines daily. Some of the side effects include changes in appetite and taste, constipation, weakness, and nausea.

I   *Involuntary weight gain or loss:* Changes in weight (more than just a few pounds) should always be seen as a warning sign that a person's nutrition status may be compromised.

N   *Needs assistance in self-care:* Older people who need help with walking, shopping, cooking, and feeding are at risk for decreased nutritional status.

E   *Elder years past age 80:* Increasing age brings increased risk of health problems. Be sure to see your physician regularly, at least on an annual basis.

Adapted from: The Nutrition Screening Initiative, a project of the American Academy of Family Physicians, the American Dietetic Association, and the National Council on Aging; 1989.

and the MNA include an assessment of weight, muscle mass (mid-arm or calf circumference), and mobility or functional capacity. These criteria have been recommended in a consensus statement from the Academy of Nutrition and Dietetics and the American Society for Parenteral and Enteral Nutrition.[8] A diagnosis of malnutrition includes two or more of the following six characteristics:

- Insufficient energy intake
- Weight loss
- Loss of muscle mass
- Loss of subcutaneous fat
- Localized generalized fluid accumulation that may mask weight loss
- Diminished functional status as measured by handgrip strength

UNDERNUTRITION: WEIGHT LOSS AND MALNUTRITION

Because the population of older adults is so heterogeneous, the prevalence of malnutrition will vary depending on age distribution and living situation, among other variables. A review of the results of the MNA survey that included countries in Europe, the United States, and South Africa showed that the prevalence of malnutrition in older adults was 22.8%. The highest rates of malnutrition were found among individuals living in institutional settings (50.5%) and the lowest among people living in the community (5.8%).[9]

Decreases in body weight are common in adults ages 65 to 90, and this should always be seen as a warning sign that the individual may be at nutritional risk. There is a clear relationship between undernutrition and increased morbidity and mortality.[10]

Involuntary **weight loss** may be caused by inadequate dietary intake, loss of appetite, muscle atrophy, and/or the inflammatory effects of disease. Many older adults may experience a combination of these factors, resulting in nutritional deficiencies in addition to weight loss.

Inadequate Dietary Intake   Many older adults live and eat alone. Social isolation is associated with decreased food intake. Several studies have shown that food intake can be improved when older adults are able to eat with others.[11,12] Older adults are often on fixed incomes, which may limit their ability to purchase food. Chronic disease and the medications associated with managing these conditions may also increase the financial burden for older adults, forcing them to choose between food and medications.

Inadequate nutritional intake and unexplained weight loss in older adults is often associated with malignancy (cancer) or depression. Several small studies of patients with unexplained weight loss showed that malignancy was a factor in between 16% and 36% of the patients evaluated.[13-15] Depression is associated with decreased food intake. This is a factor in both the nursing home and institutional environment, as well as for community-dwelling older adults. Wilson et al. reviewed the charts of over 1,000 medical outpatients and found that depression was a cause of weight loss in 30% of the older patients.[13] In comparison, only 15% of the younger patients were found to have weight loss associated with depression.[13]

Dysphagia, the decreased ability or inability to swallow, is a common result of stroke and is also associated with Parkinson's disease or other motility or structural disorders of the esophagus. It is estimated that 7–10% of older adults suffer from dysphagia and the consequent negative impact on nutritional intake.[16,17] Dementia also is associated with poor nutritional intake. In fact, inadequate energy and **protein** intake are commonly seen in persons with Alzheimer's disease; this lack of proper caloric intake is a predictive factor of morbidity and mortality.[18]

The physiological changes associated with aging also can result in decreased appetite or **anorexia**. There is a general reduction in gastrointestinal motility. Prolonged satiety from a decrease in the rate of gastric emptying can inhibit food intake.[19] Decreased gastrointestinal motility may also be a factor in the development of constipation, a frequent complaint of older adults.

A decrease in appetite can be the result of declines in the senses of taste and smell.[20] Age raises the threshold for odor detection and for recognition of salt and other specific tastes. Reduced taste and smell acuity also can be caused by certain drugs and medications. **Table 7-1** presents a summary of the effects of certain categories of drugs on appetite. Additionally, zinc deficiencies can lead to loss of taste.

There is a normal decrease in food intake associated with aging.[21,22] This is appropriate because the basal metabolic rate decreases with age, resulting in a decrease in energy needs. However, the regulation of food intake through hormones involved in satiety and neurotransmitters involved in appetite can be impaired in the older adult, resulting in further reduced food intake[23] and inappropriate weight loss. An extreme example of this would be **cachexia**, which is defined as a "complex metabolic syndrome associated with underlying illness and characterized by loss of muscle with or without loss of fat mass."[24] This is

TABLE 7-1   Drugs That Affect Appetite

Examples of Drugs That Increase Appetite	Examples of Drugs That Decrease Appetite
Alcohol	Antibiotics
Antihistamines	Bulk agents
Corticosteroids	Indomethacin
Insulin	Digoxin
Thyroid hormone	Glucagon
Psychoactive drugs	Morphine
	Fluoxetine

Source: Beers, MH, Porter, RS, Jones, TV, Kaplan, JL, Berkwits, M. Nutrition: General considerations. *The Merck Manual* (18th ed.). Whitehouse Station, NJ: Merck & Co.; 2006.

associated with the production of inflammatory cytokines that stimulate fat and muscle breakdown as well as anorexia. This condition is often resistant to nutritional intervention and must be treated by addressing the illness leading to the production of the cytokines.[25,26]

Sarcopenia or Loss of Muscle Mass   Aging is also associated with the loss of muscle mass or **sarcopenia**. Loss of muscle mass is obviously associated with a loss of strength, which can be severe enough to interfere with the ability to perform activities of daily living (ADLs). Causes of sarcopenia include changes in endocrine function such as low estrogen and testosterone levels,[27] or chronic diseases associated with insulin resistance[28] and inadequate dietary protein intake.[29] Physical activity frequently decreases with age, which also is associated with the decrease of lean muscle tissue.[30] In one study, sarcopenia was identified in more than half of men and women over the age of 80.[31] It occurs in overweight individuals as well as individuals who are of normal weight or underweight. Increasing and maintaining physical activity levels in older adults may be one of the most effective methods to prevent or treat sarcopenia.[32]

Decreased Absorption of Nutrients   Other gastrointestinal changes that can affect food intake and absorption include **lactose intolerance** resulting from decreased lactase production. Lactase is an enzyme that converts lactose to the absorbable sugars glucose and galactose. Without the enzyme, lactose cannot be absorbed, and instead becomes food for intestinal bacteria, resulting in intestinal disturbances such as gas, bloating, diarrhea, and cramping. Lactose intolerance is more common in Native Americans as well as certain ethnic groups originating from Asia, Africa, and the Mediterranean. When the condition is severe, it can cause malabsorption of other nutrients, but the primary problem is decreased **calcium** intake due to decreased intake of dairy products.

Celiac disease is also more common in the elderly than was first recognized. About 25% of newly diagnosed patients are over the age of 60. Individuals have a sensitivity to the protein gliadin, which is a component of **gluten** found in wheat and some other grains. For those with celiac disease, consumption of gliadin or gluten results in damage to intestinal villi and malabsorption, especially of fats, fat-soluble vitamins such as vitamin D, and minerals such as calcium and iron.[33]

Vitamin B_{12} absorption decreases with age. In addition, medications for heartburn, gastroesophageal reflux, or diabetes, which are commonly taken by older adults, can interfere with its absorption. Patients on these medications should have their vitamin B_{12} levels measured by their physician.

The ability to synthesize **vitamin D** in the skin by sunlight decreases with aging. In addition, older adults, especially those who are homebound, are less likely to get outdoors so exposure to sunlight is limited. Low vitamin D levels may increase the risk of falls and fractures and contribute to the development of osteoporosis.

With aging comes a change in sense of thirst and diminished activity in the hormonal regulation of fluid balance. Together these changes may make **dehydration** more likely, and severe dehydration can lead to confusion and hospitalization.[8]

Dehydration causes several specific signs and symptoms:

- Dry lips
- Sunken eyes
- Swollen tongue
- Increased body temperature
- Decreased blood pressure
- Constipation
- Decreased urine output
- Nausea
- Confusion

Chewing difficulty related to poor dental health also increases the risk for malnutrition and weight loss for the older adult. Individuals with missing teeth or poorly fitting dentures or for whom chewing is painful often limit their food choices to soft foods and liquids. A limited variety of foods in the diet increases the risk for nutrient deficiencies in addition to lowered caloric intake. Poor nutrition can contribute to poor dental health, so it is important to encourage appropriate dental care for the older individual.

TREATMENT OF WEIGHT LOSS AND OTHER NUTRITIONAL PROBLEMS RELATED TO AGING

WEIGHT LOSS

Conducting regular body measurements in older adults is one of the simplest ways to assess nutritional adequacy. When an older adult loses 5% or more of his or her body weight in 1 month or 10% or more in 6 months, healthcare providers need to identify the cause for the weight loss. Once the cause has been identified, it is important to treat the condition and provide appropriate nutritional support to return the person to their ideal weight. Reversible causes of weight loss in the elderly are described by the mnemonic MEALS ON WHEELS, developed by Morley.[34]

M: medications
E: emotional (depression)
A: alcoholism, anorexia tardive, or abuse of elders
L: late-life paranoia
S: swallowing problems (dysphagia)
O: oral problems
N: no money (poverty)

W: wandering and other dementia-related problems

H: hyperthyroidism, pheochromocytoma

E: enteric problems (malabsorption)

E: eating problems

L: low-sodium, low-**cholesterol** diet

S: shopping and meal preparation problems

A referral to a registered dietitian can provide appropriate intervention when the weight loss is due to inadequate food intake. In cases where dietary restrictions, such as sodium restrictions for **hypertension** or **carbohydrate** restriction for diabetes, are associated with weight loss, modification of the dietary restrictions can be considered. The need for feeding and shopping assistance may also need to be assessed. Meals can be planned and foods purchased to meet the individual's preferences. Nutrient supplements can be considered. The nutrient density of foods can be increased by adding egg whites, tofu or milk powder, or healthy oils to foods like puddings, sauces, vegetables, grains, and pasta. Healthy snacking and high-calorie nutritional supplements may be helpful.

TREATMENT OF GASTROINTESTINAL PROBLEMS

Constipation   Constipation can often be treated by increasing the intake of fluid and fiber. These two components must be considered together. Older adults often limit their intake of fluids. This may be unintentional and related to changes in the ability to sense thirst or intentional because of concerns about incontinence. The potential of limited fluid intake must be recognized because **dietary fiber** absorbs fluid and the combination of fiber and fluid aids in moving waste material through the large intestine. The hydrated fiber softens the stools and makes them much easier to pass.[35] It is absolutely critical that any recommendation to increase dietary fiber intake be accompanied by a recommendation to increase fluid intake. Failure to do so increases the risk for fecal impactions. Ensuring adequate fiber intake also reduces the incidence of diverticulosis and may also lessen the risk of certain types of colon cancer.[36]

Malabsorption   The two most common **malabsorption** problems in older adult are lactose intolerance and celiac disease.

Lactose intolerance, or lactose malabsorption, is treated by eliminating lactose from the diet. Lactose is a sugar found in all dairy products. If all dairy products are avoided, care must be taken to include other calcium-rich or calcium-fortified foods in the diet. Dairy products treated with the enzyme lactase, which converts the lactose to glucose and galactose that can be absorbed, are also an option. There are many commercially treated dairy products available on the market. Yogurt with active cultures and acidophilus milk may also be well tolerated by some individuals. In spite of the availability of these products, individuals with lactose intolerance may have difficulty meeting their calcium needs, so calcium supplements might need to be considered.

Individuals with celiac disease, also known as gluten-induced enteropathy, must avoid all products containing gluten in order to avoid intestinal damage and the accompanying malabsorption. Gluten is found in the cereal grains wheat, barley, and rye. Any products containing these grains or their derivatives must be avoided. Fortunately there are many gluten-free products available commercially, so the diet is much less restrictive today than it was before these products became readily obtainable.

Inadequate Intake or Absorption of Vitamins and Minerals   Routine multivitamin and mineral supplementation in the absence of compromised nutritional status is controversial. There is very little clinical evidence to support this practice. In addition, the 2006 National Institutes of Health Consensus Conference on the use of multivitamins and minerals found insufficient evidence to recommend for or against the use of multivitamins or minerals for the prevention of chronic disease in the general population.[37] A multivitamin supplement should be used to ensure adequate intake of nutrients whenever there is the suspicion of poor or inadequate food intake, laboratory results reveal a deficiency, or there is some other reason why an individual may not be getting enough nutrients through diet. Older adults are most at risk of developing deficiencies of vitamin B_{12}, vitamin D, and calcium.

Because of the age-related, decreased ability to absorb vitamin B_{12}, all older adults will benefit from supplemental B_{12}. This could be in the form of a multivitamin and mineral supplement or fortified foods such as fortified breakfast cereals. Supplemental vitamin B_{12}, including what is added to fortify foods, is more easily absorbed than B_{12} found naturally in food.[38] Daily recommended intake is 10–15 micrograms.[39]

There is also an age-related decrease in the ability to synthesize vitamin D. Older adults at highest risk for vitamin D deficiency include those who are institutionalized, homebound, or have limited sun exposure.[40] Inadequate vitamin D status has been associated with muscle weakness, functional impairments, depression, and an increased risk of falls.[41] The daily recommended intake of vitamin D for adults up to age 70 years is 600 international units; this increases to 800 international units after age 71.[42] Many older adults will not meet their vitamin D requirements, especially if dairy intake is limited, so vitamin D supplements should be considered.

Calcium is another nutrient whose absorption also decreases with age. Because dairy products are a major source of calcium in the U.S. diet, individuals with lactose intolerance or those who avoid dairy products should be evaluated for the need for calcium supplements. The recommendation for adults over age 51 is 1,200 mg per day.[42] In most cases a multivitamin and mineral supplement will not include enough calcium to meet the requirement, so additional supplementation will be needed.

OVERNUTRITION

Overnutrition is a condition of excess nutrient and energy intake over time. It can be considered a form of malnutrition when it leads to morbid obesity. In the general population, overnutrition (i.e., a body mass index [BMI] of 25.1 to 29.9, signaling overweight, or a BMI of 30 or greater, signaling obesity) is associated with an increase in all causes of mortality, as well as morbidity related to hypertension, dyslipidemia, type 2 diabetes, and other chronic diseases. However, some data suggest the mortality risk of obesity may decrease with age. There may even be a slight advantage to being overweight for men and women over age 65.[43] Recommendations for older adults regarding weight loss must be made on an individual basis. Those with a high-risk profile for cardiovascular disease or diabetes, or those who are experiencing a decrease in the quality of life due to excess weight, may benefit from losing weight. Any weight loss should be pursued cautiously, with care taken to provide adequate calcium and vitamin D supplementation as well as exercise in order to prevent loss of muscle mass and a decrease in bone density.

CARDIOVASCULAR DISEASE

Although weight loss in the elderly remains controversial, there is mounting evidence to support the positive effect of making dietary changes for the primary prevention of **cardiovascular disease** in older adults. Most recently, data from the PREDIMED trial showed a relative risk reduction for cardiovascular disease of 30% in both men and women who were consuming a **Mediterranean diet** supplemented with either nuts or olive oil, as compared to a low-fat control diet. The subjects in the study ranged in age from 55 to 80 years, and 92% were overweight or obese. The participants had either type 2 diabetes or at least three major risk factors for cardiovascular disease such as smoking, hypertension, dyslipidemia, being overweight, or a family history of premature coronary heart disease. The diet was energy (calorie) unrestricted, and participants did not lose significant amounts of weight. The Mediterranean diet is consistent with the U.S. Dietary Guidelines discussed later in this chapter.[44]

DIABETES

Care for the older adult with **diabetes** should include a medical nutritional evaluation by a dietitian. The dietitian can tailor a nutrition prescription based on the medical, lifestyle, and personal needs of the older adult. The older person who has diabetes needs regular help in adhering to a diet to manage blood glucose levels, whether or not she or he is insulin dependent. The individual needs to work with his or her physician and dietitian to formulate a diet plan and develop workable menus that provide good control, as well as take into consideration the person's food preferences and lifestyle habits. The emphasis should be on foods that are low on the glycemic index and the diet should be rich in fruits, vegetables, and minimally processed carbohydrates. The obese older adult with diabetes may benefit from modest weight loss; however, because weight loss in older adults increases the risk of morbidity and mortality, this should be addressed in the medical nutrition evaluation.[45] The Mediterranean diet and the **DASH (Dietary Approach to**

Stop Hypertension) diet, as recommended in the 2010 Dietary Guidelines for Americans, are good models to follow.

GENERAL NUTRITION RECOMMENDATIONS

The most important thing to consider when making general nutrition recommendations for the older adult is the heterogeneity of this population. Any dietary recommendations must be made after consideration of each older adult's individual needs. A good place to start is with the 2010 **Dietary Guidelines for Americans**,[46] which emphasizes the need to balance calories in order to maintain a healthy weight. The guidelines also include recommendations about foods that should be increased in the diet such as fruits and vegetables, whole grains, and low-fat or fat-free dairy products, as well as foods that should be reduced, such as processed foods high in sodium and sugary drinks. Diet plans consistent with these recommendations would include the DASH diet and the Mediterranean diet. Both of these diet plans are rich in fruits and vegetables, low-fat or nonfat dairy, and whole grains. They tend to be higher in fiber, low to moderate in fat, and rich in potassium, calcium, and magnesium. The meal plans are consistent with dietary recommendations for the treatment of hypertension, heart disease, and diabetes. Sample meal plans with recommended servings from each group are shown in **Table 7-2**. The appropriate caloric level will be based on individual needs and should be chosen in order to maintain a healthy weight.

There are many resources available on the Internet to assist healthcare professionals as they help their clients or patients implement these recommendations. For example, MyPlate is part of a communications initiative from the U.S. Department of Agriculture to help Americans adopt healthier eating habits based on the 2010 Dietary Guidelines for Americans. MyPlate uses a graphic of a place setting to illustrate the five food groups—dairy, protein, fruits, vegetables, and grains. The food groups are arranged on the plate to emphasize the importance of choosing a diet rich in fruits and vegetables; these two groups cover half of the plate. MyPlate is part of a larger communications initiative that includes the website ChooseMyPlate.gov, which is a good resource for healthcare professionals as well as consumers. Two groups have produced adaptations of MyPlate for older adults. Both of these modified resources include graphics to emphasize important messages for older adults, such as maintaining adequate fluid intake and consuming fiber-rich foods and foods fortified with or rich in vitamins B_{12} and D.

The University of Florida resource (http://fycs.ifas.ufl.edu/Extension/HNFS/ENAFS/MyPlate.php) includes an example of a food plan at a lower calorie level more appropriate to the decreased energy needs of older adults (see **Figure 7-1**). Drawings of older adults engaging in physical activity are included to emphasize the value of physical activity for weight control and maintenance of muscle mass and strength.

TABLE 7-2   Dietary Guidelines for Americans

The number of daily servings in a food group vary depending on caloric needs.

Food Group	1,200 Calories	1,400 Calories	1,600 Calories	1,800 Calories	2,000 Calories	2,600 Calories	3,100 Calories	Serving Sizes
Grains	4–5	5–6	6	6	6–8	10–11	12–13	1 slice bread 1 oz dry cereal ½ cup cooked rice, pasta, or cereal
Vegetables	3–4	3–4	3–4	4–5	4–5	5–6	6	1 cup raw leafy vegetable ½ cup cut-up raw or cooked vegetable ½ cup vegetable juice
Fruits	3–4	4	4	4–5	4–5	5–6	6	1 medium fruit ¼ cup dried fruit ½ cup fresh, frozen, or canned fruit ½ cup fruit juice
Fat-free or low-fat milk and milk products	2–3	2–3	2–3	2–3	2–3	3	3–4	1 cup milk or yogurt 1½ oz cheese
Lean meats, poultry, and fish	3 or less	3–4 or less	3–4 or less	6 or less	6 or less	6 or less	6–9	1 oz cooked meats, poultry, or fish 1 egg
Nuts, seeds, and legumes	3 per week	3 per week	3–4 per week	4 per week	4–5 per week	1	1	⅓ cup or 1½ oz nuts 2 Tbsp peanut butter 2 Tbps or ½ oz seeds ½ cup cooked legumes (dried beans, peas)
Fats and oils	1	1	2	2–3	2–3	3	4	1 tsp soft margarine 1 tsp vegetable oil 1 Tbsp mayonnaise 1 Tbsp salad dressing
Sweets and added sugars	3 or less per week	3 or less per week	3 or less per week	5 or less per week	5 or less per week	<2	<2	1 Tbsp sugar 1 Tbsp jelly or jam ½ cup sorbet, galatin dessert 1 cup lemonade
Maximum sodium limit	2,300 mg/day	2,300 mg/day	2,300 mg/day	2,300 mg/day	2,300 mg/day	2,300 mg/day	2,300 mg/day	

Source: Data from U.S. Department of Agriculture and U.S. Department of Health and Human Services. *Dietary Guidelines for Americans, 2010,* 7th Edition. Washington, DC: U.S. Government Printing Office, December 2010.

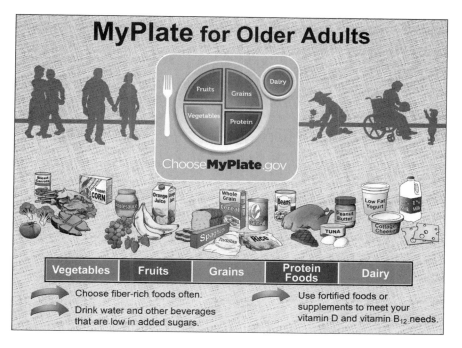

Figure 7-1   MyPlate for Older Adults: University of Florida Version.
Courtesy of University of Florida Family, Youth, and Community Sciences.

The adaptation by the nutrition scientists at Tufts University (www.nutrition.tufts .edu/research/myplate-older-adults) includes no text, but uses images to reinforce the healthy choices for older adults (see **Figure 7-2**). The following foods, fluids, and physical activities are represented on the Tufts University MyPlate for Older Adults:

- Bright-colored vegetables such as carrots and broccoli
- Deep-colored fruit such as berries and peaches
- Whole, enriched, and fortified grains and cereals such as brown rice and 100% whole wheat bread
- Low- and nonfat dairy products such as yogurt and low-lactose milk
- Dry beans and nuts, fish, poultry, lean meat, and eggs
- Liquid vegetable oils, soft spreads low in saturated and trans fat, and spices to replace salt
- Fluids such as water and fat-free milk
- Physical activity such as walking, resistance training, and light cleaning

Both of these adaptations emphasize some of the important factors discussed earlier in the chapter, including the need for exercise, plenty of fluid intake, and the use of

MyPlate for Older Adults

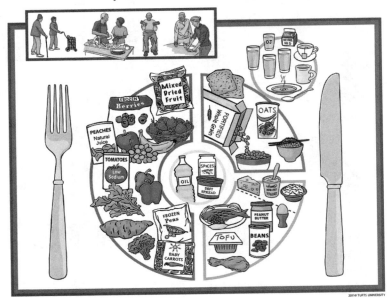

Figure 7-2 MyPlate for Older Adults: Tufts University Version.
© 2011 Tufts University. For details about the MyPlate for Older Adults, please see http://nutrition.tufts.edu/
research/myplate-older-adults.

fortified foods or supplements to meet needs for vitamins B_{12} and D. In addition, tips to adapt the MyPlate eating plan for a vegetarian diet can be found on the ChooseMyPlate .gov website (www.choosemyplate.gov/healthy-eating-tips/tips-for-vegetarian.html).

Additional nutrition information for older adults can be found at these websites:

- Nutrition.gov: Nutrition Information for You, Seniors: www.nutrition.gov/life-stages /seniors
- NIH SeniorHealth, Eating Well as You Get Older: http://nihseniorhealth.gov /eatingwellasyougetolder/benefitsofeatingwell/01.html
- National Institute on Aging, Healthy Eating After 50: www.nia.nih.gov/health /publication/healthy-eating-after-50

DRUG AND NUTRIENT INTERACTIONS

More than 90% of older adults aged 57 to 85 regularly take at least one medication daily. Prescription medication use is the most prevalent, used by about 81% of this population. Over-the-counter medications or dietary supplements also are used by almost half of this population. More than half of older adults use five or more prescription medications, over-the-counter medications, or dietary supplements every day. The most widely used medications are cardiovascular drugs including antihyperlipidemic agents and anticoagulants. **Nutritional supplements** including multivitamins and individual vitamins and minerals were the most commonly used over-the-counter medications.[47] This extensive use of medications in the population of older adults creates the potential for not only drug–drug interactions, but also drug–nutrient interactions. Antihyperlipidemic drugs such as statins can interact with niacin, a nutritional supplement (vitamin B_2), increasing the risk of myopathy and rhabdomyolysis. Garlic interacts with Coumadin (warfarin), an anticoagulant, and increases the risk of bleeding. Vegetables high in vitamin K may decrease the effectiveness of Coumadin and increase the risk of clotting. Grapefruit juice affects the metabolism of a large number of drugs including the statins. It increases the bioavailability of these drugs and can result in higher serum levels.[48] These are only a few examples, but they illustrate the necessity for older adults to consult a physician, dietitian, and/or pharmacist to avoid complications related to drug and nutrient interactions.

ALCOHOL

Continued use and abuse of alcohol in later life may be brought on by the many social changes that older adults experience, such as death of a spouse, loss of friendship, and feelings of loneliness and isolation. Healthcare professionals need to be sensitive to these problems and be ready to make referrals to other appropriate healthcare professionals and community support groups. Nutritionally speaking, alcohol abuse compromises health and leads to malnutrition for several reasons. First, alcohol replaces food in the diet. Alcohol is a source of empty calories, and when older people spend their limited resources on alcohol instead of healthy foods, they can compromise their health. Second, alcohol interferes with the normal absorption of vitamin B_{12}, folic acid, and vitamin C. Alcohol also interferes with the metabolism of vitamins D and B_6 and increases the need for B vitamins and magnesium. All of these may result in multiple deficiencies that can impair health.

SUMMARY

The value of appropriate nutrition screening and intervention cannot be overestimated in providing quality care for older adults. Good nutrition not only optimizes health and well-being, but also helps prevent the onset of many chronic diseases.

It is imperative that healthcare providers be sensitive to the many changes that occur with aging and to the ways in which nutrition can affect the quality of life of older people. The first step is to understand the basic principles of nutrition and how these can be applied to encourage healthy eating. Second, healthcare professionals need to be aware of how the aging process can alter nutritional status. With careful screening, counseling, and referral if necessary, healthcare professionals can be certain that older persons' nutritional well-being is optimal. Ensuring quality nutrition is a crucial component of providing the best health care possible for the older population.

Review Questions

1. An important factor to consider when working with the older adult population is that
   A. It is a heterogeneous population.
   B. All suffer from chronic diseases.
   C. It is an economically disadvantaged population.
   D. All are underweight.

2. According to the Academy of Nutrition and Dietetics and the American Society for Parenteral and Enteral Nutrition, nutrition screening tools should include an assessment of
   A. Weight
   B. Muscle mass
   C. Functional capacity
   D. All of the above

3. In which of the following groups is the prevalence of malnutrition highest?
   A. Residents of long-term care facilities
   B. Residents of retirement communities for active older adults
   C. Older adults ages 60–80 living in a small town
   D. Attendees of a college program for seniors

4. Poor dietary intake is associated with
   A. Depression, dysphagia, and dementia
   B. Poverty, living with a spouse, and hypertension
   C. Constipation, diabetes, and Alzheimer's disease
   D. Dyslipidemia, lack of exercise, and alcohol

5. One of the most effective treatments for sarcopenia is
   A. A high-protein diet
   B. The Mediterranean diet
   C. Physical activity
   D. Bed rest

Learning Activities

1. You have just met with a patient who will be included in your caseload. The patient is an 82-year-old man whose wife died last year. He has no family members who live in the community. He was referred to you by his physician, who is concerned because he has lost 20 pounds in the past year. The patient is 5'10" and his current

weight is 158 pounds. What additional information do you need to assist this patient? What could be the potential causes of his weight loss? What are your recommendations? To whom would you refer him?

2. You have just met with a new patient at the practice where you work as a medical assistant. Your new patient is a 75-year-old woman who is 5'4" and weighs 105 pounds. She has a medical history of chronic pain caused by arthritis. She reports that she has recently lost interest in cooking for herself and her husband. She adds that she has a poor appetite and often forgets to eat. What would you suggest?

3. You are asked by your employer to give a presentation to a senior citizen women's group that regularly meets at their local church for evening meals financed by the church and prepared by volunteers. You agree to join them, and note that the meal consists of roast beef, mashed potatoes and gravy, biscuits with butter, coffee, and apple pie. During dinner you ask and find that most of their meals are similar to this one. You present your talk on osteoporosis and agree to come back in a month for another talk. What would you want to focus on next time? Why?

4. Discuss either how your current diet will be appropriate as you age or how it might need to change to improve your chances for optimal aging. Given the current weight status of your age group (and other cohorts), what will likely be the issues with regard to nutrition in the future? What can be done now to ensure future well-being to the highest degree possible?

REFERENCES

1. Allen, JE. *Assisted Living Administration: The Knowledge Base.* 2nd ed. New York: Springer, 2004: 300.

2. Reuben, DB, Yoshikawa, TT, Besdine, RW (Eds.). *Geriatrics Review Syllabus Supplement.* New York: American Geriatrics Society, 1993: 172.

3. Centers for Disease Control and Prevention, Merck Company Foundation. *The State of Aging and Health in America 2007.* Whitehouse Station, NJ: Merck Company Foundation, 2007. Retrieved April 12, 2012, from http://www.cdc .gov/aging/pdf/saha_2007.pdf

4. U.S. Department of Health and Human Services, Administration on Aging. Older Americans Act. 2006.

5. Institute of Medicine. *The Role of Nutrition in Maintaining Health in the Nation's Elderly: Evaluating Coverage of Nutrition Services for the Medicare Population.* Washington, DC: National Academy Press, 2000.

6. Dwyer, JT. *Screening Older Americans' Nutritional Health: Current Practices and Future Possibilities.* Washington, DC: Nutrition Screening Initiative, 1991.

7. Skipper, A, et al. Nutrition screening tools: An analysis of the evidence. *Journal of Parenteral and Enteral Nutrition,* 2012;36:292.

8. White, JV, et al. Consensus statement: Academy of Nutrition and Dietetics and American Society for Parenteral and Enteral Nutrition: Characteristics recommended for the identification and documentation of adult malnutrition (undernutrition). *Journal of Parenteral and Enteral Nutrition,* 2012;36:275.

9. Kaiser, MJ, et al. Frequency of malnutrition in older adults: A multinational perspective using the Mini Nutritional Assessment. *Journal of the American Geriatrics Society,* 2010;58:1734.

10. Sullivan, DH. Impact of nutritional status on health outcomes of nursing home residents.

Journal of the American Geriatrics Society, 1995;43:195.

11. de Castro, JM, Brewer, EM. The amount eaten in meals by humans is a power function of the number of people present. *Physiology and Behavior,* 1992;51:121.

12. Locher, JL, et al. The effect of the presence of others on caloric intake in homebound older adults. *Journals of Gerontology Series A: Biological Sciences and Medical Sciences,* 2005;60:1475.

13. Wilson, MM, et al. Prevalence and causes of undernutrition in medical outpatients. *American Journal of Medicine,* 1998;104:56.

14. Thompson, MP, Morris, LK. Unexplained weight loss in the ambulatory elderly. *Journal of the American Geriatrics Society,* 1991;39:497.

15. Rabinovitz, M, et al. Unintentional weight loss. A retrospective analysis of 154 cases. *Archives of Internal Medicine,* 1986;146:186.

16. Achem, SR, Devault, KR. Dysphagia in aging. *Journal of Clinical Gastroenterology,* 2005;39:357.

17. Keller, HH. Malnutrition in institutionalized elderly: How and why? *Journal of the American Geriatrics Society,* 1993;41:1212.

18. White, H. Weight change in Alzheimer's disease. *Journal of Nutrition, Health and Aging,* 1998;2:110–112.

19. Horowitz, M, et al. Changes in gastric emptying rates with age. *Clinical Science (London),* 1984;67:213.

20. Rolls, BJ. Do chemosensory changes influence food intake in the elderly? *Physiology and Behavior,* 1999;66:193.

21. Roberts, SB. A review of age-related changes in energy regulation and suggested mechanisms. *Mechanisms of Ageing and Development,* 2000;116:157.

22. Morley, JE. Decreased food intake with aging. *Journals of Gerontology Series A: Biological Sciences and Medical Sciences,* 2001;56(2):81.

23. Parker, BA, Chapman, IM. Food intake and ageing—the role of the gut. *Mechanisms of Ageing and Development,* 2004;125:859.

24. Evans, WJ, et al. Cachexia: A new definition. *Clinical Nutrition,* 2008;27:793.

25. Martinez, M, Arnalich, F, Hernanz, A. Alterations of anorectic cytokine levels from plasma and cerebrospinal fluid in idiopathic senile anorexia. *Mechanisms of Ageing and Development,* 1993;72:145.

26. Oldenburg, HS, et al. Cachexia and the acute-phase protein response in inflammation are regulated by interleukin-6. *European Journal of Immunology,* 1993;23:1889.

27. Joseph, C, et al. Role of endocrine-immune dysregulation in osteoporosis, sarcopenia, frailty and fracture risk. *Molecular Aspects of Medicine,* 2005;26:181.

28. Rasmussen, BB, et al. Insulin resistance of muscle protein metabolism in aging. *FASEB Journal,* 2006;20:768.

29. Garry, PJ, et al. Nutritional status in a healthy elderly population: Dietary and supplemental intakes. *American Journal of Clinical Nutrition,* 1982;36:319.

30. Rantanen, T, Era, P, Heikkinen, E. Physical activity and the changes in maximal isometric strength in men and women from the age of 75 to 80 years. *Journal of the American Geriatrics Society,* 1997;45:1439.

31. Lindle, RS, et al. Age and gender comparisons of muscle strength in 654 women and men aged 20–93 yr. *Journal of Applied Physiology,* 1997;83:1581.

32. Montero-Fernández, N, Serra-Rexach, JA. Role of exercise on sarcopenia in the elderly. *European Journal of Physical and Rehabilitation Medicine,* 2013;49(1):131–143.

33. Holt, PR. Intestinal malabsorption in the elderly. *Digestive Diseases,* 2007;25:144–150.

34. Morley, JE. Anorexia of aging: Physiologic and pathologic. *American Journal of Clinical Nutrition,* 1997;66:760–773.

35. Slavin, JL. Position of American Dietetic Association: Health Implications of Dietary Fiber. *Journal of the American Dietetic Association,* 2002;102(7):993–1000.

36. Giovannucci, E, et al. Relationship of diet to risk of colorectal cancer adenoma in men. *Journal of the National Cancer Institute,* 1992;84:91–98.

37. National Institutes of Health State-of-the-Science Panel. National Institutes of Health state-of-the-science conference statement: Multivitamin/mineral supplements and chronic disease prevention. *Annals of Internal Medicine,* 2006; 145:364.

38. Baik, HW, Russell, RM. Vitamin B$_{12}$ deficiency in the elderly. *Annual Review of Nutrition*, 1999;19:357–377.

39. Institute of Medicine, Food and Nutrition Board. *Dietary Reference Intakes: Thiamin, Riboflavin, Niacin, Vitamin B-6, Vitamin B-12, Pantothenic Acid, Biotin, and Choline*. Washington, DC: National Academy Press, 1998.

40. MacLaughlin, J, Holick, MF. Aging decreases the capacity of human skin to produce vitamin D$_3$. *Journal of Clinical Investigation*, 1985;76:1536.

41. Gerdhem, P, Ringsberg, KA, Obrant, KJ, Akesson, K. Association between 25-hydroxy vitamin D levels, physical activity, muscle strength and fractures in the prospective population-based OPRA study of elderly women. *Osteoporosis International*, 2005;16:1425.

42. National Research Council. *Dietary Reference Intakes for Calcium and Vitamin D*. Washington, DC: National Academies Press, 2011.

43. Sui, X, et al. Cardiorespiratory fitness and adiposity as mortality predictors in older adults. *Journal of the American Medical Association*, 2007; 298:2507.

44. Estruch, R, et al. Primary prevention of cardiovascular disease with a Mediterranean diet. *New England Journal of Medicine*, 2013;368: 1279–1290.

45. Wedick, NM, Barrett-Connor, E, Knoke, JD, Wingard, DL. The relationship between weight loss and all-cause mortality in older men and women with and without diabetes mellitus: The Rancho Bernardo study. *Journal of the American Geriatrics Society*, 2002;50:1810.

46. U.S. Department of Agriculture, U.S. Department of Health and Human Services. *Dietary Guidelines for Americans, 2010*. 7th ed. Washington, DC: U.S. Government Printing Office, December 2010.

47. Qato, DM, Alexander, GC, Conti, RM, Johnson, M, Schumm, P, Lindau, S. Use of prescription and over-the-counter medications and dietary supplements among older adults in the United States. *Journal of the American Medical Association*, 2008;300(24):2867.

48. Leibovitch, ER, Deamer, RL, Sanderson, LA. Food–drug interactions: Careful drug selection and patient counseling can reduce the risk in older patients. *Geriatrics*, 2004;59:19–33.

CHAPTER 8

AN ORAL PERSPECTIVE ON HEALTHY AGING AND PREVENTION FOR THE OLDER ADULT

MARJI HARMER-BEEM, RDH, MS

Every tooth in a man's head is more valuable than a diamond.
—Miguel de Cervantes, *Don Quixote*, 1605

Chapter Outline

Behavioral Objectives

Upon completion of this chapter, the reader will be able to:

1. Explain and discuss *Oral Health in America: A Report of the Surgeon General*, highlighting themes that relate to the oral health and well-being of older adults.
2. Identify the percentages of periodontal disease, edentulism, and oral and pharyngeal cancers in the elderly.
3. Recognize dry mouth (xerostomia) and describe the risk factors it poses for the well-being of the older adult.
4. List dental changes of aging versus signs of a disease state.
5. Review oral health of the older adult and its correlates to well-being.
6. List societal and personal barriers for the older adult seeking dental care.
7. Describe common oral conditions the healthcare professional may encounter.

8. Describe a simple oral screening procedure that the healthcare professional can do.
9. Name the basic role of the interprofessional healthcare provider in assisting the older person with oral health concerns.
10. List new models for oral health care to help alleviate oral health disparities.

Key Terms

Attrition	Oral screening
Dental caries	Periodontal disease
Dental plaque (biofilm)	Root caries
Edentulism	Stereognosis
Fluoride gel	*Streptococcus mutans*
Fluoride varnish	Xerostomia
Oral and pharyngeal (throat) cancers	

As the relative proportion of elderly increases in society, so will the need for the healthcare provider to have knowledge of all the systems that affect the well-being of this burgeoning and diverse segment of the population. The oral cavity is no exception. The older adult will present with wide and varied medical and dental histories. This segment of the population has a disproportionate number of chronic conditions and diseases that are managed rather than cured (e.g., cardiovascular disease, arthritis, visual impairment). These conditions can limit an individual's daily choices and impair their functioning throughout the day.[1]

Rarely does the average person reflect on how important the mouth is to daily life, functioning, and health. General health and oral health are concepts that should be interpreted as a single entity and should not be separated.[2] Oral health means more than healthy teeth to the older adult. Damage to the craniofacial complex, whether from illness, injury, or disorder, can result in the loss of health, self-esteem, and well-being.[2]

Healthy aging is as individualized as the person's whole lifestyle, culture, social history, and family history. The goal of healthy aging from the oral perspective is to recognize the difference between aging and disease, retain more natural teeth, preserve health and function, and provide the elderly seeking oral care with effective disease preventive measures. Preventive measures can be managed by the knowledgeable interprofessional team. Using simple provider-based and self-initiated daily measures like effective toothbrushing, flossing, and a fluoride regime can prevent dentally related disease.[2]

ORAL HEALTH IN AMERICA: A REPORT OF THE SURGEON GENERAL

The oral structures, much like the rest of the body, show signs of aging. An understanding of the significance of the oral cavity to a person's general well-being is vital for the healthcare professional. In the 2000 report *Oral Health in America*, then-Surgeon General David Satcher was the first person ever to alert Americans to the full implication of oral health and its link to general health.[2] The increasing evidence that oral disease impacts endocrine (e.g., diabetes), cardiovascular, and pulmonary health, particularly in frail elders, may provide many older people the needed incentive to seek care.[1] The oral cavity, with its bacterial plaque and biofilm, is a portal for infection, and may lead to aspiration pneumonia.[3] Bacteria traveling via the blood to remote sites from the oral cavity can infect artificial joints or the heart with endocarditis.[4] The report stresses the importance of overarching themes, such as the "silent epidemic" of oral diseases that affect older people, as well as being free of needless pain and suffering by keeping a clean and healthy oral cavity, thus preventing the associated physical, financial, and social costs, which can be especially devastating for the country's most vulnerable population.[2]

Oral health is fundamental to general health. In the early 1900s most Americans could expect to lose their teeth by middle age amid pain and suffering. Older people today have lived through some of the most technologically advanced discoveries of all time and unprecedented biomedical progress. This is reflected in the oral restorative materials used, from acrylic dentures designed to last 50 years to porcelain, composite (resin) white fillings, amalgam (silver) fillings, and titanium implants. The first wave of the baby boomer generation was the first group to grow up in the age of dental prevention. Public health measures, such as fluoride in municipal water supplies, have decreased **dental caries** (dental decay) rates over the past 50 years. Toothpastes, mouth rinses, and sonic toothbrushes also have contributed to positive results.[1]

ORAL STRUCTURES AND CHRONIC ORAL DISEASES

Oral structures of the craniofacial complex include the vermillion border (lips); oral mucosa, which is the lining of the cheeks; gums; tongue; and oral pharynx[3] (see **Figure 8-1**). Structures that are not readily seen include the salivary glands, the muscles of mastication, and the upper and lower jaws. The health of these structures is integral to psychosocial well-being. Emotions are expressed using the oral structures, food is enjoyed, and communication is enhanced.[2] **Figure 8-2** shows occurrences that may be encountered in the oral cavity of the older adult, such as wear on the teeth and restoration of the teeth.

The healthcare professional has a responsibility to support oral health in the older adult. Chronic oral disease in older adults includes periodontal disease, edentulism, oral and pharyngeal cancers, decreased saliva flow, and caries. All impact the person's quality of life and their well-being. Tooth loss has been highly correlated with a lower self-perceived quality of life.[5]

Periodontal disease is the inflammatory reaction and dissolution of the bony structures that hold the teeth within the jaws. Bad breath, food pocketing in the gums, gum recession, pus, and loose teeth are all problems that can accompany this disease (**Figure 8-3**). **Dental plaque (biofilm)**, which is an accumulation of pathogenic bacteria,

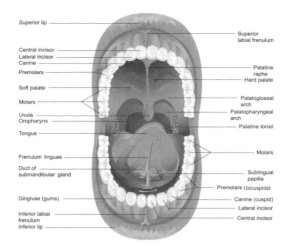

Figure 8-1   Normal structures of the mouth.
Source: © stockshoppe/ShutterStock, Inc.

combined with the individual's immune response, can cause periodontal disease. All of the following are related to periodontal disease and have a significant impact on general health:

- Pain
- The inability to chew food

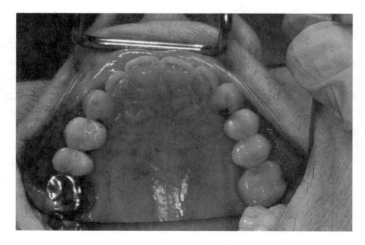

Figure 8-2   Many restorations, including posterior porcelain and metal full-coverage crowns, and wear (incisal attrition) of anterior teeth of an 83-year-old woman.
Source: Courtesy of Natalie Lavoie, University of New England

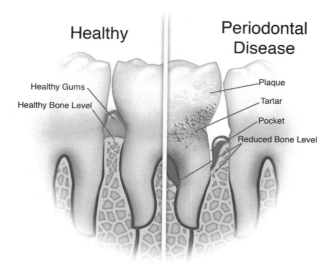

Figure 8-3   Periodontal disease.
Source: © Highforge Solutions/ShutterStock, Inc.

- Decreased caloric intake and subsequent loss of weight
- Root caries due to recession of the gum tissue
- Loose teeth
- Tooth loss
- Speech difficulties
- Decreased self-esteem
- Chronic systemic inflammation

Twenty-three percent of 65- to 74-year-olds have severe periodontal disease.[2] Inflammatory periodontal disease has been associated with poor cardiovascular health, ischemic stroke,[2] and dementia.[6] Inflammatory mediators, such as cytokines, may facilitate these diseases.[4] In the Nun Study to investigate dementia, longitudinal dental records were reviewed, and the researchers found that the subjects with the fewest teeth had the highest risk of both prevalence and incidence of dementia.[6] Periodontal bone loss is also a known risk factor for osteoporosis.[7]

The causes of **edentulism**, or toothlessness, are multifactorial. Currently about 30% of adults 65 years and older are edentulous, having lost all of their teeth, compared to 46% in the 1980s.[2] Clearly, there is a trend that people are keeping their teeth longer. The states with the greatest prevalence of toothlessness are also the states with the greatest poverty rate.[8,9] Edentulism greatly affects food choices, which impacts nutritional state. Diet plays a pivotal role in general health as well as oral health in that a good diet can slow the degenerative progression of oral tissue disease.[10]

Dental caries, also known as cavities or tooth decay, is a bacterial infection attributed to *Streptococcus mutans*. The process of decay entails dental biofilm metabolizing food particles through fermentation to produce an acid substrate, which in turn demineralizes the hard (mineral) structure of the tooth, turning the surface to which the dental biofilm adheres into dark cavitations. Untreated caries is a major cause of tooth loss. **Root caries** in older individuals pose a unique problem because root surfaces that are left exposed as a result of recessed gums from periodontal disease are at greater risk for decay.[11] Caries often go untreated due to lack of sensitivity in the vulnerable teeth; without symptoms, the older adult may not perceive a need to visit the dentist.

Oral and pharyngeal (throat) cancers are primarily diseases found in the elderly. These have a poor prognosis. Approximately 31,000 cases are diagnosed each year, mostly in older people.[12] Survival rates at the 5-year mark are 62.9% for whites and 37.2% for African Americans.[12] Early diagnosis and treatment can do much to allay suffering, and to preserve the form and function of the oral cavity. (See **Table 8-1**.) The survival rate for all races increases to 82.4% when even localized lesions are included, so healthcare providers should be acutely aware of these diseases and recommend regular examinations of the oral cavity. Smoking is often the cause of these cancers. It is well known that smoking is a detriment to health at any age, and smoking cessation should be encouraged.

SEPARATING ORAL AGING FROM DISEASE

Xerostomia is dry mouth associated with decreased saliva flow. Saliva is important in many ways. It protects against excess wear on tooth surfaces, aids in cleansing the oral cavity of debris, flushes acids, maintains oral pH, and makes minerals like calcium and phosphorus available to remineralize early carious lesions on enamel and root surfaces of teeth.[13,14] Dry mouth can lead to uncomfortable swallowing, speech difficulties, mouth sores, and the cavitation of the hard tooth structure, resulting in tooth decay. With

TABLE 8-1   Oral Cancer Survival Rate at 5 Years Based on Stage of Disease

Stage at Diagnosis	Stage Distribution (%)	5-Year Relative Survival (%)
Localized (confined to primary site)	31	82.7
Regional (spread to regional lymph nodes)	47	59.2
Distant (cancer has metastasized)	17	36.3
Unknown (unstaged)	6	49.3

Source: Reproduced from SEER Stat Fact Sheets: Oral Cavity and Pharynx, http://www.seer.cancer.gov/statfacts/html/oralcav.html; Young JL Jr, Roffers SD, Ries LAG, Fritz AG, Hurlbut AA (eds). SEER Summary Staging Manual—2000: Codes and Coding Instructions, National Cancer Institute, NIH Pub. No. 01-4969, Bethesda, MD, 2001.

xerostomia, the clearance of food particles is more difficult. The most common cause of dry mouth in older adults is the use of prescription and over-the-counter medicines. Over 400 commonly used medications cause dry mouth.[15] Five out of six persons 65 and older are taking at least one medication, and almost half take three or more.[5] Individuals living in long-term care facilities are prescribed an average of eight drugs.[1] The risk is high that at least one medication will cause pharmaceutical inhibition of salivary flow, making it difficult to swallow, speak, and wear dentures.

Severe xerostomia is life altering. For older adults with medication-related xerostomia whose drug therapy cannot be changed, drug schedules should be modified if possible to achieve maximum drug effect during the day, because nighttime xerostomia is more likely to cause caries.[16] Custom-fitted acrylic night guards carrying **fluoride gel** may also help limit caries in older adults.[16] For all drugs, easy-to-take formulations, such as liquids, should be considered, and regular sublingual dosage forms should be avoided. Recommendations include lubricating the mouth and throat with water before swallowing capsules and tablets or before using sublingual nitroglycerin.[16] The older adult with xerostomia should avoid decongestants and antihistamines.[16] Dry mouth without an obvious cause needs to be investigated.

As older people keep their teeth into old age, tooth decay (caries) and gum disease (periodontal disease) become lifelong concerns.[5] **Table 8-2** lists common oral conditions

TABLE 8-2 Summary of the Most Common Oral Conditions and Treatment Considerations

Condition	Treatment Consideration
Oral lesions	Oral lesions that do not heal should be biopsied by an oral surgeon.
Dental caries	Tooth restoration, fillings, and crowns; extraction for severe unrestorable teeth with caries.
Edentulism	Prevention of tooth loss, fabrication of prostheses (dentures), dental implants, regular check-ups to reduce the risk of mouth sores, ulcers, and tissue overgrowths.
Periodontal disease	Daily toothbrushing and flossing after every meal, water irrigation, antimicrobial rinses, systemic antimicrobial therapy, tooth scaling and root debridement, surgical periodontal therapy.
Xerostomia	Preventive therapy, fluoride therapy, frequent oral hygiene visits, salivary substitutes, medications that stimulate saliva.
Candidiasis/thrush infection	Topical antifungal agents; patients using inhaled steroids should rinse mouth after use of inhaler.

Source: Adapted from: Rai, S, Kaur, M, Goel, S, Bhatnagar, P. Moral and professional responsibility of oral physician toward geriatric patient with interdisciplinary management—the time to act is now! *Journal of Midlife Health.* 2011;2(1):18–24.

and treatments for older adults that the healthcare professional may encounter during their work.

Dry mouth is not a sign of aging; most frequently it is related to pharmacological inhibition, or other disease states such as uncontrolled diabetes, Sjögren's syndrome, or autoimmune diseases.[16] Tooth wear and breakdown over time can be related to dry mouth, because lubrication prevents wear. Tooth loss also is not a sign of aging, and currently there is an increasing trend for tooth preservation.[17]

Other facial structures undergo atrophy,[18] and the temporomandibular joint (TMJ) may be susceptible to arthritic changes, making chewing and opening the mouth more difficult.[4] Just like in other parts of the body, oral motor functions are often mildly diminished in older people. Tongue **stereognosis**, or the ability to sense objects by the touch of the tongue, allows one to perceive problems or alterations in the mouth.[4] This sensory system declines with age. Healthy natural dentition is associated with good oral stereognostic ability, whereas edentulous subjects usually show a decreased oral stereognostic ability.[19]

Taste disorders are common among older people. Taste disorders often go unrecognized and underestimated. The most widespread reasons for taste complaint are medication use (21.7%), zinc deficiency (14.5%), and oral and systemic diseases (7.4% and 6.4%, respectively).[20] Considering taste and gustatory function should be part of any comprehensive geriatric assessment.[20]

Color changes in the teeth with age may arise from the long-term intake of food with coloring agents or from prolonged tobacco use. Occlusal or incisal **attrition** (see Figure 8-2) may be derived from long-term dietary habits, occupational factors, bruxism (grinding the teeth), or xerostomia. Teeth displaying attrition may be more brittle, and more prone to chipping and loss of surface detail. Loss of tooth imbrications, which are the ridges or seams of tissue on the tooth, is a sign of the aging tooth.[4]

The aging of the dental pulp and the resulting loss of sensitivity can contribute to undetected disease because the older person may not perceive pain until the dental disease is far advanced. The pulp becomes smaller with the physiologic laying down of secondary dentin, probably in response to trauma and the wear and tear of continued use over time.[21]

The mouth is a mirror to overall health, so when the oral cavity is pink, moist, and clean and lacks signs of inflammation, this can be a predictor of general good health. Healthy teeth lack bacterial film, the progenitor of dental disease. The tongue is velvety in appearance and breath is not unpleasant. Unpleasant breath (halitosis) may be a sign of disease. Diseases other than dental disease that can cause halitosis include alcoholism, uncontrolled diabetes, kidney failure, bowel obstruction, and sinusitis. Many systemic diseases also have primary signs and symptoms in the oral cavity, for example blood diseases such as leukemia and anemia.

Oral health is directly related to quality of life of the older adult.[4] The relationship between oral health and well-being is being established in the literature and is highlighted by the report of the surgeon general mentioned previously.[2] Poorer scores on quality-of-life ratings in people who are homebound, irrespective of gender, correlate to the presence of oral problems such as dry mouth and tooth decay. Well-being correlates linked to oral health include the number of missing teeth and years of education.[22] Most older people viewed limitations (including dental disease) as a consequence of aging and not as problems that can be solved.[5] The healthcare professional can make a difference to the older adult by recognizing oral problems and referring the adult to the proper professional for treatment.

RECOGNIZING BARRIERS TO CARE

There are a number of reasons why older adults do not access dental and preventive care. Not having the money to pay for services seems like an apparent cause, but this may be more related to the value placed on dental care than true lack of funds. Values are instilled in an individual and are carried throughout life. Not perceiving the need for dental care is a barrier to attaining proper dental care. Lifestyle behaviors can also inform the elder's choice. For example, if an older adult is informed of a diagnosis that is not covered by insurance and costs more than the person can comfortably spend, or would require charity, the elder may choose not to opt for the prescribed dental treatment. The lack of affordable care is a barrier. Those who recognize their health needs and seek care do so because they not only value their well-being, but also perceive that they can afford care.

Another factor is the accessibility of care. Millions of elders live in rural and inner city areas where dentists choose not to practice, so even with the ability to pay, dental care may not be readily available, especially for older people for whom transportation is not readily available.[23] Physical access is particularly a problem for older people who are disabled and homebound.[22] Disability was identified as second only to financial challenges as a barrier to receiving dental care.[22] Homebound elderly with moderate to substantial supportive care needs, including needing assistance with oral care routines, reported a lower general quality of life.[22] In-home prevention and care are options worth considering, as more older people "age in place" and are being cared for at home rather than in long-term care facilities. The options for in-home preventive care come from dentists and dental hygienist professionals affiliated with home health organizations.

Financial and economic barriers to oral health are well cited in the literature as a reason for the lack of dental care. Loss of dental insurance at retirement or not having access to dental insurance has affected older adults' dental health outcomes.[2] Access to affordable health care, including dental care, has yet to be a reality in the United States for those over 65. Reimbursements for dental and medical services are low.[2] Socioeconomic status, the number of oral symptoms, and where the older adult lives are all associated with general health status.[24,25] However, independent of socioeconomic status, poor oral health was associated with worse general health as well as the need for dental prostheses or dentures.[26,27]

THE INTERPROFESSIONAL ROLE IN ORAL CARE AND PREVENTION

The 21st century offers the healthcare professional an opportunity to reassess current curricular structures and practice models to begin dissolving traditional disciplinary barriers and to begin including an interprofessional healthcare team approach for health education, health promotion, and disease prevention.[28] Oral health professionals are vital members of the healthcare team. Proper education and training should encourage students in dental sciences to act as team members who can use their expertise in the realm of oral care and education to improve the overall quality of life for the older adults of the future.[28]

PREVENTION

Caregivers and oral health professionals can promote straightforward and safe measures to reverse, arrest, and prevent oral disease in older adults.[2] Preventive regimes for the older adult include antimicrobial mouth rinses (e.g., chlorhexidine gluconate 0.12%), fluoride rinses, gels, or toothpastes, and removal of biofilm and hard deposits that are retentive to biofilm. Five percent sodium **fluoride varnish** is used in extended and/or long-term care facilities and the private homes of people who are medically compromised and home-bound to arrest or decrease the development of dental caries for this high-risk population.[29] Educating older adults about the manual removal of disease-causing biofilm by toothbrushing two or three times a day with a soft-bristle toothbrush is important, as is the consistent and effective use of dental floss. Older adults with arthritis may appreciate an electric toothbrush or built-up handles and grips to better manipulate the tools to promote oral cleanliness.

Approximately 5% of Americans aged 65 and over live in nursing homes where oral care can be problematic.[2] Nursing homes and other long-term care facilities have limited capacity to deliver needed oral healthcare services, even though most residents are at risk for oral diseases.[2] Conducting risk assessments and implementing anticipatory guidance management (i.e., teaching ahead of need) can make inroads towards realizing true oral prevention outcomes.

Caregivers of older adults must consider the functional capacity of the care recipient when planning for oral hygiene. Higher-level functioning capacity is a factor for successful independent living and is an indicator for effectively completing crucial oral hygiene behaviors.[30] Otherwise, it is the caregiver's duty to provide basic oral hygiene to the older adult whose functioning will not allow for self-initiated dental hygiene practices. Education and motivation of the family, other caregivers, and long-term care facility staff are essential if oral diseases are to be avoided.[31]

Oral prostheses (or removable dentures) require removing and rinsing the dentures after eating. The older adult, caregiver, or healthcare professional needs to clean the mouth with gauze or a soft-bristle brush to remove film from the gum tissues. The person should also scrub the dentures at least once per day. Dentures need to be handled carefully. Most types of dentures need to remain moist to keep their shape. The dentures should be placed in water or a mild denture-soaking solution overnight,[32] and then rinsed thoroughly. Denture adhesives may increase bite strength but are not a substitute for a well-fitting denture.[33] The older adult needs to consistently wear the dentures to ensure continued proper fit.

SIMPLE ORAL SCREENING

Recognizing oral conditions through a simple **oral screening** procedure may save an elder's life and provide early detection of oral or pharyngeal cancers and other oral conditions needing attention. Risk factors for oral and pharyngeal cancer include alcohol and tobacco use, older age, excessive sun exposure, human papilloma virus (HPV), and a diet low in fruits and vegetables. Oral candidiasis can appear as a red or white lesion, and as cracks at the corners of the mouth. **Table 8-3** outlines simple procedures and what to look for during a straightforward screening. It should take no longer than a few minutes, with a flashlight and a tongue depressor to aid visualization. To promote the well-being of the older adult, the healthcare team can examine the oral cavity, take a history, inform the person of the results, and recommend follow-up for a diagnosis as needed.

TABLE 8-3 Six Steps to Examining the Oral Cavity

Steps	What to Look For
Examine head, neck, face, and lips	Look for asymmetry, crusts, fissuring, growths, or color change. Palpate lymph nodes.
Labial and buccal mucosa	Pull upper lip up toward nose, and observe gums, teeth, and inner lips. Repeat for the lower lip, pulling toward chin. Observe for color, texture, and swelling abnormalities.
Gums	Stretch the mouth, looking at the gums for bleeding, pus, or growths; perform from back to front in all sections.
Tongue	Observe the back, sides, and undersurface of the tongue, looking for swelling, coating, or variation in size, coloration, or texture. Gauze squares may assist full protrusion of the tongue, pulling laterally.
Floor of the mouth	With the tongue elevated and tip to the roof of the mouth, observe the floor of the mouth for color changes, swellings, and surface abnormalities.
Oral pharynx	Have the patient tilt their head back and say "ah" while you observe the palate, tonsil area, uvula, and back of the throat for swellings and red or white lesions.

Data from Detecting Oral Cancer: A Guide for Health Care Professionals. National Institutes of Health, National Institute of Dental and Craniofacial Research. http://www.nidcr.nih.gov/oralhealth/topics/oralcancer /detectingoralcancer.htm.

NEW MODELS OF CARE

New models of care include healthcare teams that are interprofessional in nature. Interprofessional teams deliver more flexible care with shared learning from other professions. Different health professionals can come together to learn about gerontology, sharing strengths and gaining knowledge from one another to provide better care for the older adult. There are many interprofessional programs referenced in the literature, such as the Program for Outreach to Interprofessional Services and Education (POISE) and Area Health Education Centers (AHEC). These programs aim to develop, implement, evaluate, and sustain interprofessional education and training for healthcare learners, while emphasizing improved access to health services for the geriatric population in medically and dentally underserved areas.[25]

There is also room for community- and home-based programs[34] for the rapidly increasing older population. Suggested public health priorities include the better integration of oral health into medical care, implementing community programs to promote healthy behaviors and improve access to preventive services, developing a comprehensive strategy to address the oral health needs of the homebound and long-term care residents, and assessing the feasibility of ensuring a safety net that covers preventive and basic restorative services to eliminate pain and infection.[35]

Because many physicians and dentists resist low or no reimbursement rates, burdens are shifted downward to the clients themselves, or care is not sought at all. Prevention makes sense as a method to keep older people performing at optimal functional levels. Relying on well-trained mid-level providers is one answer to keeping costs affordable and accessible, and could offer a viable alternative to the present system.[23,36] Examples of mid-level providers are the physician assistant, nurse practitioner, and advanced dental hygiene practitioner or dental therapist. Other models include training the workforce to specifically work with older adults and other underserved populations. Allowing mid-level practitioners or independently practicing allied health and dental hygiene professionals to treat the elderly in their homes would fill a serious gap in services.[23,36]

SUMMARY

It is imperative for healthcare professionals of every type to realize that oral health cannot be separated from general health. Each professional should be able to differentiate between age-related and disease-related physiologies. Social issues such as poverty affect oral health and general health. Oral health is highly correlated to the older adult's nutritional status and their general quality of life. The importance of dental health to well-being cannot be overstated. Preventive oral health measures, such as mechanical control of pathogenic biofilm and the use of safe fluorides, are effective for older people. Being aware of the directions of change, such as trends toward less edentulism in older adults and the link between oral health and general health, will better inform priorities and planning for the health and comfort of the diverse older population.

CASE STUDY 1

Ms. May, age 80, grew up in Kingston, New York, which became fluoridated in the 1940s. By the time she entered college she had a full upper denture. She was majoring in sociology. In her time it was remarkable for a woman in her family to go to college. She went to the dentist only if something hurt, so by the time Ms. May reached retirement her lower teeth were restored with many fillings and crowns, and her dentist recommended that she have routine cleanings every 3 months to control the biofilm causing her red swollen gums. Tragically, Ms. May had a stroke (right cerebrovascular accident [CVA]) with left hemiplegia. She was sent to the rehabilitation hospital.

Break into interprofessional groups, if possible, and use personal data devices to research the following: any terms with which the group is unfamiliar, the effects of lifelong fluoride use, dental concerns of stroke, and other questions the group may have. Answer the following questions:

1. What preventive factors were not available when Ms. May went to college?
2. What dental restorative materials could have been used to help Ms. May regain function from her edentulism?
3. What is happening to Ms. May's gums?
4. Which types of heathcare professionals could contribute to Ms. May's care? List as many as you can.
5. How should she care for her denture?
6. What types of adaptive oral care devices could the healthcare professional recommend, or with whom could he or she consult to decide best practice?

CASE STUDY 2

Mrs. Jones's daughter usually brings Mrs. Jones to her dental appointments, but has not accompanied her today. Mrs. Jones is 15 minutes late for her appointment. She has never been late before; she said she was daydreaming and lost her way. She seems slightly disoriented. She has forgotten her medications. Her blood pressure is 142/94.

Last year, Mrs. Jones was on medication for osteoporosis. Her periodontal pockets have worsened from 4 mm to 6 mm. It appears she may have a small area of bone sequestration on the lingual of #30. The dental hygienist evaluates Mrs. Jones's oral hygiene and finds it has slipped terribly; it had been very good. She seems apathetic. It looks like her upper denture has not been cleaned in a while. The hygienist takes the denture out and sees red, pebble-shaped projections on the palate, within the bony ridges. The patient seems socially withdrawn; she lost her sister to Alzheimer's disease last year.

Break into interprofessional groups, if possible. Use personal data devices to research the following: any terms with which the group is unfamiliar, dementia, stages of Alzheimer's disease, interprofessional concerns for communication with the older adult, and other questions the group may have. Answer the following questions:

1. What is an oral side effect of medication used to treat osteoporosis?
2. Which healthcare professionals may be involved in Mrs. Jones's care? Identify as many as you can.
3. What is the probable cause of the pebble-shaped lesions on Mrs. Jones's palate? How can they be treated and prevented?

Review Questions

1. Examining the oral cavity entails six steps. Which of the following is not a part of those six steps?
   A. Palpating the lymph nodes
   B. Stretching the mouth to look for bleeding
   C. Having the person say "ah" to observe the palate
   D. Having the person touch tongue to nose

2. What percentage of those over 65 have severe periodontal disease?
   A. 10%
   B. 23%
   C. 45%
   D. 73%

3. Recession of gum tissue causes all of the following except:
   A. Weight gain
   B. Pain
   C. Root caries
   D. Decreased self-esteem

4. The ability to sense objects by the touch of the tongue in the mouth is essential for the perception of oral self-cleanliness. The lack of touch sense in the mouth is called
   A. Periodontal disease
   B. Sjörgren's syndrome
   C. Astereognosis
   D. Taste disorder

5. Taste disorders are common among the elderly, and often go unrecognized and underestimated. Which of the following is *not* a widespread reason for taste complaint?
   A. Medication use
   B. Mineral deficiency

C. Systemic diseases

D. Lack of interest in food

Learning Activities

1. Examine classmates' mouths with a flashlight and tongue depressor for signs of oral health. Compare and contrast color, texture, moisture, and lack of inflammation (redness), being mindful of infection control. The goal is to have an interprofessional perspective of oral well-being.
2. Interview elderly family members and friends about attitudes regarding oral health, access to preventive oral health, disparities that affect the older adult, and policies that the elder thinks could help oral health outcomes and disparities, if they are identified. Class members will report the findings to the larger group, categorizing similar answers.
3. Search online for the keywords *periodontal disease* and *general health*. Create a bibliography in class that shows the link between oral health and general health.
4. Search the web for professionals who treat the older population, and create an interprofessional referral base for potential senior dental patients in your area.

REFERENCES

1. Shay, K. The evolving impact of aging America on dental practice. *Journal of Contemporary Dental Practice*, 2004;5(4):101–110.
2. U.S. Department of Health and Human Services. *Oral Health in America: A Report of the Surgeon General—Executive Summary.* Rockville, MD: U.S. Department of Health and Human Services, National Institute of Dental and Craniofacial Research, National Institutes of Health, 2000.
3. Shay, K, Scannapieco, FA, Terpenning, MS, Smith, BJ, Taylor, GW. Nosocomial pneumonia and oral health. *Special Care in Dentistry*, 2005;25(4):179–187.
4. Rai, S, Kaur, M, Goel, S, Bhatnagar, P. Moral and professional responsibility of oral physician toward geriatric patient with interdisciplinary management—the time to act is now! *Journal of Midlife Health,* 2011;2(1):18–24.
5. Haikal, DS, Paula, AM, Martins, AM, Moreira, AN, Ferreira, EF. Self-perception of oral health and impact on quality of life among the elderly: A quantitative-qualitative approach. [Abstract.] *Ciência & Saúde Coletiva*, 2011;16(7):3317–3329.
6. Stein, PS, Desrosiers, M, Donegan, SJ, Yepes, JF, Kryscio, RJ. Tooth loss, dementia and neuropathology in the Nun study. *Journal of the American Dental Association,* 2007;38(10):1314–1322; quiz 1381–1382.
7. Koduganti, RR, Gorthi, C, Reddy, V, Sandeep, N. Osteoporosis: "A risk factor for periodontitis." *Journal of Indian Society of Periodontology,* 2009; 13(2):90–96.
8. Christie, L. America's Wealthiest (and Poorest) States. *CNN Money.* Sept. 16, 2010. Retrieved June 28, 2013, from http://money.cnn .com/2010/09/16/news/economy/Americas_ wealthiest_states/index.htm
9. Centers for Disease Control and Prevention (CDC). *Behavioral Risk Factor Surveillance System Survey Data.* Atlanta, GA: U.S. Department of Health and Human Services, Centers for Disease Control and Prevention, 2004.
10. Schwartz, N, Kaye, EK, Nunn, ME, Spiro, A 3rd, Garcia, RI. High fiber foods reduce periodontal disease progression in men aged 65 and older: The Veterans Affairs normative aging study/

dental longitudinal study. *Journal of the American Geriatrics Society,* 2012;60(4):676–683.

11. Shay, K. Infectious complications of dental and periodontal diseases in the elderly. *Clinical Infectious Diseases,* 2002;34(9):1215–1223.

12. National Cancer Institute. Surveillance Epidemiology and End Results (SEER). SEER Stat Fact Sheets: Oral Cavity and Pharynx, Stage Distribution and 5-Year Relative Survival by Stage at Diagnosis for 2003–2009, All Races, Both Sexes. Retrieved from http://www.seer.cancer.gov /statfacts/html/oralcav.html

13. Llena-Puy, C. The role of saliva in maintaining oral health and as a diagnostic aid. *Medicina Oral, Patologia Oral, Cirugia Bucal,* 2006;11(5):449–455.

14. Shay, K, Ship, JA. The importance of oral health in the older patient. *Journal of the American Geriatrics Society,* 1995;43(12):1414–1422.

15. Centers for Disease Control and Prevention, Division of Oral Health. Oral Health for Older Americans. Dec. 2006. Retrieved June 28, 2013, from http://www.cdc.gov/OralHealth /publications/factsheets/adult_older.htm

16. Merck Manual for Healthcare Professionals. Xerostomia. 2012. Retrieved June 28, 2013, from http://www.merckmanuals.com/professional /dental_disorders/symptoms_of_dental_and_ oral_disorders/xerostomia.html

17. Qualtrough, AJ, Mannocci, F. Endodontics and the older patient. *Dental Update,* 2011;38(8):559–562, 564–566.

18. Penna, V, Stark, GB, Esienhardt, SU, Bannasch H, Iblner, N. The aging lip: A comparative histological analysis of age-related changes of the upper lip complex. *Plastic and Reconstructive Surgery,* 2009;124(2):624–628.

19. Jacobs, R, Bou Serhal, C, van Steenberghe, D. Oral stereognosis: A review of the literature. *Clinical Oral Investigations,* 1998;2(1):3–10.

20. Imposcopi, A, Inelmen, EM, Sergi, G, Miotto, F, Manzato, E. Taste loss in the elderly: Epidemiology, causes and consequences. *Aging Clinical and Experimental Research,* 2012, July 24. [Epub ahead of print].

21. Morse, DR. Age-related changes of the dental pulp complex and their relationship to systemic aging. *Oral Surgery, Oral Medicine, Oral Pathology,* 1991;72(6):721–745.

22. Stromburg, E, Holmen, A, Hagman-Gustafsson, ML, Gabre, P, Wardh, I. Oral health-related quality-of-life in homebound elderly dependent on moderate and substantial supportive care for daily living. *Acta Odontologica Scandinavica,* 2012, Nov. 13. [Epub ahead of print].

23. American Dental Hygienists' Association. Access to Care Position Paper, 2001. Retrieved July 28, 3013, from http://www.adha.org/resources-docs/7112_Access_to_Care_Position_Paper.pdf.

24. Brennan, DS, Singh, KA. Dietary, self-reported oral health and socio-demographic predictors of general health status among older adults. *Journal of Nutrition, Health and Aging,* 2012;16(5):437–441.

25. Toner, JA, Ferguson, KD, Sokal, RD. Continuing interprofessional education in geriatrics and gerontology in medically underserved areas. *Journal of Continuing Education in the Health Professions.* 2009;29:157–160.

26. de Andrade, FB, Lebrao, ML, Santos, JL, Teixeira, DS, de Oliveira Duarte, YA. Relationship between oral health-related quality of life, oral health, socioeconomic, and general health factors in elderly Brazilians. *Journal of the American Geriatrics Society,* 2012;60(9):1755–1760.

27. Rouleau, T, et al. Receipt of dental care and barriers encountered by persons with disabilities. *Special Care Dentistry,* 2011;31(2):63–67.

28. Dounis, G, Ditmyer, NM, McClain, MA, Cappelli, DP, Mobley, CC. Preparing the dental workforce for oral disease prevention in an aging population. *Journal of Dental Education,* 2010;74(10):1086–1094.

29. Hong, L, Watkins, CA, Ettinger, RL, Wefel, JS. Effect of topical fluoride and fluoride varnish on in vitro root surface lesions. American Journal of Dentistry. 2005;18(3):182–187.

30. Moriya, S, et al. Relationships between higher-level functional capacity and dental health behaviors in community-dwelling older adults. *Gerontology,* 2012. doi: 10.1111/j.1741-2358. [Epub ahead of print].

31. Niessen, LC, Fedele, DJ. Aging successfully: Oral health for the prime of life. *Compendium of Continuing Education in Dentistry,* 2002;23(10 Suppl):4–11.

32. Carr, A. Denture care: How do I clean dentures? Mayo Clinic. 2011. Retrieved June 28,

2013, from http://www.mayoclinic.com/health/denture-care/AN02028

33. Kalra, P, Nadiger, R, Shah, FK. An investigation into the effect of denture adhesives on incisal bite force of complete denture wearers using pressure transducers—a clinical study. *Journal of Advanced Prosthodontics,* 2012;4(2):97–102.

34. Shahidi, A. Casado, Y, Friedman, PK. Taking dentistry to the geriatric patient: A home visit model. *Journal of the Massachusetts Dental Society,* 2008;57(3):46–48.

35. Griffin, SO, Jones, JA, Brunson, D, Griffin, PM, Bailey, WD. Burden of oral disease among older adults and implications for public health priorities. *American Journal of Public Health,* 2012;102(3):411–418.

36. American Dental Hygienists Association, Division of Communications. Mid-level oral health providers: An update. *Access,* Nov. 2012, 12–15.

SEXUALITY AND AGING

NANCY MACRAE, MS, OTR/L, FAOTA, and
JESSICA J. BOLDUC, DrOT, MS, OTR/L

Chapter Outline

Behavioral Objectives

Upon completion of this chapter, the reader will be able to:

1. Recognize the importance of intimacy in feelings of sexuality.
2. Define sexuality.
3. Describe gender differences in sexual functioning caused by aging.
4. Recognize complications from common diseases that can interfere with the expression of sexuality.
5. List techniques to ameliorate complications in the expression of sexuality.
6. Understand the causes of inappropriate client/patient sexual behavior and be able to choose appropriate responses.

7. Recognize the role prescription drugs can play in sexual expression.
8. Identify two approaches to deal with sexuality issues.
9. Recognize the ethical and policy dilemmas for sexuality for institutionalized older adults.

Key Terms

Estrogen replacement therapy
Gay
Intimacy
Lesbian

Menopause
PLISSIT model
Sexuality

The demographics of the United States underscore the graying of the American population, with 55 million older adults (65 years or older) predicted in 2020. This is a 36% increase of the older adult population from 2010 to 2020.[1] Issues of aging must be faced. Providing accurate information about the effects of time and development on the body, mind, and spirit is crucial to keep people informed about what to expect and, perhaps more important, what can be done to prolong health and to become a successful ager. Healthcare practitioners need to be vigilant about remembering that only a small portion of older adults are institutionalized. The vast majority of older adults are leading active lives. Each succeeding cohort has benefited from more education and better healthcare practices. It will be fascinating to see what more knowledgeable and demanding older adults will require of themselves and their healthcare practitioners in terms of health in the future decades.

With a high quality of life potentially continuing longer, we can expect older adults to remain active in every significant area of their life. One wellness perspective artificially divides life into occupational, intellectual, spiritual, social, physical, and emotional (includes sexuality and relationships) dimensions.[2] The individually determined balance among these areas dynamically changes as people mature. Physical activities may decrease in importance as spiritual and social ones increase, for example. Changes likely will occur in the sexual area, if only because of decreased opportunities.

However, an awareness of each of these areas and how one can participate in each throughout life can enrich life. This chapter provides information about sexuality and aging, knowledge about specific acute and chronic conditions older adults experience, and information on inappropriate client/patient sexual behavior and discusses how these topics can be combined using two recommended approaches to help healthcare practitioners deal with the sexuality issues of their older clients. Addressing these issues may well help these clients regain intimacy and a sense of autonomy or control in their lives, both crucial for a meaningful existence.

SEXUALITY

Sexual innuendo pervades our society. We see sexual images and stereotypes portrayed in our daily lives in advertisements, in print, in songs, in movies, on television, and on the Internet. Jokes with sexual connotations are also a frequent occurrence in our day-to-day activities. Yet as prevalent as sex is within our society, little time or attention is devoted to sexuality. **Sexuality** is much more than a nine-letter word. It is a core characteristic of who we are; it is a state of mind; it is a holistic concept. We can be sexual without engaging in sex. Learning about sexuality is a lifelong process, a lifelong adventure. What we learn about sexuality, whether explicit or not, frames how we perceive ourselves and can greatly influence how we act. Taking stock of what constitutes sexuality can help us realize how very basic it is to our sense of self.

Sexuality includes the ability to be intimate with another person in a mutually satisfying manner. Obvious components of sexuality are our feelings and beliefs about what it is to be male or female; how we relate to people of our own or the opposite gender; how we establish relationships, especially close and intimate ones; and how we express our feelings. The familial, cultural, and religious environments in which we develop influence the development of sexuality. If we were loved and nurtured and our sense of competence was fostered and strengthened by those we love, it is likely we have healthy self-images and a fair amount of success in both initiating and sustaining personal relationships. If abuse of any sort was present in our background, conversely, it is likely that we will not develop a positive sense of self-worth and may have difficulty with trusting relationships.

How our first exposure to overtly sexual feelings was handled by others also colors our perception of ourselves as sexual beings. Embarrassment, ridicule, or censure as reactions to sexual expressions can leave lasting scars. Acceptance, encouragement, and enjoyment of such feelings obviously lead to a different conclusion. Fostering the ability to say no and accepting the responsibility that accompanies the expression of sexuality can only strengthen one's feeling of self-efficacy.

AGING AND SEXUALITY

Deeply embedded in our youth-oriented society is the assumption that sex and sexuality are provinces of only the young. Aging men are depicted as "dirty old men" if they show any interest in sex, whereas aging women are characterized as sexless old hags. Yet the feelings of sexuality do not disappear as the years pass. These feelings change and can grow as other aspects of our beings change and grow. As age increases, older adults may have fewer sexual encounters, but may find more pleasure and satisfaction, as sex is linked to quality of life.[3] Satisfaction with sexual behavior therefore is not associated with age, but with health.[3]

Betty Friedan, in her book *The Fountain of Age*,[4] challenges us to look at how social values victimize both sexes: women by the feminine mystique, men by a lifetime of machismo. Images of youthful erection always leading to intercourse and an excessive emphasis on performance are a heavy burden for both older men *and* women to bear, because these youthful sexual measures impose barriers to intimacy for those who are aging. Pleasuring, cuddling, and touching have been found to be more important among older adults,[5-7] who tend to view the total sexual experience through a qualitative rather than a quantitative lens.

A 2007 study of sexuality by Lindau and colleagues in the *New England Journal of Medicine* defines sexual activity as "any mutually voluntary activity with another person that involves sexual contact, whether or not intercourse or orgasm occurs."[8(p.762)] Successful sexuality experiences are more than meeting or exceeding a standard of performance. First, the two people involved in a sexual relationship define the parameters. Second, an infinite variety of possibilities may prove satisfying to one or both partners.

Lindau and colleagues' groundbreaking national representative probability study of sexuality and health among older U.S. community-dwelling adults[8] found a strong association between physical health and sexual activity.[7] Older adult sex can have a number of beneficial aspects for the participants: improved health (both mental and physical), increased life span, more solid relationships, and a bona fide escape from reality.[9] This association is stronger than the association between age alone and sexual activity. The majority of surveyed older adults reported sexuality to be an important component of their lives and engaged regularly in spousal or other intimate sexual relationships. Despite various sexual problems, sexual activity only began to substantially decrease after the age of 74. The difficulty of women having a partner/spouse with whom to be intimate was substantiated.[5,7] Older adults involved in this study welcomed the opportunity to discuss sexuality, something rarely brought up by their physicians. Fifty percent of the sexually active older adults indicated at least one "bothersome" problem, often erectile dysfunction for males and low desire and vaginal lubrication and climax difficulties for females.

Another U.S. study by Laumann, Das, and Waite analyzed data from the 2005–2006 National Social Life, Health, and Aging Project (NSHAP) with a sample of women and men aged 57–85 years.[10] Lindau and colleagues' findings that biological aging does not result in increased sexual issues for either gender, excepting men's erectile and orgasmic problems, were validated. The NSHAP study found sexual problems among older adults were in response to multiple stressors in their lives from physical health, mental health, and intimate relationships. Stress, anxiety, and depression, along with poor mental health, are strongly associated with women's reports of sexual problems, less so with men's problems. Results on intimate relationships suggest that sexual health is relational and jointly produced.[10]

A British study in 2003 by Gott and Hinchliff on the views of older adults about the importance of sex in their lives relied on a combination of quantitative and qualitative data.[11] Again, these adults welcomed the chance to discuss sex. Findings underscore sex as an important part of a close relationship. Health problems and widowhood can lead to a reprioritization of the role of sex in older adults' lives, and maintaining physical intimacy, even when intercourse is no longer possible, is centrally important.

In a study of lower-income older adults, Ginsberg, Pomerantz, and Kramer-Felley found that participants wanted to engage in sexual activities more frequently than they did, but could not often because of a lack of partners.[12] Touching and kissing were desired, whereas mutual stroking, masturbation, and intercourse were less often experienced or desired. Age and health status, again, were found to be predictive of preferences for sexual activity.

INTIMACY

What becomes clear in the recent literature on sexuality and older adults is the importance of **intimacy**.[5,13] Sexual intimacy requires self-acceptance and risk taking. It involves purposely losing control of oneself and acquiescing to what is happening. When the result of sexual intimacy is a satisfying one, feelings of self-esteem and trust are reinforced.

Intimacy needs to be included as a component of meaningful sexuality. Women, as kin keepers, have traditionally nurtured a capacity for connection and engagement with others in all forms of intimacy. Men may have many friends, but deep and honest disclosure, so vital to intimacy, may not be a part of these friendships. Jung,[14] in describing the years after 40, called them the "afternoon" and "evening"[15] of life, and suggested that each gender comes to know its polarities, the sexually opposite side of their nature: for the male, his feminine qualities; for the female, her male traits.[16] Coming to grips with these unused and unfamiliar characteristics can involve stress and anxiety, but ultimately their emergence can lead to a freedom of expression previously unknown.[13] This "crossover" may be a key to vital aging. "Disengagement from the roles and goals of youth and from activities and ties that no longer have any personal meaning may, in fact, be necessary to make the shift to a new kind of engagement in age."[4] It can enhance sexual activity, with the woman showing more initiative but also expecting more closeness and disclosure from her partner. Couples who persevere through these growth trials can find a new depth and richness in their relationships.[17] They will then be ready to reinvest in different ways of communicating with each other. They continue to want to genuinely touch, know, and love each other. Such renewed ties of intimacy can lead to a sense of control of life and an acceptance, rather than a fear, of aging.[18]

PHYSIOLOGIC CHANGES IN WOMEN

Undeniable changes occur in both men and women in the physiologic aspects of their sexual functioning as they age. The effects of gravity begin to be seen in both men and women as bodies begin to sag and waistlines begin to widen. The changes each gender encounters do not need to preclude sexual activity because reduced sexual hormones affect only response time and perhaps the intensity of the physical response. Knowing about and understanding the effect of these changes, combined with appropriate adaptations, can actually enhance rather than deter sexual satisfaction.

Menopause, a natural consequence of getting older, is the cessation of menstruation. It is part of the climacteric, a period of time lasting from 6 to 15 years that leads up to and follows the experience of the last menstrual period. It is usually accepted as the beginning of a woman's second half of life and is a physiologic marker for changes in her sexual functioning. The average age of the last period of American women is approximately 52 years, with an average range from ages 45 to 55.[19,20]

Much has been written in feminist texts[4,19,21,22] about the "medicalization" of sex and menopause, with large portions of the medical field viewing it as a "deficiency" disease. This medicalization has intruded into the lives of younger women with the creation of a new category of disease: female sexual dysfunction, which often has the support of researchers associated with drug companies.[23] How menopause is approached and dealt with by women is significantly influenced by a combination of cultural, religious, and family experiences, as well as whether the women accept or deny the aging process.

Ironically, during the first half of the 20th century in the United States, medical intervention was seldom used for menopause because it was viewed as a natural event. Now that 50 million women are nearing menopausal age, an incredible market for manufactured hormones exists.[6] **Estrogen replacement therapy** (ERT) or hormone replacement therapy is recommended by physicians to treat this "deficiency disease," with its accompanying hot flashes, sweating, and vaginal dryness, and to reduce the likelihood of developing osteoporosis or heart disease. Debates regarding the necessity for ERT abound because of an increased likelihood of developing uterine or breast cancer, heart disease, stroke, and cognitive decline with this treatment.[24] In the WHI Memory Study, women over the age of 65 undergoing estrogen plus progestin therapies had twice the rate of dementia; women using estrogen replacement therapy were at higher risk of mild cognitive impairment.[25] The final decision must be made by the individual woman based on her particular health status and unique family medical history. More natural approaches (e.g., use of homeopathic and herbal remedies, diet, and mind and body practices, such as yoga, t'ai chi, and acupuncture) are also now preferred to help women experience the menopausal years.[26–30]

Women's sexual dysfunction does increase with age, yet older adults do regularly engage in and enjoy sex.[7] Decreased hormones, such as estrogen, and medical and psychiatric illnesses can impact sexual functioning. Interestingly, Trompeter, Bettencourt, and Barrett-Connor researched sexual activity and satisfaction in healthy community-dwelling older women.[31] They focused on sexual satisfaction rather than sexual dysfunction, leading to some surprising findings. Despite some of the concerns surrounding menopause, the majority of sexually active women reported frequent arousal, lubrication, and orgasm into old age, even with low sexual desire. Additionally, sexual activity was not necessary for sexual satisfaction in old age, supporting a nonlinear model of sexuality in older women. This suggests women engage in sexual activity for reasons other than sexual desire, like sustenance of a relationship, validation, and nurturance; touching, caressing, and the like were utilized.[32,33] This study reaffirmed that good physical and emotional health were related to engagement in sexual activity.

Decreasing amounts of estrogen account for many of the signs exhibited at menopause. These signs include the following:

- Vaginal changes
  - Thinning of walls
  - Decreased lubrication
  - Foreshortening of vagina
  - Delayed and reduced expansion of the vagina[17]
- Vasomotor changes leading to hot flashes or flushes
  - Blood flows to skin, causing a 4–8°F skin temperature increase
  - Sweating
  - Increased heart rate
  - Chills
  - Tingling of skin
- Less rapid and extreme vascular responses to sexual arousal
  - Waning of flush
  - Reduced increase in breast volume during arousal[26]
- Orgasm with fewer contractions
- Bladder and urethral changes
  - Increased need to urinate, particularly immediately after intercourse
  - Irritability—a variant of "honeymoon cystitis"[26]
- Diminished fatty tissue of mons
  - Labia majora become susceptible to mechanical trauma from repetitive bumping or rubbing during intercourse
- Clitoral area is more susceptible to irritation by forceful manipulation[20,34]

An obvious omission from this list of changes is a decrease in libido. Sexual desire and activity do not need to decrease during this period because "sex drive is *NOT* related to estrogen levels."[23] Not all aging women are concerned about decreased libido.[7,31] Basson suggests women's desires arise from intimacy needs, not biological urges.[35] Libido can actually increase postmenopausally because of the elimination of pregnancy fears, decreased child care responsibilities, an increase in energy and a zest for life, and improved self-knowledge. Yet, if desire does decrease it may be the result of health problems, medications, and a lack of available partners.[36] Women age 65 and older report one or more sexual concerns, a similar number to younger women, and they also report that their partner's sexual difficulties are a significant barrier. Despite this, physicians often do not initiate a discussion about sexuality concerns with female patients, and when they do, they seldom include partners' difficulties, which can directly affect women's sexual satisfaction.

PHYSIOLOGIC CHANGES IN MEN

Sexual functioning also changes for men as they age. From midlife on changes occur, but they are less dramatic than those experienced by women perimenopausally. A gradual decrease in circulating testosterone after 60 years of age accounts for these changes;[17] they do not signal a decrease in potency. Changes include the following:

- Arousal
  - Delayed and less firm erection with longer intervals to ejaculation
  - Less clear sense of impending orgasm
- Orgasm
  - Abbreviated ejaculation
  - Decreased expulsive urethral contractions
  - Decreased force of seminal fluid expulsion
  - Reduced amount of semen ejaculation; ejaculation may not occur with every intercourse
- Postorgasm
  - Rapid loss of erection
  - Longer time needed between erections
- Extragenital
  - Decreased swelling and erection of nipples
  - Absence of flush
  - Reduced elevation of testicles[26,29,30]

Knowing about these changes can diminish a man's fears of performance and can, in fact, contribute to increased sexual pleasure. Realizing the need for more prolonged and direct stimulation can lead to lengthened and more engaging lovemaking sessions, sessions that may offer a more profound sense of pleasure than when the partners were younger. The technique of "stuffing," when a partially erect penis is stuffed into the vagina and the woman tightens her vaginal muscles rhythmically to stimulate both partners, can be an effective technique.

GENDER DIFFERENCES

New meanings regarding sexuality may emerge as one ages. Despite the fact that men and women develop distinctive sexual styles and gender differences persist throughout life, some older women have been affected by the current cultural expectations for sexual behavior. These cultural changes may include different sexual scripts,[37,38] whereby the woman can assume the lead, asking for dates or paying her share of expenses on dates. Occupational accomplishments can lead to secure jobs, increased self-esteem, role transitions (loss or change of partner), and an increase in sexual agency, including the ability to choose and have control over one's sexual life.[39]

Masturbation, sexual self-stimulation, is a normal part of human sexuality. It is a safe way to relieve sexual tension and avoid both pregnancy and sexually transmitted diseases. About 90% of men and 65% of women practice masturbation.[40] Masturbation often continues throughout the life span, in private. Occurrences increased significantly over time for unmarried women, according to a nonrandomized sample of 102 respondents ages 60 to 85 in a 1985 Adams and Turner study.[39] In a more recent study, participants' average age was 60 (N = 1,974), with 63% of men and 46% of women reporting masturbating in the last year.[41] Besides preserving sexual functioning when a partner is not available, masturbation may enhance feelings of autonomy. However, masturbation was not a favored sexual activity of the majority of those, both men and women, who engaged in it. It was viewed as a substitute sexual activity. In this same study, 85% of women and 89% of men preferred interpersonal rather than solo sexual activity if given a choice. Additionally, 66% of men and 67% of women reported engaging in sexual intercourse a few times a month.[41] Adams and Turner conclude their article on a hopeful note: A substantial minority of women in the study experienced an increase in the frequency of orgasm, subjective pleasure, and overall satisfaction.[39] These changes in sexuality occurred in late middle life and beyond.[42] In the more recent Ginsberg, Pomerantz, and Kramer-Felley study, masturbation was not wanted by most of the participants,[43] yet the Lindau and colleagues study[8] found the masturbation rate to be higher among men (52%) than among women (25%) with a spouse or other intimate partner in the previous year.

Interviews with older adults reveal a lasting difference in how men and women view sexual activity. Duke Longitudinal Studies have found sexual activity is more stable over time than previously thought.[44,45] They found three-quarters of men in their 70s engaged in intercourse at least once a month; more than a third of men in their early 60s and nearly 30% of men in their late 60s reported engaging in weekly intercourse. The majority of women were not sexually active, primarily because of a paucity of partners or their male partners' decreased desire, which can be termed "voluntary celibacy."[33] However, the same Duke University Studies found nearly one-half of married 66- to 71-year-old women were sexually active. Nearly 30% of those close to age 80 were sexually active.[44,45] The 2005 AARP and 2007 Lindau et al. studies reconfirm these findings: Even in the oldest age group, those closer to age 80 who were sexually active adults stated that they engaged in sexual activity 2–3 times a month, with 23% reporting once a week or more.[8,42] Oral sex was more frequent among younger respondents, likely an indication of the cohort effect.

In interviews with 10 high-functioning, healthy, active, divorced or single women older than 60 years, Crose and Drake found a decrease in incidence but a constant or increased level of sexual satisfaction from when they were younger.[46] These women also felt that they displayed more positive sexual attitudes over time, sexual encounters had become less pressured, pregnancy was no longer a fear, and seeking pleasure for themselves was an acceptable goal. Masturbation was increasingly used by these women to relieve sexual tension. They indicated a stimulating relationship was a prerequisite to sex. Women maintain and renew ties of intimacy (with both men and women), and this may help them to maintain a sense of control in their later lives.[4]

PHYSICAL DISABILITIES AND SEXUALITY

Nosek and her colleagues performed a national study of women with physical disabilities that contained both quantitative and qualitative parts.[47] They found out about such issues as sense of self, relationships, sexuality, and healthcare concerns. Their study, with information found in three articles, found that:[48–50]

- Women with disabilities were less satisfied with frequency of dating and constraints in attracting partners.
- Women with disabilities were less likely to have friendships evolve into romantic relationships.
- Over 80% had experienced at least one serious relationship or marriage.
- They had experienced emotional, physical, or sexual abuse as frequently as nondisabled women, but for longer periods of time.
- They had as much sexual desire as women in general, but not as much opportunity for sexual activity.
- They had significantly lower levels of sexual response and satisfaction with their sexual lives.
- They did not have adequate information about how disability affects sexual functioning.
- They were less likely to have received information about sexuality after injury.

The national study by Nosek and colleagues underscores the importance of psychosocial factors in sexual functioning.[48–50] A 2005 study by Taleporos and McCabe found differences in the relationship between severity and duration of physical disability and body esteem in men and women.[51] Men with physical disabilities devalued the lower parts of their bodies more than women, threatening their body image because it contradicts the masculine ideal of strength and masculinity. Age uniquely predicted self- and body esteem in women, with women more likely to possess poorer body image as they age. An earlier study by these authors found body esteem in women to be more closely related to self-esteem, whereas for men it was related to sexual esteem.[52]

For racially and ethnically diverse women, sexual functioning was of interest, but lack of partners was a strong contributor to sexual inactivity in this population. Women's ethnic background and sociocultural factors can influence interest in and expectations about sexual activity. Biological differences, environmental factors, and cultural differences in expectations also affect willingness to discuss sexual activity and function.[53]

Couples, "two people in a committed relationship which may include but is not exclusive to heterosexual married and cohabiting couples"[54(p.268)] are also greatly affected when one partner becomes disabled. A majority report a decline in sexual activity frequency, a necessary change in its pattern, as well as a decline in both satisfaction and interest. Yet a desire for more satisfaction was expressed.[55] Fear, feelings of discomfort, and increased stress affecting their roles and personal boundaries are the reasons for these limitations. Those with postdisability-formed relationships report greater satisfaction (both with frequency and variety of sexual activity).[56] The longer a partner acts as a caretaker in a predisability-established relationship, the more difficult achieving intimacy can become.[57] Furthermore, when one sustains a disability in older age (permanent or transient), the ability to adjust and form a new identity as a sexual being is challenged, potentially leading to dissatisfaction with sexual activity or a latency period before reengaging.[58] Associations with other people and activities appear to be the strongest predictor of positive marital adjustment.[59] Education and counseling also can help.

Recognition of the importance of continuing sexuality in the lives of older adults can help people to enhance self-esteem and increase their options for intimacy. Combined with more realistic expectations about age and disability-related changes, this recognition can assist in the development of adaptive coping strategies.

OLDER LESBIANS AND GAY MEN

Older **lesbian** and **gay** people are a diverse group—a group whose popular image is often a negative one. Their issues with sexuality are both similar to those heterosexuals confront and different. Ageism added onto homophobia increases the challenges faced by aging lesbians and gays as they deal with their changing and developing sexuality. Negative stereotypes of lonely, depressed, oversexed, unattractive, and unemotional older lesbians and gay men are myths. Friend's 1991 article on older lesbian and gay people found them to be "psychologically well-adjusted, self-accepting, and adapting well to the aging process," and a majority of older lesbian women studied were found to be happy and well adjusted.[60]

Friend, using a social construction theory, proposed that the concept of heterosexuality has shaped or constructed the homosexual identity as one of sickness.[60] The current older lesbian and gay cohorts have had to manage heterosexism for the greater part of their lives. They have had to reconstruct the meaning of a homosexual identity in an attempt to control their own sexuality. Cass identifies the developmental stages that gays and lesbians progress through as identity, confusion, comparison, tolerance, acceptance, pride, and synthesis.[61] Stages mastered at appropriate ages facilitate maturity, whereas inability to master certain stages leads to immaturity and feelings of incompetence.[62] Reconstructing their identities often involves conflicts with family and friends and active attempts to initiate social change. They may be the only group who needs to inform their family of origin about their changed group membership status—their "coming out."[63] Efforts to find a niche in society often lead to high levels of adjustment where lesbians and gays develop skills that facilitate their ability to manage the aging process. Such experience develops a "crisis competence" flexibility in gender role and a redefinition of family that provide a unique perspective on other crises in their lives.[60,64] The fact that they may not be able to count on family in old age has encouraged this group to plan more carefully for older age.

Lesbian women can and do experience sexual difficulties. Instead of one woman undergoing menopausal changes in the relationship, there may be two, and at the same time. One may experience a decreased interest in sex.[37] Same-gender relationships can, because of a certain closeness that comes from being the same gender, become extremely close and confining, necessitating the establishment of a healthy balance between togetherness and aloneness. Expectations, because of being the same gender, that the other will intuitively know what is wanted and needed may be unrealistic and, as with hetero-sexual relationships, require good communication between partners. Sexual health can also be affected, due to reduced access to care and reduced screenings. Discrimination or perceived discrimination can account for this reduction in care and access.

Older gays and lesbians fear discrimination by healthcare professionals and not being treated respectfully and with dignity. This fear is particularly high among lesbians.[64] Pope made a number of recommendations for healthcare practitioners in their interactions with older lesbians and gays: take a nonjudgmental approach, assess their identity development stage, develop an awareness of their cultures, develop an awareness of the societal dis-crimination they face, understand the importance of sex for older gay men and relation-ships for older lesbians, understand there will be a variety of sexual behaviors to satisfy older gays and lesbians, and develop a positive, or at least nonjudgmental, view of sexual activity in this population.[65] If physicians are not able to appropriately deal with gay, lesbian, and transsexual people, they have the responsibility to realize this and to refer them to alterative services for their sexual care.[66]

ADDRESSING SEXUAL ISSUES

Because sexuality is such a primal core of our lives, it is a necessary part of a functional evaluation throughout the life span, even in end-of-life situations.[67] It is identified as an activity of daily living and falls within the domain of practice of many healthcare practi-tioners.[68] Because the issue of sexuality is viewed as another aspect of the day-to-day activities in which a client will be involved and its psychosocial importance is understood, it needs to be regularly included in assessment procedures. Mentioning it to clients as yet another aspect of daily life to be considered provides an open door and an opportunity for clients to talk about their functioning in this area and to pursue any desired intervention.

It is crucial for practitioners to have a clear comprehension of their own comfort level in dealing with issues of sexuality. An obvious prerequisite is an acceptance of one's own sexuality, which requires a level of maturity and a period of introspection. A helpful tool is Annon's four-level **PLISSIT model**,[69] which not only identifies the level of intervention needed by a client, but also assists the practitioner in understanding the level at which he or she can comfortably provide intervention.

Annon's model is a conceptual scheme for differentiating and treating sexual problems and concerns. His schema can help distinguish those who are likely to respond to sex education and brief sex therapy from those who need intensive psychotherapy. Each descending level requires more expertise from practitioners so the approach can be geared to their own level of competence. Knowledge of resources available within their treatment site or community is a necessary component of this approach so that referrals can be handled smoothly and with no embarrassment or anxiety.

The four levels of treatment within the PLISSIT model are as follows:

- *Permission*: The client is given permission to discuss any concerns and is reassured as a sexual being. This level affords an opportunity for practitioners to provide a non-judgmental and relaxed environment in which to share their knowledge.
- *Limited information*: Specific factual information directly relevant to the particular sexual concern is provided on a one-on-one basis; myths and misconceptions, particularly about disabilities, can be dispelled.
- *Specific suggestions*: Strategies or alternatives are provided to change or influence the specific problem behavior. The partner needs to be involved at this level. Positioning and adaptive equipment are examples of what might be discussed.
- *Intensive therapy*: Long-term treatment for chronic sexual problems is provided.

Healthcare practitioners need to proceed only to the level at which they feel comfortable and for which they feel prepared. Many will feel able to deal effectively with the first three levels. Inherent in this is preparation for the requisite referral information and knowledge about myths, various disabilities, and cultural sensitivity. What is crucial, however, is being able to calmly relay information in an accepting and nonjudgmental manner and smoothly refer to others, such as occupational therapists and psychologists, for their expertise when necessary.

Potentially helpful questions that may assist an older adult to specify sexuality issues are:

- How do you express your sexuality?
- Do you have any concerns or questions about fulfilling continuing sexual needs?
- How has your sexual relationship with your partner changed as you have aged?
- What (information or interventions) can I provide to help you fulfill your sexuality?

For practitioners to be able to help clients deal with their sexual concerns they need to exhibit the following characteristics:

- Sensitivity
- Understanding of the effect of losses on the mind, spirit, and body
- Knowledge of the processes of diagnoses, as well as knowledge of available resources
- Respect for cultural and gender differences in sexual expression
- Familiarity with a wide number of possible strategies for intervention

They also need to be aware of the following assumptions:

- The client will bring up sexuality issues.
- Chronological age may indicate an increased or decreased libido.
- The client's sexual preference fits with the practitioner's views of morality.
- The client is monogamous.
- The client shares the practitioner's views on morality.

In other words, practitioners may need to make the first move and be aware of indirect attempts on the part of the client (jokes, for example) to bring up the topic.

Inappropriate client/patient sexual behavior (ISB) can interfere with client care and intervention. Definitions of ISB vary and depend on personal sensitivity to appropriateness. Inappropriate sexual behavior can range from offensive jokes and flattering comments, to asking for a date and/or deliberate touching, to exposure and attempts at sexual fondling.[70] These types of behaviors are common in the healthcare field and occur along a continuum of mild to severe.[71–73] Disinhibition from neurological conditions (such as dementia), longstanding sexual dysfunctions, fear of loss of sexual function, a diversion from treatment, and an attempt to gain power or control are possible causes of this behavior. ISB can be defined as sexual harassment, or "unwelcome sexual advances, requests for sexual favors, and other verbal or physical harassment of a sexual nature," because of its unwelcome nature, its possible interference with an individual's work performance, and the creation of a hostile, offensive work environment.[74] Ignoring the behavior may be the practitioner's response, but this accomplishes nothing. There are more effective ways to respond. Although each case must be viewed individually and contextual clues are of paramount importance, practitioners can be assertive and provide nonthreatening feedback to the client, while being honest and clear. Discussing the issue with the client can lead to a positive therapeutic relationship.[75] Friedman recommends that practitioners not ignore this behavior.[70] Practitioners should not accept any behavior from a client they would not accept from anyone else.[17] Immediate reporting of repeated behavior must occur, and an interprofessional behavioral plan may need to be developed, which is often appropriate for clients with decreased inhibition.

With aging comes an increase in both chronic and acute physical problems and disabilities. Typical older adults have a number of chronic conditions that can affect them not only physically, but also emotionally and sexually. Some of the most prevalent chronic conditions of those 65 years and older are arthritis, hypertension, heart disease, deformity or orthopedic impairment, and diabetes.[76]

Another approach to addressing sexual issues is to look at the areas of sexual concern for those who are physically challenged, whether from a recent injury or because of chronic problems. These areas fall into four general categories:[77]

- Self-esteem
- Body image
- Relationships
- Family

Questions about continued worthiness as a man or woman can arise soon after the disability occurs or they may appear gradually as a chronic condition worsens with age. Issues about whether one's body can be trusted or respected again are likely to coincide with questions regarding self-esteem. Anxiety about the ability to maintain or initiate new relationships, from social to intimate, also surfaces. Options for sexual relations and for continuing to fulfill family roles effectively may also need to be addressed.

Practitioners prepared with a foundation of healthy acceptance of their own sexuality and a desire to holistically treat those who are aging can effectively use their clinical knowledge and skills to help in the recovery of a client and/or the client's ability to learn to live with one or more disabilities. Approaching sexuality from a positive viewpoint, based on what does work rather than on what the person cannot do, and from a base of open communication and intimacy can make a crucial difference.[78] Additionally, healthcare practitioners should be knowledgeable about sexuality and the aging population in order to support a positive and healthy outlook.[79]

EXEMPLAR DIAGNOSTIC CATEGORIES

Knowledge—about specific diagnostic categories likely to be associated with being older as well as the coexistence of multiple chronic illnesses—is necessary to deal with sexuality issues effectively and sensitively. Building on psychosocial issues that were mentioned earlier using Annon's PLISSIT model and taking into account the areas of sexual concern for those who are physically challenged can help a healthcare practitioner assist a client. A combination of these two approaches is used to demonstrate how sexual issues can be dealt with in the following three diagnostic categories, chosen for their prevalence in older adults.

Arthritis   Limitations imposed by arthritis and rheumatism affect more than 50% of people age 65 and older.[80] Arthritis, including osteoarthritis, rheumatoid arthritis, gout syndrome, and fibromyalgia, occurs most frequently in women, obese people, and those who do not exercise regularly.[81] Sore joints, range-of-motion limitations, loss of mobility, and pain or discomfort with movement can impede sexual performance and affect psychosocial and quality of life issues. Yet regular sexual activity can lead to adrenal gland production of cortisone and production of endorphins that can decrease stress and lead to less pain, discomfort, and depression.[78,82] The following are suggestions for older adults to deal with the problems a diagnosis of arthritis may cause:

- Rest prior to sexual activity to prevent fatigue or engage at times when you have the most energy (energy conservation).
- Place a pillow under painful limbs.
- Use aspirin prophylactically, if medically allowed, for pain before sexual activity.
- Use a hot shower or other thermal heat source before sexual activity or use a warm waterbed.
- Experiment with alternative positions that do not put prolonged pressure on involved joints (joint protection).
- Use alternatives to intercourse such as mutual masturbation or oral sex.
- Empty bladder before sexual activity to increase comfort.
- Exercise regularly to increase or maintain joint mobility.
- Communicate with the partner about fears

Heart Disease   Heart disease can lead to anxiety about and avoidance of sexual activity. However, the energy expenditure of the average sexual act approximates walking rapidly or climbing one or two flights of stairs. Four to five weeks after a coronary attack an individual is usually ready to resume these activities. However, it is not uncommon for men to have sexual difficulties for up to 6 to 12 months after recovery. Fear of sudden death during sex, low endurance, and medication-induced erectile problems feed a man's anxiety. In fact, death during coitus accounts for less than 1% of sudden coronary deaths, and, of these, 90% typically occur in men involved in extramarital relations, due to the stress and unfamiliar location.[83–85] Women with heart disease are less likely to develop subsequent sexual problems. However, coitus in general is regarded as a positive physical activity that can contribute to good physical health, much like walking or other daily activities.[83]

Suggestions for dealing with the effects of heart disease include the following:

- Taking a less active role in the sexual act
- Learning and using relaxation or destressing techniques
- Masturbating as an alternative
- Taking time for foreplay to allow the heart to warm up slowly
- Avoiding sexual activity when one is anxious or fatigued or when the weather is extremely hot, cold, or humid
- Using positions that both conserve energy and are non-weight-bearing (sitting or side-lying, for example)[86]
- Using an activity configuration to determine energy and desire to participate in sexual activity[81]

Cerebrovascular Accidents   Cerebrovascular accidents (CVAs or strokes) can lead to sensory losses, perceptual problems, loss of strength and mobility, visual problems, and/or communication problems. Suggestions for older people with this diagnosis can include using touch, smell, and vision rather than speech, as well as the following:

- Experimenting with comfortable positions
- Having your partner stay within the visual field
- Using a waterbed
- Using a vibrator to compensate for weakness or incoordination
- Stimulating areas that remain responsive to touch[86]

An alternative way to present helpful possibilities is one that does not rely on diagnostic categories but rather on symptomatology. The chart in **Table 9-1** is self-explanatory.

THE INFLUENCE OF MEDICATIONS

Knowledge of how medications can affect sexual functioning is also important for effective intervention for clients with sexuality concerns. Honest reporting of concerns to the

TABLE 9-1   Presenting Problems and Potential Solutions

Presenting Problem	Possible Diagnoses	Precautions	Potential Solutions
Decreased endurance	Arthritis Cardiac disease Post-CVA Parkinson's disease Multiple sclerosis	Avoid extreme temperatures, heat, cold, and humidity. Avoid anxiety and fatigue. Avoid sexual activity until 1 hour after a large meal. Avoid alcohol.	Rest prior to sexual activity. Schedule sexual activity for the best energy time during the day. Utilize sexual positions and techniques that require less energy: • Affected partner lying on back (no energy expended to support weight on arms) • Both partners in spoon side-lying position with back of one to front of another (no overworking of muscles to support weight) • Ample direct genital foreplay • Masturbation as an alternative
Pain, stiff joints, or decreased range of motion	Arthritis	Respect pain. Support painful area. Do not continue painful motion. Avoid staying in one position for too long. Be well rested.	Place pillow under affected limbs. Precede sexual activity with a warm bath, hot shower, or other heat source. Take aspirin prophylactically for pain prior to sexual activity. Exercise regularly to increase or maintain joint mobility. Use a warm waterbed. Use relaxation techniques. Experiment with alternative positions that do not put prolonged pressure on involved joints: • Rear entry supported by woman • Nonaffected partner on top Use prescribed muscle relaxants to manage high tone (stiff muscles) prior to sexual activity.

(Continues)

TABLE 9-1 **Presenting Problems and Potential Solutions (*Continued*)**

Presenting Problem	Possible Diagnoses	Precautions	Potential Solutions
Contractures	Arthritis Post-CVA	Avoid stress to contractures.	Use comfortable positions. Work within pain-free range of movement.
Tremors	Parkinson's disease Medication-related side effect		Use positions that incorporate weight bearing on affected limbs. Either decrease or increase movement, depending on which produces fewer tremors.
Bladder/bowel dysfunction	Post-CVA Spinal cord injury	Have towels nearby in advance.	Discuss fears and concerns with partner before sexual activity. Determine safest time during urinary schedule for sexual activity. Use protective covering on mattress. Man can wear condom for small amounts of urinary incontinence during sexual activity. Empty bladder before sexual activity. If on a catheterization program, catheterize and empty bladder before sexual activity. Secure indwelling catheter prior to sexual activity (woman, to abdomen; man, to penis) Use extension on tubing for bedside drainage bag for more maneuverability.

Data from: Laflin, M. Sexuality and the elderly. In CB Lewis (Ed.), *Aging: The Health Care Challenge*, 3rd ed. Philadelphia: F. A. Davis; 1996:364; Leiblum, SR. Sexuality and the midlife woman. *Psychology of Women Quarterly*, 1990;14:495; Lewis, CB (Ed.). *Aging: The Health Care Challenge*. Philadelphia: F.A. Davis; 1985:293; Montgomery, EA, Hogan, LS. *A New Beginning: Sexuality and Rehabilitation*. Boston: Spaulding Rehabilitation Hospital; 1992; Siegal, DL, et al. *Menopause: Entering Our Third Age*. In PB Doress, DL Siegal (Eds.), *Ourselves Growing Older*. New York: Touchstone Books; 1987:116.

physician is necessary. Alternative medications, ones that may eliminate or reduce any sexual problems, may be available. A list of commonly used drugs and their possible side effects is included in **Table 9-2**. Additionally, some of the drugs used to treat sexual dysfunction are listed.

TABLE 9-2 Drug-Induced Sexual Dysfunction

Drug	Potential Effects
Alcohol (ethanol)	Libido enhanced at low doses; dose-related progressive decline due to central nervous system depressant effects; can result in failure of erection in men and reduced vaginal vasodilation and delayed orgasm in women; can also cause disinhibition, impaired judgment, and decreased ability to enjoy sexual encounter
Amphetamines	Libido enhanced at low doses; possible erectile dysfunction in men with higher doses; may cause hyperexcitability, tremulousness, and anxiety
Anticonvulsants	Reduced libido; can cause drowsiness, irritability, dizziness, confusion, ataxia, and slurred speech, as well as nausea, constipation, and/or diarrhea, which may interfere with sexual activity
Antidepressants	
Tricyclics; monoamine oxidase inhibitors (MAOIs)	Decreased libido, erectile dysfunction, impotence, delayed and/or painful ejaculation, and anorgasmia in men; decreased libido, delayed orgasm, and anorgasmia in women
Selective serotonin reuptake inhibitors	Drugs that cause delayed orgasm or no orgasm at all.
Trazodone	Priapism, increased libido in women
Antihypertensives	
Diuretics	Decreased libido, erectile dysfunction, impotence, gynecomastia
Beta-blockers	Erectile dysfunction, decreased libido, impotence
Alpha-blockers	Erectile dysfunction, priapism (i.e., prolonged erection)
Calcium-channel blockers and methyldopa, clonidine, hydralazine	Erectile dysfunction
Barbiturates and benzodiazepines	Libido enhanced at low doses; progressive decline with higher doses due to central nervous system depressant effects
Cocaine	Erectile dysfunction, ejaculatory dysfunction, anorgasmia

Data from: Nolin, TD, Aldridge, SD. Drug-induced sexual dysfunction. *Clinical Pharmacy*, 1982;1:141–147; Lee, M, Sharfi, R. More on drug-induced sexual dysfunction. *Clinical Pharmacy*, 1982;1:397; Smith, RJ, Talbert, RL. Sexual dysfunction with antihypertensive and antipsychotic agents. *Clinical Pharmacy*, 1986;5:373–384; Thompson, JF. Geriatric urologic disorders. In LY Young, MA Koda-Kimble (Eds.), *Applied Therapeutics: The Clinical Use of Drugs.* Vancouver, WA: Clinical Therapeutics, 1995:103–111; Troutman, WG. Drug-induced sexual dysfunction. In PO Anderson, JE Knoben (Eds.), *Handbook of Clinical Drug Data.* Stamford, CT: Appleton & Lange, 1997:686.

SEXUALITY ISSUES FOR THOSE WHO ARE INSTITUTIONALIZED

When older adults become dependent and are institutionalized, their need for intimacy and sexual expression does not disappear. Their needs for intimacy and personal validation may, in fact, increase as they make efforts to cope within a constrained environment. Kaplan has said "sex is among the last pleasure-giving biological processes to deteriorate, it is potentially an enduring source of gratification at a time when these are becoming fewer and fewer, and a link to the joys of youth."[87(p.204)] People who are institutionalized may suffer from what Ghusen terms "emotional malnutrition."[88] Long-term care residents report they support the sexual rights of their peers, whether or not they personally are sexually active.[45] Healthcare providers must acknowledge these needs and rights, as well as maintain a client-centered focus, and take steps to accommodate them as important signs of respect; this is normally done on a case-by-case basis. The need to address sexual relations in nursing homes will become more prevalent with the increase in baby boomers; inclusion of this act may be needed in advanced directives in the future.[89] Some institutions have set aside one room where couples may spend time alone to pursue whatever course of intimacy they choose; other organizations help schedule time alone for couples in shared rooms when the roommate is regularly out of the room, and help assure privacy.[90,91] Staff are educated to be accepting of expressions of intimacy and sexuality (masturbation, hand holding, kissing, touching, petting)[45] and to know when to guide the involved people into more private areas. Furthermore, the rights of all persons (heterosexual or homosexual) must be respected.[89]

Ghusen offers several strategies to enhance sexuality expression for institutionalized older adults.[88] Practitioners need to be aware of the myths and realities of sexuality, to be educated about older adults' sexual needs, to help shield residents from abuse, to reexamine their own prejudices, and to work to change restrictive or old-fashioned policies into ones that promote a high quality of life for residents and help families not to impose their own biases on their older family members. Finally, he recommends alternate outlets for sexual expression that maintain and restore ego strength.

Special needs may also be apparent in the community partners of those who are institutionalized. Providing time and space for intimacy when it is desired is important, as is offering counseling and understanding from the medical staff.[92]

A primary issue of concern in this area is of competence. Determining whether an older adult is capable of making a choice and not being taken advantage of is crucial. Guidelines have been proposed by Lichtenberg for use in long-term care settings.[17,92] They are based on having a Mini Mental State Examination[93] score of at least 14 and a subjective interview that addresses the client's awareness of others, capacity to decline uninvited sexual contact, and realization that a relationship may be time limited.[94] However, such formulaic approaches may not appropriately apply to sex, where passion and sentiment are prominent, or to cultural differences. These approaches tend to be overly restrictive, because they do not account for changes in one's mind, the context, and the effects dementia can have on personality. Capacity for sexual decision making should be assumed until proven otherwise, with staff needing to prove a person does *not* have capacity. This also brings into focus the dignity of risk, which is another human right.[95] Sexual decision making poses many ethical and legal dimensions for healthcare providers. It obviously requires thoughtful discussions and consideration on a case-by-case basis within an inter-professional team.[17] If such discussion occurs within the parameters of a client/person-centered philosophy and the belief that decisions can be made by the concerned individual, better and more humane decisions can be provided. Borrell advocates for a specific process: assembling key stakeholders, learning about the issues, conducting focus groups for values clarification, reviewing sample policies, creating working definitions of key concepts, identifying interventions, drafting a working policy document that defines consent and risk, and implementing and evaluating the policy.[96]

RESPONSIBLE SEXUAL BEHAVIOR

Age is not an excuse for failure to follow safe sex practices. Sexually transmitted diseases and human immunodeficiency virus (HIV) cases do exist in the older adult population. Sexually transmitted diseases in older adults appear to exist at a comparable rate to those who are younger.[17] However, approximately one-fourth of HIV/acquired immune deficiency syndrome (AIDS) cases in the United States are in people 50 years of age and older. There has been a particularly steep rise in cases of women of color over 50.[97] Statistics from the Centers for Disease Control and Prevention show that approximately 27.4% of the newly diagnosed cases of HIV are among Americans 50 years or older.[97] The incidence of HIV is rising faster among this age group than it is in younger age groups, with a male to female ratio of approximately 9:1.[97,98]

This older group differs from those who are younger with HIV/AIDS. By 2015, 50% of those with HIV will be 50 years or older.[99] This is due to doctors not always testing older adults for HIV, shame on the part of the older adults, no preventive efforts aimed at this age cohort, and physicians not asking older adults about their sex lives or drug use.[100] However, homosexual or bisexual behavior remains the predominant risk factor for HIV infection up to the age of 70.[101] The number of older adults diagnosed with AIDS, and those living with HIV, is increasing because nonspecific symptoms can frequently be overlooked because of the high level of chronic illnesses in the older population, and may be due to ageist beliefs on the part of the practitioner.[17] HIV infection among older adults is associated with faster disease progression, leading to higher rates of morbidity and mortality than those infected at a younger age.[102] This delay in diagnosis can shorten survival time, as can the addition of comorbidities older adults may also have.[103]

AIDS dementia complex may be the initial manifestation of HIV infection, and needs to be part of any differential diagnosis of older adults with diffuse cognitive dysfunction.[104] Evidence now suggests that older adults with HIV are at higher risk for developing cognitive impairments.[105] This type of dementia tends to progress more rapidly than that of Alzheimer's disease. New criteria for determining the presence of cognitive impairment have been developed and assess executive functions, episodic memory, speed of information processing, motor skills, attention/working memory, language, and sensory perception using tools such as the HIV Dementia Scale.[106,107]

Educational efforts regarding safe sexual practices have been almost exclusively directed to younger cohorts. This is at least partially explained by the societal stereotype that older adults are no longer sexual. Consequently, safe sex practices often are not subscribed to by this age group, and this cohort is at greater risk because they often know less about HIV/AIDS and other sexually transmitted diseases. In the study by Schick et al., two-thirds of the subjects (aged 50+) reported not using a condom.[41] Additionally, atrophic vaginal tissue changes and decreased lubrication in older women make them particularly susceptible to lesions that may readily admit HIV.[101,108] Although little is known about older adult sexual behavior, few secondary HIV interventions have targeted HIV-positive older adults. One such program is Project ROADMAP (Re-educating Older Adults in Maintaining AIDS Prevention), which focuses on reducing high-risk sexual behavior among HIV-positive older adults in primary care clinics.[109]

Recommendations to improve safe sex practices in this group include fostering an increased awareness on the part of healthcare practitioners, particularly physicians, of the need to routinely make sexual histories a part of their medical examinations.[101,104] The 2007 Lindau study supports the willingness of older adults to talk about sexuality in their lives.[8] This process also involves demystifying the stereotype that older adults are sexually inactive. Healthcare practitioners also need to be aware of the different ways sexually transmitted diseases (STDs) may be transmitted among older adults and the appropriate modes of treatment, and have sensitivity as to how safe sex information is acknowledged by clients and shared with significant others.[100] Support, in all forms, must be provided for this group, as for any age group.

SUMMARY

Acknowledging the sexual rights of older adults and the importance sexuality plays in all of our lives, as well as displaying sensitivity to the personal nature of this component of our lives, can help healthcare practitioners assist older adults to effectively deal with sexuality issues. Providing empathy and appropriate information, devising adaptations, and encouraging experimentation to find resolutions can provide invaluable services to clients. Advocating for humane and respectful policies in institutions for older adults can facilitate older adults remaining sexual beings. Tact, discretion, and judicious use of humor also can be useful tools upon which healthcare practitioners can rely. When healthcare practitioners routinely discuss sexuality as another one of the activities of daily living, it can open the door for clients to talk about and deal with any issues in this area. Collaborative problem solving can help to empower the client to gain control over this most intimate of areas. The resulting feelings of wholeness and connectedness to another are gifts we can offer to ensure a more fully lived later life.

Review Questions

1. Sexuality is not only a nine-letter word. It can best be defined by which of the following phrases?
   A. Sexual intercourse
   B. Basic to our sense of self
   C. Intimacy is a prerequisite
   D. A dynamic concept defined in a mutually satisfying way by both partners

2. Choose the statement that is *not* true:
   A. Aging causes physiologic changes in both genders.
   B. Aging precludes sexual activity.
   C. For women, aging has become medicalized (in its treatment of menopause).
   D. Aging causes a decrease in testosterone in men, but not necessarily a decrease in potency.

3. Choose the *true* statement that best completes the following sentence: For women, sexuality changes in later life can include
   A. An increase in orgasm frequency, subjective pleasure, and overall satisfaction
   B. Masturbation as a favored sexual activity
   C. Increased lubrication of the vaginal walls
   D. Few vasomotor changes

4. Choose the *false* statement that best completes the following sentence: For men, sexuality changes in later life can include
   A. A rapid loss of erection
   B. A reduced amount of ejaculate
   C. An increase in potency
   D. Less dramatic changes than those experienced by premenopausal women

5. Which of the following issues do older lesbian and gay people face that heterosexuals do not encounter?
   A. Homophobia
   B. Ageism
   C. Aging bodies
   D. Negative stereotypes

Learning Activities

1. Describe your first discoveries of sexual feelings.
2. How have your family, culture, and religion affected:
   a. Your own sexuality?
   b. Your views on the sexuality of others?

3. What effects has peer pressure had on your sexuality?

4. How can cohort effects influence one's sexuality?

5. Using the PLISSIT model, and considering the four areas of sexual concern, develop a plan that addresses the specific diagnosis, age, and concerns of the following clients. Also discuss who might be involved in their care using a team approach:

   a. A woman, age 72, with a total hip replacement and arthritis who is interested in continuing sex with her partner.

   b. A 65-year-old man with congestive heart failure who is very concerned about continuing his sexual relationship with his 55-year-old wife.

   c. A 70-year-old man post right cerebrovascular accident who is experiencing both sensory changes (decreased sensation on the left side, decreased left visual field) and decreased endurance. Despite these, he wishes to maintain an intimate relationship with his wife of more than 50 years.

6. Bring in advertisements and/or jokes that depict older adults and sexuality in both positive and negative ways. Discuss their veracity and the stereotypes they defy or confirm.

REFERENCES

1. Administration on Aging (AoA), Department of Health and Human Services. A Profile of Older Americans: 2011. Retrieved May 13, 2013, from http://www.aoa.gov/Aging_Statistics/Profile/2011/docs/2011profile.pdf

2. Test Well. *Wellness Inventory.* Stevens Point, WI: National Wellness Institute, 2008.

3. Jian-Kang, C, et al. Relationship among sexual desire, sexual satisfaction, and quality of life in middle-aged and older adults, *Journal of Sex and Marital Therapy,* 2011;37(5):386–403.

4. Friedan, B. *The Fountain of Age.* New York: Simon and Schuster, 1993.

5. Boston Women's Health Book Collective. *Our Bodies, Our Selves,* New York: Touchstone, 2005.

6. Starr, BD, Weiner, MB. *The Starr–Weiner Report on Sex and Sexuality in the Mature Years.* New York: Stein and Day, 1981.

7. Wilkins, KM, Warnock, JK. Sexual dysfunction in older women. *Primary Psychiatry,* 2009;16(3): 59–65.

8. Lindau, ST, et al. A study of sexuality and health among older adults in the United States. *New England Journal of Medicine,* 2007;357(8): 762–766.

9. Block, J, Smith, M, Segal, J. Better Senior Sex: Tips for Enjoying a Healthy Sex Life as You Age. 2012. Retrieved from http://www.helpguide.org/elder/sexuality_aging.htm

10. Laumann, EO, Das, A, Waite, LJ. Sexual dysfunction among older adults: Prevalence and risk factors from a nationally representative US probability sample of men and women, aged 57–85 years of age. *Journal of Sexual Medicine,* 2008;5(10):2300–2311.

11. Gott, M, Hinchliff, S. How important is sex in later life? The views of older people. *Social Science and Medicine,* 2003;56:1617–1628.

12. Ginsberg, TB, Pomerantz, SC, Kramer-Felley, V. Sexuality in older adults: Behaviours and preferences. *Age and Ageing,* 2005;34:475–480.

13. Butler, RN, Lewis, MI, Hoffman, E, Whitehead, ED. Love and sex after 60: How physical changes affect intimate expression. A roundtable discussion: Part 1. *Geriatrics,* 1994; 49(9):21–27.

14. Bruce, MA, Borg, B. *Frames of Reference in Psychosocial Occupational Therapy.* Thorofare, NJ: Slack, 1987.

15. Kelleher, K. The afternoon of life: Jung's view of the tasks of the second half of life. *Perspectives in Psychiatric Care*, 1992;28(2):25–28.

16. Rossman, I. The Duke Longitudinal Studies of Normal Aging 1955–1980: Overview of history, design, and findings. *JAMA*, 1986;256(20):2887. doi:10.1001/jama.1986.03380200125042

17. Miracle, AW, Miracle, TS. Sexuality in late adulthood. In BR Bonder, V Dal Bello-Haas (Eds.), *Functional Performance in Older Adults.* Philadelphia, PA: F.A. Davis, 2009: 409–426.

18. Comacho, ME, Reyes-Ortiz, CA. Sexual dysfunction in the elderly: Age or disease? *International Journal of Impotence Research*, 2005;17:S52–S56.

19. Northrup, C. *Women's Bodies, Women's Wisdom.* New York: Bantam, 1994.

20. Northrup, C. *Women's Bodies, Women's Wisdom: Creating Physical and Emotional Health and Healing.* Rev ed. New York: Bantam, 2010.

21. Siegal, DL, et al. Menopause: Entering our third age. In PB Doress, DL Siegal (Eds.), *Ourselves Growing Older.* New York: Touchstone Books, 1987, 116–126.

22. Cacchioni, T, Tiefer, L. Why medicalization? Introduction to the special issue of medicalization of sex. *Journal of Sex Research*, 2012;49(4): 307–310.

23. Moynihan, R. The making of a disease: Female sexual dysfunction. *British Medical Journal*, 2003; 326:7379:45–47.

24. MedlinePlus. Hormone Therapy. 2011. Retrieved June 28, 2013, from http://www.nlm .nih.gov/medlineplus/ency/article/007111.htm

25. National Institutes of Health. Facts About Menopausal Hormone Therapy. 2005. Retrieved June 28, 2013, from http://www.nhlbi.nih.gov /health/women/pht_facts.pdf

26. Weed, SS. *Menopausal Years: The Wise Woman Way.* Woodstock, NY: Ash Tree, 1992.

27. Brett, K, Keenan, NL. Complementary and alternative medicine use among midlife women for reasons including menopause in the United States: 2002. *Menopause*, 2007;14(2):300–307.

28. National Center for Complementary and Alternative Medicine. Menopausal Symptoms and Complementary Health Practices. 2012. Retrieved June 28, 2013, from http://nccam.nih .gov/health/menopause/menopausesymptoms

29. Northrup, C. *Women's Bodies, Women's Wisdom.* New York: Bantam, 1994.

30. Northrup, C. *Women's Bodies, Women's Wisdom: Creating Physical and Emotional Health and Healing.* Rev ed. New York: Bantam, 2010.

31. Trompeter, SE, Bettencourt, R, Barrett-Connor, E. Sexual activity and satisfaction in healthy community-dwelling older women. *American Journal of Medicine*, 2012;125(1):37–43.

32. Bancroft, JHJ. Sex and aging. *New England Journal of Medicine*, 2007;357:820–822.

33. Bradford, A, Meston, CM. Senior sexual health: The effects of aging on sexuality. In L Vande-Creek, FL Peterson, JW Bley (Eds.), *Innovations in Clinical Practice: Focus on Sexual Health.* Sarasota, FL: Professional Resources Press, 2007: 35–45.

34. Masters, WH. Sex and aging—Expectations and reality. *Hospital Practice*, 1986, Aug. 15, 175.

35. Basson, R. The female sexual response: A different model. *Journal of Sex and Marital Therapy*, 2000;26:51–65.

36. Nusbaum, MRH, Singh, AR, Pyles, AA. Sexual healthcare needs of women aged 65 and older. *Journal of the American Geriatrics Society*, 2004;52(1):117–122.

37. Leiblum, SR. Sexuality and the midlife woman. *Psychology of Women Quarterly*, 1990;14:495.

38. McCormick, NB. Sexual scripts: Social and therapeutic implications. *Sexual and Relationship Therapy*, 2010;25(1):96–120.

39. Adams, CG, Turner, BE. Reported change in sexuality from young adulthood to old age. *Journal of Sex Research*, 1985;21(2):126.

40. Aetna/IntelliHealth. Masturbation. 2008. Retrieved June 28, 2013, from http://www .intelihealth.com/IH/ihtIH/WSIHW000 /23414/23451/266765.html?d=dmtContent

41. Schick, V, et al. Sexual Behaviors, Condom Use, and Sexual Health of Americans Over 50: Implications for Sexual Health Promotion for

Older Adults. *Journal of Sexual Medicine,* 2010;7(Suppl 5):315–329.

42. Sharpe, TH. Introduction to sexuality in late life. *The Family Journal,* 2004;12(2):199–205.

43. Ginsberg, TB, Pomerantz, SC, Kramer-Felley, V. Sexuality in older adults: Behaviors and preferences. *Age and Ageing,* 2005;34:475–480.

44. Pfeiffer, E, et al. Sexual behavior in middle life. *American Journal of Psychiatry,* 1972;128(10):82.

45. Steinke, EE. Sexuality in aging: Implications for nursing facility staff. *Journal of Continuing Education in Nursing,* 1997;28(2):59–63.

46. Crose, R, Drake, LK. Older women's sexuality. *Clinical Gerontologist,* 1993;12(4):51.

47. Nosek, MA, et al. Sexual functioning among women with physical disabilities. *Archives of Physical Medical Rehabilitation,* 1996;77:107.

48. Nosek, MA, Foley, CC, Hughes, RB, Howland, CA. Vulnerabilities for abuse among women with physical disabilities. *Sexuality and Disability,* 2001;19(3):177–189.

49. Nosek, MA, Howland, C, Rinala, DH, Young, ME, Chanpong, GF. National study of women with physical disabilities: Final report. *Sexuality and Disability,* 2001;19(1):5–39.

50. Nosek, MA, Hughes, RB, Swedlund, N, Taylor, HB, Swank, P. Self-esteem and women with disabilities. *Social Science and Medicine,* 2001;56(8):1737–1747.

51. Taleporos, G, McCabe, MP. The relationship between the severity and duration of physical disability and body esteem. *Psychology and Health,* 2005;20(5):637–650.

52. Taleporos, G, McCabe, MP. The impact of sexual esteem, body esteem, and sexual satisfaction on psychological well-being in people with physical disability. *Sexuality and Disability,* 2002;20(3):177–183.

53. Huang, AJ, et al. Sexual function and aging in racially and ethnically diverse women. *Journal of the American Geriatrics Society,* 2009;57: 1362–1368.

54. Esmail, S, Esmail, E, Munro, B. Sexuality and disability: The role of health care professionals in providing options and alternatives for couples. *Sexuality and Disability,* 2001;19(4): 267–282.

55. Sadoughi, W, Leshner, M, Fine, HL. Sexual adjustment in a chronically ill and physically disabled population: A pilot study. *Archives of Physical Medicine and Rehabilitation,* 1971; 52(7):311–317.

56. Kreuter, M, Sullivan, M, Siosteen, A. Sexual adjustment after spinal cord injury (SCI) focusing on partner experiences. *Paraplegia,* 1994; 32:225–235.

57. Miller, L. Sex and the brain-injured patient: Regaining love, pleasure and intimacy. *Journal of Cognitive Rehabilitation,* 1994;12(3):12–20.

58. Parker, MG, Yau, MK. Sexuality, identity and women with spinal cord injury. *Sexuality and Disability,* 2012;30(1):15–27. doi: 10.1007/ s11195-011-9222-8

59. Urey, JR, Viar, V, Henggeler, SW. Prediction of marital adjustment among spinal injured persons. *Rehabilitation Nursing,* 1987;12(1):26–27.

60. Friend, RA. Older lesbian and gay people: A theory of successful aging. *Journal of Homosexuality,* 1991;20(3–4):99.

61. Cass, V. Homosexual identity formation: A theoretical model. *Journal of Homosexuality,* 1979;4:219–235.

62. Coleman, JC, Butcher, JN, Carson, RC. *Abnormal Psychology and Modern Life.* 7th ed. Glenview, IL: Scott, Foresman and Company, 1984.

63. Elliot, JE. Career development with lesbian and gay clients. *Career Development Quarterly,* 1993;41(3): 210–226.

64. MetLife Mature Market Institute. Out and Aging: The MetLife Study of Lesbian and Gay Baby Boomers. 2006. Retrieved August 2, 2013, from https://www.metlife.com/assets /cao/mmi/publications/studies/mmi-out-aging-lesbian-gay-retirement.pdf

65. Pope, M. Sexual issues for older lesbians and gays. *Topics in Geriatric Rehabilitation,* 1979; 12(4):53–60.

66. Hinchliff, S, Gott, M, Galena, E. "I daresay I might find it embarrassing": General practitioners' perspectives on discussing sexual issues with lesbian and gay patients. *Health and Social Care in the Community,* 2005;13(4):345–353.

67. Stausmire, JM. Sexuality at the end of life. *American Journal of Hospice and Palliative Care,* 2004;21(1):33–39.

68. Friedman, JD. Sexual expression: The forgotten component of ADL. *OT Practice,* 1997;2(1), 20–25.

69. Annon, JS. The PLISSIT model: A proposed conceptual scheme for the behavioral treatment of sexual problems. *Journal of Sex Education and Therapy*, 1976;2(2):1–15.

70. Friedman, JD. Inappropriate patient sexual behavior: Part I: Understanding this prevalent situation. *Advance for Occupational Therapy Practitioners*, 2007;23(19):46–47.

71. McComas, J, Hebert, C, Geacomin, C, Kaplan, D, Dulberg, C. Experiences of students and practicing physical therapists with inappropriate patient sexual behaviour. *Journal of Physical Therapy*, 1993;73:762–769.

72. Schulte, HM, Kay, J. Medical students' perceptions of patient-initiated sexual behavior. *Academic Medicine*, 1994;69:842–846.

73. Zook, R. Sexual harassment in the workplace. *American Journal of Nursing*, (2000);100(12):24AAAA–24CCCC.

74. Equal Employment Opportunity Commission. Guidelines on discrimination because of sex. *Federal Register*, 1980:74676–74677.

75. Schneider, J, Wierakoon, P, Heard, R. Inappropriate client sexual behaviour in occupational therapy. *Occupational Therapy International*, 1999;6(3):176–194.

76. Adams, PF, Benson, V. Current estimates from the National Health Interview Survey. National Center for Health Statistics. *Vital Health Statistics*, 1991;10(184):1–239.

77. Fox, S. Dismissing taboos: OTs integrate sexuality into "whole reason" treatment approach. *Advance for Occupational Therapists*, June 18, 1990:13–17.

78. Joe, BE. Coming to terms with sexuality. *OT Week*, Sept 19, 1996:214–216.

79. Langer-Most, O, Langer, N. Aging and sexuality: How much do gynecologists know and care? *Journal of Women and Aging*, 2010;22(4):283–289.

80. Centers for Disease Control and Prevention (CDC). Arthritis-Related Statistics. 2011. Retrieved June 28, 2013, from http://www.cdc.gov/arthritis/data_statistics/arthritis_related_stats.htm

81. Hattjar, B. *Sexuality and occupational therapy: Strategies for persons with disabilities*, Bethesda, MD: AOTA Press, 2012.

82. Doheny, K. 10 Surprising Health Benefits of Sex. 2012. Retrieved June 28, 2013, from http://www.webmd.com/sex-relationships/guide/10-surprising-health-benefits-of-sex

83. Chen, X, Zhang, Q, Tan, Q. Cardiovascular effects of sexual activity. *Indian Journal of Medical Research*, 2009;130:681–688.

84. Lewis, CB. (Ed.). *Aging: The Health Care Challenge*. Philadelphia, PA: F. A. Davis, 1985.

85. Parzeller, M, Raschka, C, Bratzke, H. Sudden cardiovascular death in correlation with sexual activity—results of a medicolegal postmortem study from 1872–1998. *The European Society of Cardiology*, letters to the editor. 2001:610–611.

86. Laflin, M. Sexuality and the elderly. In CB Lewis (Ed.), *Aging: The Health Care Challenge*. 3rd ed. Philadelphia, PA: F. A. Davis, 1996: 364–390.

87. Kaplan, HS. Sex, intimacy, and the aging process. *Journal of the American Academy of Psychoanalysis*, 1990;18(2):185–205.

88. Ghusen, H. Sexuality in institutionalized patients. *Physical Medicine and Rehabilitation*, 1995;9(2):475–486.

89. Tenenbaum, E. Sexual Expression and Intimacy Between Nursing Home Residents with Dementia: Balancing the Current Interests and Prior Values of Heterosexual and LGBT Residents. 2012. Retrieved June 28, 2013, from http://papers.ssrn.com/sol3/papers.cfm?abstract_id=2149841

90. Galindo, D, Kaiser, FE. Sexual health after 60. *Patient Care*, 1995;29:25–38.

91. Roach, SM. Sexual behavior of nursing home residents: Staff perceptions and responses. *Journal of Advanced Nursing*, 2004;48(4)372–379.

92. McCartney, JR, et al. Sexuality and the institutionalized elderly. *Journal of the American Geriatrics Society*, 1987;35:331–333.

93. Folstein, M, Folstein, SE, McHugh, PR. "Mini Mental State" a practical method for grading the cognitive state of patients for the clinician. *Journal of Psychiatric Research*, 1975;12(3):189–198.

94. Lichtenberg, PA. *A Guide to Psychological Practice in Geriatric Long-Term Care*. New York: Haworth Press, 1994.

95. Tarzia, L, Fetherstonhaugh, D, Bauer, M. Dementia, sexuality and consent in residential aged care facilities, *Journal of Medical Ethics*, 2012;38:609–613.

96. Borrell, LJ. Too Much or Too Little Care, Closeness and Love: How to Establish Boundaries and Guidelines for Intimacy, Sexuality and Sexual Behavior in Assisted Living and Nursing Home Environments (*Senior Psychiatric Connection Continuing Education Series #5*). Retrieved June 28, 2013, from http://www.seniorpsychiatry.com/articles/toomuchtoolittle.pdf

97. National Institute on Aging. Study Sheds New Light on Intimate Lives of Older Americans. Retrieved August 7, 2013, from http://www.nih.gov/news/pr/aug2007/nia-22.htm

98. Feldman, MD, et al. The growing risk of AIDS in older patients. *Patient Care*, 1994;10:61–71.

99. High, KP, et al. HIV and aging: State of knowledge and areas of critical need for research. *Journal of Acquired Immune Deficiency Syndrome,* 2012;60:S1–S18.

100. Stall, R, Catania, J. AIDS risk behaviors among late middle-aged and elderly Americans: The national AIDS behavioral surveys. *Archives of Internal Medicine*, 1994;154:57–63.

101. Whipple, B, Scura, KW. The overlooked epidemic: HIV in older adults. *American Journal of Nursing*, 1996;96(2):23–28.

102. Smith, RD, Delpech, VC, Brown, AE, Rice, BD. HIV transmission and high rates of late diagnoses among adults aged 50 years and over. *AIDS,* 2010;24(13):2109–2115. doi: 10.1097/QAD.0b013e32833c7b9c

103. Goodroad, BK. HIV and AIDS in people older than 50. A continuing concern. *Journal of Gerontological Nursing*, 2003;29(40):18–24.

104. Wallace, JI, et al. HIV infection in older patients: When to suspect the unexpected. *Geriatrics*, 1993;48(6):61–70.

105. Gorman, AA, Foley, JM, Ettenhofer, ML, Hinkin, CH, van Gorp, WG. Functional consequences of HIV-associated neuropsychological impairment. *Neuropsychology Review*, 2009;19(2):186–203. doi: 10.1007/s11065-009-9095-0.

106. Power, C, Selnes, OA, Grim, JA, McArthur, JC. HIV dementia scale: A rapid screening test. *Journal of Acquired Immune Deficiency Syndromes and Human Retrovirology*, 1995;8:273–278.

107. Woods, SP, Moore, DJ, Weber, E, Grant, I. Cognitive neuropsychology of HIV-associated neurocognitive disorders. *Neuropsychology Review*, 2009;19(2):152–168. doi: 10.1007/s11065-009-9102-5.

108. Centers for Disease Control and Prevention. 2008. HIV/AIDS among persons aged 50 and older. Retrieved July 29, 2013, from http://www.cdc.gov/hiv/pdf/library_factsheet_HIV_among_PersonsAged50andOlder.pdf

109. Illa, L, et al. Project ROADMAP: Reeducating older adults in maintaining AIDS prevention: A secondary intervention for older HIV-positive adults. *AIDS Education and Prevention,* 2010;22(2):138–147.

Chapter 10

LIVING OPTIONS AND THE CONTINUUM OF CARE

REGULA H. ROBNETT, PhD, OTR/L, and
ANN O'SULLIVAN, OTR/L, LSW, FAOTA

Home is a place you grow up wanting to leave, and grow old wanting to get back to.
John Ed Pearce *(1917–2006),* Pulitzer Prize–winning journalist

Chapter Outline

Behavioral Objectives

Upon completion of this chapter, the reader will be able to:
1. Describe housing options for people who are able to live independently, including advantages and disadvantages.
2. List group housing options and relate these to older adults' needs.
3. Define assisted living.
4. Describe how home health care and rehabilitation fit into the healthcare continuum.

5. Discuss how technology interfaces with aging in gerontechnology.
6. Discuss past and current perceptions of long-term care.
7. List factors associated with long-term care needs.
8. Discuss how healthcare professionals can help facilitate a supportive environment for older clients.
9. Discuss factors that contribute to older adult health and well-being in any setting.
10. Identify the importance of family caregivers for older adults, and discuss contributions and needs of this group and their role in providing long-term care.

Key Terms

Activities of daily living (ADLs)
Adaptation
Adult day services
Agencies on aging
Aging in place
Assisted living facility
Board and care facilities
Cohousing
Congregate housing
Continuing care retirement community (CCRC)
Eden Alternative
Empowerment
Family caregiver
Gerontechnology
Home health care
Homelessness
Hospice
Independence
Instrumental activities of daily living (IADLs)

Long-term care
Long-term care insurance
Medicaid
Medicare
Naturally occurring retirement community (NORC)
Physiatrists
Program of All-Inclusive Care for the Elderly (PACE)
Rehabilitation
Residential care facilities
Reverse mortgage
Shared housing
Single-room occupancy (SRO) units
Skilled nursing facility
Telehealth
Universal design
Village to Village Network

One's health is intimately related to one's living environment. Physically and cognitively able older adults may continue to live independently in their own homes, whereas those with physical and/or cognitive disabilities may need assistance or a more supportive environment. This chapter explores the continuum of options for older people, looking at different living environments, along with their limitations and advantages, and relates these options to the healthcare requirements of older adults. This chapter also covers the basic tenets of universal design and physical adaptations. Adapting activities or the environment can be an important component of an individual's safety and support independent functioning in all settings.

THE HOUSING AND HEALTH CONNECTION

Many factors can influence choices of where and how to live; in turn, a person's living situation can influence their overall abilities and quality of life. **Figure 10-1** illustrates the complexity of the living environment and its health connection. For example, physical abilities certainly influence the choice of where one lives. For someone who uses a wheelchair, the optimal living situation does not involve a three-story home with numerous staircases (and no elevator). On the other hand, going up and down stairs several times a day actually can help a person maintain endurance and vital physical skills. Another example involves the **activities of daily living (ADLs)**; by completing tasks such as self-care (safely within the supportive environment), one is able to maintain these skills longer. If we expect decline because we have reached a certain age, we may be more likely to experience that decline, and this decline certainly impacts where and how we live.

INDEPENDENCE

The term *independent*, when discussing living arrangements, is a relative term. Unless one lives "off the grid," nobody is truly independent. Therefore, when working with older people and considering living arrangements, the first order of business is to define specifically what independent living means to your clients. In a study researching the link

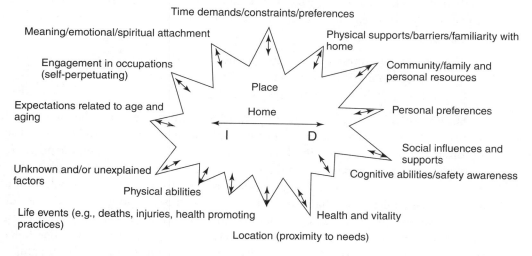

Figure 10-1 The housing continuum ranges from completely independent living (I) to totally dependent living (D).

between health and housing, MacDonald and associates[1] found that the desire for **independence** was extremely strong among the older adults who participated in their study. However, independence was interpreted in a number of different ways. Whereas some viewed it as living comfortably without needing regular assistance from anyone else, others viewed independence as living in one's own apartment or home rather than in a nursing home, and/or as the ability to make one's own decisions. Certain participants viewed independence as not being a burden to their family, whereas others viewed being independent as being able to manage with just the help of their families, not outside resources. Independence was on a relative scale, not an all-or-nothing construct, at least to this group of senior citizens.

As healthcare practitioners, our job is to promote the level of independence sought by older people. We must first seek to understand the meaning of independence to the person and respect his or her particular viewpoint, even if it differs from our own. Then those of us who assist people in gaining and maintaining their independence (e.g., therapists, nurses) must use all our creative and scientific resources to promote the kind of life the older adult is seeking.

EMPOWERMENT

Empowerment is closely related to independence, or perhaps more aptly stated, freedom. It relates not only to people's abilities, but also to the right to make choices affecting their own lives. Decisions made by a competent person of any age should garner our respect, as stated earlier, even if these choices do not fit in with our own comprehension of what is right for the person.

Participants in the study by MacDonald and colleagues[1] clearly stated that they sought control over, and thereby wanted to make choices about, their own lives, particularly in three areas:

1. The type of environment in which they live (housing in general)
2. Where they would go if they needed additional care (continuum of care)
3. Control over their day-to-day lives (reflecting their personal view of independence)

Healthcare professionals need to keep the idea of empowerment at the forefront when working with and for older people, respecting and encouraging choices whenever possible. Too often as people get older, the fact that they are old seems to empower others (e.g., healthcare providers or family members, such as their children) to take over decision making, even when this is not necessary. We may need to remind older people who have forgotten that choices exist that it is the right of all competent adults to guide the course of their own daily lives to the extent they wish. Making choices does come with a certain amount of responsibility. At the very least, each person should be given the choice of whether to accept this level of responsibility. Indeed many of the problems of aging may be directly related to what theorists call the "environmentally induced loss of control."[2] Respecting freedom of choice supports people to "gain mastery over their lives."[2]

On a community or national level, the results of older people taking control can be dramatic. People come together through support groups, coalitions, organizations, and associations to reach common goals by working collectively. These goals can be as diverse as improving housing conditions or access to health care or even lowering the local crime rate. Old age is not a stage when one must simply become a victim of fate, but rather a time when older adults can offer years of valuable past experience and current free time to significantly improve the quality of their own and others' lives. As an example, many localities nationwide have formed *triads* to bring law enforcement, older adults, and the community together to promote senior safety and to reduce unwarranted fear of crime. Groups are organized at the grassroots level, with national support. They conduct organized programs and activities, such as distributing emergency cell phones, offering daily phone check-in programs, and providing community education relating to safety.[3]

Empowerment is also a key idea behind the **Village to Village Network**. According to the network's website (www.vtvnetwork.org), the purpose of villages is to promote **aging in place**—to foster a person's ability to continue to live in his or her home safely, as independently as possible, and comfortably, regardless of age, income, or ability level. It means living in a familiar environment and being able to participate in family and other community activities.[4] The promoters of the village concept believe that older people working together are a powerful force that can take control over their own lives, and that as a cohesive group they can design and implement the future they want for themselves. Villages are starting up all over the country.[5] Although each village has its own business plan and way of doing things, they all work on promoting aging in place through the coordination of affordable services and offering social support. They promote a sense of community and older people taking care of one another through creative ideas such as time banking, during which members can volunteer for another member or the village, and bank those hours in case they need help later.[5] Every year there is a National Village Gathering, during which members of various villages can share ideas and concerns. Given the importance so many people place on staying at home as long as possible,[6] this movement is likely to snowball as baby boomers reach old age.

ENGAGEMENT IN PERSONALLY MEANINGFUL ACTIVITIES

Engagement in enjoyable and productive activity is paramount to productive aging.[7] Longevity is associated with being active,[8] and successful aging includes maintaining physical activity and pursuing cognitive challenges.[9] Continued participation involves reassessing one's needs and desires. Older people may need to refocus to remain engaged when life changes, such as in the event of retirement or the death of a spouse. The choice of purposeful activity may need to be altered to accommodate changing strengths and abilities.

Nevertheless, as healthcare practitioners, we can promote an optimal level of participation through our own particular healthcare provider roles. A significant lack of interest in day-to-day activities or life in general may indicate clinical depression, which is not a normal part of aging. Encourage the older person to seek assistance from a physician if this seems to be the case. At other times the person may need assistance in finding meaningful activities or hobbies. A referral to a recreational or occupational therapist may be appropriate if the person can no longer participate in or enjoy past occupations (including hobbies, home management, and work activities).

Many communities offer opportunities for older adults to volunteer using the skills they have developed over a lifetime. The Retired Senior Volunteer Program (RSVP) is an example of a national program that matches volunteers with community needs. Local **agencies on aging** can be a resource for learning how older adults can connect with opportunities for service. Agencies can be found through the Eldercare Locator website (www.eldercare.gov) maintained by the Administration on Aging.

An important consideration in fostering the involvement of older adults is to engage them in the choice and planning of the activity as well. Although encouragement and enthusiasm for participation may be appreciated, individuals should never be forced to attend an event, and neither should anyone's activity preferences be assumed without consulting with that person.

SOCIAL AND EMOTIONAL SUPPORT

All of these realms—independence, empowerment, purposeful activities, social and emotional support—are hardly distinct from one another. By focusing on one, the other areas may improve as well. Numerous studies have linked the concept of social support and interaction to better health. The social support theory purports that those who are lacking adequate social support systems are more susceptible to disease because of a decrease in functioning of the body's immune system. During tense times, the love and support of other people can decrease a person's stress level and may also help to increase a person's sense of control.[2]

Marriage is correlated with a higher level of life satisfaction in older people, but one spouse (in heterosexual couples, more often the woman) is nearly always left alone after the death of the other. After losing a spouse or partner, individuals may need to find a replacement social support system. In two separate studies, Hong and colleagues[10] found that life satisfaction was positively correlated with the frequency of participation in group activities and high level of interaction with friends. Perhaps it is self-evident that close human connections are crucial in attaining and maintaining wellness for most people of all ages. People do not generally thrive in isolation. Yet as people get older, if their senses become impaired and they are less mobile, isolation becomes a greater risk. Older adults may not want to be a burden on close friends or family, or they may feel uncomfortable if they can no longer hear conversations as well or walk as quickly or as far. For whatever reason, social withdrawal can occur. This, in turn, may lead to further decline both socially and physically.

Healthcare professionals may need to intervene and stop this downward spiral. We can not only lend a listening ear, but also encourage human interaction (and animal interactions as well, if desired), either directly by setting up and becoming involved in programs or by making appropriate referrals to those who can (e.g., activity directors, social workers, nurses, recreational therapists), and by supporting efforts to create communities that are accessible to all. At least one study has found that older people value emotional support and that they feel it is important to feel "cared about" rather than just "cared for."[11]

Intergenerational programs, which bring together older adults and younger people, have gained popularity in recent years. Many school systems, universities, senior centers, and community agencies create opportunities for children and older adults to learn about each other's experiences and gain an appreciation for each other's wisdom. Some programs (such as Foster Grandparents) have been developed to promote volunteer opportunities for older adults to connect and work with children and young adults. These programs may offer a small stipend for low-income seniors. Although the youth gain valued friendships and guidance about making decisions, the older adults benefit from the social involvement and the chance to use their skills and share their vast experience. Both groups improve their awareness of issues facing the other generation. The community also benefits through the utilization of dormant resources.

HOUSING AND HEALTH SUMMARY

A Delphi study undertaken to identify the most important characteristics of "elder-friendly" communities included housing, health care, safety, transportation, and opportunities for community involvement. Older people generally want to remain active, need to feel valued, and desire to live in communities that offer both a supportive infrastructure and the needed healthcare and social services.[6] Based in the Person-Environment Fit model,[6] older people need environments that are not overly restrictive, but support and even challenge functioning to the person's highest level of ability.

FAMILY EXPECTATIONS AND CULTURE

A family's ethnic and religious background can influence the way the unit approaches aging and caregiving. Different cultures have different expectations about how a person is treated as he or she ages, how much and what types of assistance are provided by family, or where/with whom an older person will live (see **Box 10-1**). As healthcare providers, it is our responsibility to be aware of and respect these cultural factors, and to provide care that is consistent and compatible with the older adults' and families' beliefs. Although rates of caregiving vary somewhat by ethnicity,[12] **family caregivers** provide similar types of care and experience similar stresses regardless of ethnic background.[12] Professionals should avoid making assumptions about the division of caregiving duties within a family. Clarifying the amount and types of care, the caregiver's expectations of assistance from other family members, the actual extent of assistance provided by family members, and

BOX 10-1 My Children Are Coming Today

My children are coming today.
They mean well, but they worry.
They think I should have a railing in the hall.
A telephone in the kitchen.
They want someone to come in when I take a bath.
They don't really like my living alone.
Help me be grateful for their concern.
And help them to understand that I have to do what I can.
They're right when they say there are risks.
I might fall. I might leave the stove on.
But there is no challenge, no possibility of triumph, no real aliveness without risk.
When they were young and climbed trees and rode bicycles and went away to camp,
I was terrified. But I let them go.
Because to hold them would have hurt them.
Now our roles are reversed. Help them see.
Keep me from being grim or stubborn about it, but don't let them smother me.
Anonymous

Source: Reprinted with permission from *Aging Arkansas.* Arkansas Aging Foundation, Little Rock, AR, September 1995, p. 8.

the family's comfort with the caregiving arrangement will help in realistically assessing the situation.[13]

ACCESSIBILITY

Participation is difficult or impossible if activities take place in an environment that is not easily accessible. A supportive environment fosters comfort, safety, and ease of navigation and movement. Although the ideas presented here are not difficult to grasp, the process of adapting a home to fit the requirements of a particular individual with special needs usually requires technical skills and clinical reasoning. For a full home safety evaluation, a physician should refer the client to an occupational and/or physical therapist.

Environmental design that fits the needs of older people basically falls into two categories:

- Building new, accommodating structures
- Adapting existing structures

The typical newly built home is not designed with aging in mind, even though each of us is headed in that direction. With multiple living levels, narrow doorways, and inaccessible spaces (especially for those who use wheelchairs), existing homes may not be very suitable for aging in place.

UNIVERSAL DESIGN

Universal design is the design of products and environments to be usable by all people, to the greatest extent possible, without the need for **adaptation** or specialized design. The intent of universal design is to simplify life for everyone by making products, communications, and the built environment more usable by as many people as possible at little or no extra cost. Universal design benefits people of all ages and ability levels.[14]

A good example of universal design is lever door handles. Although they are easier for a person with arthritis or upper extremity weakness to use, they are also easier for anyone carrying groceries or wearing mittens.

Other design features that support people with a wide range of abilities include the following:

- Lighting that promotes functioning (people older than age 60 require twice the amount of illumination needed by a 20-year-old).[15] In her 2001 booklet, "Lighting the Way: A Key to Independence," Figueiro describes the need for older adults to have brighter, more uniform lighting, with more protection against glare and higher contrast levels. Professionals interested in this topic are encouraged to download her booklet at www.lrc.rpi.edu/programs/lightHealth/AARP/pdf/AARPbook1.pdf.[16]
- Either single-story construction or living areas easily accessed by ramp, stair glide, or elevator.
- Antislip and antiglare floor finishes.
- Doorways wide enough to allow a wheelchair or walker to pass through easily.
- Easy-to-reach switches and outlets.
- Bathroom grab bars.
- Levers on faucets.

ADAPTATION AND COMPENSATION

Even though most people wish to remain in their own homes for as long as possible, problems arise when the home can no longer offer a safe and comfortable living space. Home safety concerns warrant a full home evaluation to determine whether changes should and can be made. At times, the proposed accommodations will involve extensive remodeling such as building a bathroom on the first floor or tearing down walls to increase accessibility. Entry steps may need to be replaced by a ramp to allow for wheelchair access. Ramps are not safe unless they are built to Americans with Disabilities Act (ADA) specifications (the grade should not exceed 1 inch of height per foot of length). The document "ADA Accessibility Guidelines for Buildings and Facilities" is available at www.access-board.gov/adaag/html/adaag.htm. Doorways may need to be widened to accommodate a wheelchair, or chair lifts may need to be added to existing stairways. Kitchens may need

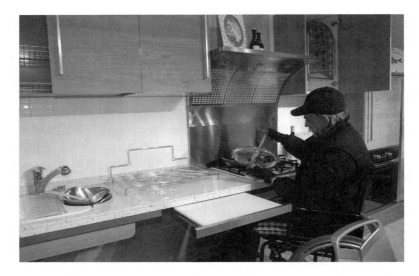

Figure 10-2   Universal design features can make kitchen tasks easier for those with physical impairments.
© paolo siccardi/age fotostock

to be remodeled to allow easy access under the counters and ease of retrieving items (**Figure 10-2**).

Many changes are less drastic and therefore perhaps more acceptable and affordable to home owners. These changes may include the following:

- Adding raised toilet seats and grab bars in the bathroom (**Figure 10-3**)
- Tacking down or eliminating scatter rugs
- Improving lighting levels
- Using shower seats or bath transfer benches
- Eliminating clutter and excess furniture
- Ensuring that smoke and carbon monoxide detectors are available and working
- Resetting the water heater to a lower temperature (not exceeding 120°F)
- Removing door thresholds
- Moving commonly used items into easily reached spaces

Not all older people need to make all of these changes to be safe, although these accommodations are unlikely to cause harm to anyone. Many other minor adjustments in the home, or small equipment purchases, may also be helpful (**Figure 10-4**). In addition to making basic alterations to accommodate the changing needs of the aging adult, the person may also learn compensatory strategies to remain as safe as possible in the

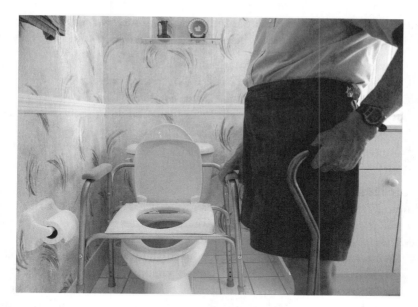

Figure 10-3   An adapted bathroom.
© Mark Gabrenya/Dreamstime.com

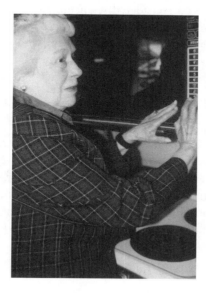

Figure 10-4   Marge, who is legally blind, has made simple adaptations to her microwave so she can continue to use it.
Courtesy of Marge's family

home. As protection from potential injury, a rehabilitation specialist, such as an occupational or physical therapist, may help an older person learn to do the following:

- Transfer into and out of the tub or shower safely
- Use a walker or cane to compensate for decreased balance or strength
- Use safer techniques when using kitchen appliances
- Use different, more effective techniques for completing their daily activities
- Use joint protection and energy conservation techniques
- Compensate for changes such as decreased eyesight, decreased memory, or decreased hearing

Gerontechnology is a term used to describe a professional field that focuses on technology specifically designed for older adults. The countries of Japan and Finland have taken the lead in technological design. These countries are two of the first worldwide to experience a higher proportion of older people among their residents, so they have embraced the use of technology, because it has the potential to help people age in place and age safely. For example, Finnish design includes a compact freezer/oven unit that holds up to a month's worth of frozen meals. All the person has to do is remove the meal, place it in the top unit, and push one button. Voilà, the person has a "home-cooked" meal. In Japan scientists have designed robotic rooms that take care of the people living in the room by monitoring their vital signs and even anticipating their needs (such as thirst or hunger).[17,18] Around the world, technological advances are making life easier in ways that would have been considered science fiction just a few decades ago.

This section has presented just a small sample of examples of accommodations and compensatory strategies that can be used on an individual basis as needed. Through these techniques and others, many people are able to remain in their environments of choice more safely and for a longer time.

INDEPENDENT LIVING

Many older adults prefer to maintain living arrangements in their lifetime homes, even when these homes may present environmental barriers, pose activity challenges, or contribute to financial hardships. These homes are often the ones in which they raised their children; the homes may offer more space than is now needed; require outdoor maintenance, such as snow shoveling or lawn mowing; or necessitate the use of stairs. The reasons to stay in place (called *pull factors*)[19] can be very compelling. A few possibilities are listed here:

- Older people may feel that by giving up their home, they are giving up their freedom and independence.
- They may feel emotionally attached to a home that holds years of cherished memories.
- They may like the neighborhood and not want to leave friends.

- They may want to maintain a large house for when family and friends visit.
- Some people fear that if they indicate a need for any additional support or assistance, they will be placed in a nursing facility.
- Many people, of all ages, either do not welcome or even may be fearful of change, or moving could just be seen as too much effort.

As healthcare professionals, we must respect competent older people's right to make their own decisions, which may include a wish to remain in their own homes, even if we do not agree. This can be difficult for families and friends to accept. Older people with disabilities overwhelmingly prefer to receive long-term care in their own home or in a community setting.[20] Studies have shown that the delivery of home or community-based long-term care services is a cost-effective alternative to nursing homes.[21] Well-meaning family members may insist that the older adult leave the familiar home, but this kind of interference may be more detrimental than helpful.

Garrett speaks to this difficulty when he describes an elderly woman, Violet, who was forced to leave her home with steep stairs, several cats over whom she regularly tripped, an outdoor toilet, and a gas stove.[22] Her children insisted that she move to a modern apartment that they believed would be much safer. However, because of Violet's hearing impairment and her lack of familiarity with the new surroundings and the way things worked in the apartment, she became isolated and depressed. Garrett contends that, although safety is crucial, the home environment should be of the person's choosing if at all possible. He states that home improvements to increase safety may be a preferred alternative to moving out of the home.

Unfortunately, the lack of adequate income may preclude some older people, especially women, from staying in their homes even if they want to and are capable of doing so. The Profile of Older Americans: 2010 indicated that 8.9% of older adults were below the poverty level in 2009, with another 5.4% being considered "near poor" (over 100% up to 125% of the poverty level). Older women had a higher poverty rate (10.7%) than did older men (6.6%) in 2009. The highest poverty rates were among Hispanic women (45%) and Black women (33%) who were living alone.[23] In 2009, 48% of older householders spent more than one-fourth of their income on housing costs.[23] Consequently, 8.4% of older people (2.5 million households) were considered *food insecure* in 2011, in that they were not confident that they would have enough money for food after paying for housing.[24] Hispanic and Black women in the southern United States are particularly vulnerable.[25]

The **reverse mortgage** program is one option that has made it possible for many older people to afford to stay in their own long-term homes. Through this program, borrowers use their home as collateral, and the bank sets up either an annuity or a line of credit to be used as needed until the home is sold or the loan repaid. This allows those with inadequate monthly income, but with substantial home equity, to continue to reside in their own homes. When the older person decides to sell, or he or she dies, the bank recovers its investment.[26] According to the National Reverse Mortgage Lenders Association, home equity conversion mortgages (HECMs), or reverse mortgages, are federally insured. This product was first offered in 1990 with approximately 150 loans being offered. The number of reverse mortgage loans peaked in 2009 with 114,692 loans. In fiscal year 2012 fewer than 55,000 loans were offered.[27]

A **naturally occurring retirement community (NORC)** is a demographic term used to describe a neighborhood or building in which a large segment of the residents are older adults. In general, they are not purpose-built senior housing or retirement communities and were neither designed nor intended to meet the particular health and social services wants and needs of older adults. Most commonly, they are simply neighborhoods where either community residents have aged in place, having lived in their homes over several decades, or a significant number of older adults has migrated into the area.[28] NORCs tend to be either vertical (e.g., in a high-rise apartment building) or horizontal (in a geographically defined neighborhood). The two types have been found to have challenges and strengths, largely dependent on the type of community they are.[29] Several of these NORCs have received federal and private grants to offer supportive services to residents, promote independence, create a sense of community, and meet unmet needs. The over-arching goal is to help older adults remain in their homes of choice and experience a high quality of life.[30] In St. Louis, the Jewish Federation partnered with Washington University to research the needs of older adults in an identified NORC. This led to regular educational (wellness) programming, social activities, resident councils, and information exchanges. A transportation program was initiated to help with grocery shopping. However, when the residents shared that they really wanted transportation to cultural events instead (because family and friends were already helping with groceries), the transportation program evolved to offer popular day trips. Ongoing funding through the National Center on Aging is supporting development of the use of resident volunteers to continue identifying needs and making services available.[31]

LIVING OPTIONS FOR OLDER PEOPLE

Although reasons for staying in one's familiar home may be compelling, for some older adults, the decision to move may be the necessary or preferred option. People may decide to move for reasons such as limited finances, social isolation, desire to be closer to family or friends, wanting fewer home management responsibilities, experiencing a loss of functional ability, and/or seeking a more moderate climate. Although there are many living options for older adults, they may not all be available to those who need them. This section highlights a range of possibilities, including those for people who are independent and across the continuum to those who need extensive assistance on a day-to-day basis.

LIVING WITH FAMILY

Many families consider the option of moving in together. Family members might move into the older adult's home, the older adult might move into a family member's home, or an in-law apartment might be made available. The number of older people who are cohabiting with their adult children is on the rise. According to the U.S. Census Bureau, in 2000, 2.3 million older adults were living with their adult children, but by 2007 that number had increased to 3.6 million, which is over a 56% increase.[32]

These arrangements work very well for some families, and not as well for others. Unfortunately, if the situation is not satisfying for everyone, it can be difficult to make changes without emotional upset. Although families most often step up to the plate to do what is necessary, before making this type of move, everyone involved likely would benefit from considering the following questions:

- Has the relationship had a history of being open and honest?
- How have past conflicts been resolved?
- Is there enough room in the home for everyone to have privacy?
- Can the home be made appropriately accessible for everyone?
- How much assistance is needed, and what is realistically available?
- Whose responsibility will it be to pay each household expense?
- Are all household members' needs being considered?
- What will be the division of labor?
- Can everyone set appropriate limits?
- If the situation does not work, what are the alternatives?

SINGLE-ROOM OCCUPANCY

Since 1988, the federal government has been supporting the development of **single-room occupancy (SRO) units**, partially funding rehabilitation of existing structures to create subsidized housing for individuals with very low incomes. These single-room units are usually found in cities and may offer shared bathroom and kitchen facilities. They are considered by some to be a substandard housing type. However, these single rooms do offer a low-cost independent living alternative, especially for those who have little money and weak family ties, and they have served as a positive alternative to homelessness.[33]

SUBSIDIZED SENIOR HOUSING

The federal government and state programs offer affordable senior housing in many areas. Rent is generally based on a percentage of a person's income. In 2008, there were more than 300,000 units in the United States, but for every available unit, there were 10 eligible older adults on a waiting list for it (average waiting time is 13.4 months).[34] For those who are able to access this option, it can offer security, a user-friendly design, affordability, and a sense of community.

COHOUSING

Cohousing is a type of collaborative housing in which residents actively participate in the design and operation of their own neighborhoods.[35] Whereas NORCs develop where people are already living, cohousing is an intentional community, with private homes and common facilities, consensus decision making, shared responsibilities, and mutual assistance. The idea originated in Denmark and began appearing in the United States in the early 1980s. In recent years, there has been interest in cohousing specifically as an option for older adults, adding elements of universal design, caregiver support, and other features to promote the ability of residents to age in place.

SHARED HOMES

Shared housing can be an alternative to moving in with family. In this arrangement, people might share expenses or exchange services for rent. For instance, a homebound homeowner might have someone do house and yard work in exchange for lodging.[36] Adults might opt to share a home to reduce expenses (such as heating), to share chores, and for companionship. This may work well in a university community, where students in human service fields may be seeking low cost housing and may welcome an opportunity to get some hands-on experience.

CONGREGATE HOUSING

Congregate housing encompasses a multitude of different options, including independent living units, adult congregate living facilities, rental retirement housing, and senior retirement centers. These units, which are sometimes subsidized by state and federal government programs, are difficult to describe comprehensively because they can vary so much from one another. Generally, they do not offer personal assistance or health services, although residents may be able to access home care services through an outside agency. These units may resemble any other apartments, with private bathrooms and kitchen facilities, and with safety features to support independent functioning. In addition, they usually offer group dining, housekeeping, and socialization opportunities.

HOMELESSNESS

Although the proportion of older persons in the total homeless population has declined, the number of homeless older adults (age 50 and older) has grown. This escalation in **homelessness** is likely to continue as increasing numbers of people reach older adulthood and the demand for affordable housing continues to outstrip supply.[37] Older homeless persons are of special concern because of their vulnerability to victimization both in shelters and on the streets, their potential frailty caused by compromised mental and physical health, and the limited resources available to them through traditional service systems for older adults.[37] Factors contributing to an older person becoming homeless may include deinstitutionalization, poverty (especially among elderly women), and the lack of affordable housing. People may become homeless for the first time after the death of a spouse, child, or friend who had been caring for them or providing financial support.[37]

VARIOUS LONG-TERM CARE OPTIONS

Long-term care is an array of long-term services and supports used by people who need assistance to function in everyday life. An estimated 70% of those over 65 will need long-term care services at some point in their lives.[38] Care services can include personal care, rehabilitation, social services, assistive technology, health care, home modifications, care coordination, assisted transportation, and more. Services may be needed on a regular or intermittent basis over a period of several months, years, or for the rest of one's lifetime. Services may be delivered in individual homes, in assisted living or supportive housing, in adult day centers, or in nursing facilities or other institutional settings. The need for long-term care is usually measured by assessing limitations in an individual's capacity to perform or manage tasks of daily living, including self-care (ADLs) and household tasks (**instrumental activities of daily living**, or IADLs).[20] Although it may be expected that most older people need lots of help, the fact is that over 88% of individuals age 75 and older do not need assistance with basic daily tasks, and over 80% have no functional limitations requiring assistance from another person for IADLs.[39]

Contrary to popular opinion, only 3.6% of those over age 65 lived in institutional settings in 2011. Although this is only 1% of those between 65 and 74, this rises to 11% for those over 85.[23] Most people who need long-term care therefore live at home or in community settings, not in institutions.[40] The vast majority of adults in the United States who receive care at home (78%) get all their care from family caregivers (unpaid family and friends). Another 14% receive some combination of family care and paid help; only 8% rely on formal (paid) care alone.[41] Family caregivers will likely continue to provide the greatest proportion of long-term care services in the United States; in fact, by 2050, we will likely have 37 million caregivers.[42]

PAYING FOR LONG-TERM CARE

Although **Medicare** pays for short-term needs, including rehabilitation, it does not generally cover the costs of long-term care such as institutionalization. Nearly 40% of long-term care spending is paid for by private funds. Medicare pays for 19%. It needs to be stressed, however, that Medicare does not pay for nonskilled nursing facility care or for ongoing personal care or housekeeping assistance at home. **Medicaid**, a program jointly run by the federal and state governments, can cover healthcare costs for individuals with limited financial resources. Medicaid currently pays for 49% of long-term care.[34] Guidelines for the program vary from state to state. Some states may cover skilled care in the home, some assisted living care, and some nursing home care for eligible individuals. In 2005, the Medicaid program spent over $300 billion; over a third of this amount was spent on long-term care services.[43]

As people survive longer, the need for ongoing care is also increasing, and paying for that care is becoming a serious national (and international) concern. Some people are purchasing **long-term care insurance** as a way to pay for services they may need in the future while protecting their financial assets. In 2010, an estimated 7 to 9 million policies were in place.[44] Depending on the individual policy purchased, long-term care insurance may cover personal care and homemaking assistance in the home, assisted living, nursing facility care, or other services.

OPTIONS FOR SERVICES AND CARE

HOME HEALTH CARE   Health services provided at home, also known as **home health care**, have existed for well over 125 years. Their purpose is to provide skilled care in the home. (Skilled care refers to services requiring a high level of skill, which can only be provided by credentialed professionals, to ensure safe and effective care.) Home health-care spending in 2011 reached $74.3 billion; over 80% of this was paid for by the Medicare and Medicaid programs.[45] There are currently 33,000 home care and hospice providers in the United States, offering an estimated 12 million patients needed nursing care, therapies (including occupational, physical, and respiratory therapies, and speech-language pathology services), home health aide services, social work intervention, and sometimes psychological and nutritional counseling.[46]

As the population ages, the number of people needing home care is expected to rise, especially as more older people who have chronic conditions are living longer. Technological developments are also allowing an array of new services to be provided in the home, from dialysis to blood pressure monitoring and reporting. In addition, **telehealth** is starting to provide opportunities to streamline the home health system, by allowing close monitoring of patients in their homes through the use of ordinary physiological assessment devices, such as stethoscopes, pulse oximeters, and blood glucose meters, which have been adapted to be capable of telecommunication. This would save the skilled medical professional, such as a nurse, a trip to every patient's home. Technologically advanced service extenders such as these may be harkening the dawn of a new age of home health care, as stated by Ron Pion, MD:

> The promise of the Internet in health care is absolutely stunning and hard to grasp as yet, particularly for home health care applications. This potential great benefit rests in connecting the relatively isolated (from in-patient-related staff and procedures) home health care population to critical information and communications with professional and informed assisters.[47]

Payers are requiring providers to collect and report data on the outcomes of the care they provide. Payment systems through Medicare and other programs are intended to encourage efficient and effective care, and support treatment accountability. Appropriate telemedicine, combined with in-home care as needed, may help to prevent hospital readmissions.[48] The Joint Commission made a statement that the delivery of home- or community-based long-term care services is a cost-effective alternative to nursing homes and is what most Americans would prefer.[49] This combination of factors suggests that we can expect continued growth and a larger number of options in this area of service delivery.

One innovative program related to long-term care that is considered a permanent part of Medicare (since 1997), but is not well known, is the **Program of All-Inclusive Care for the Elderly (PACE)**. PACE was designed in San Francisco in 1973 for people 55 or older needing a level of care normally provided in a nursing home.[50] The program entails comprehensive services including all medical and supportive services (therapies, day services, meals, counseling, respite, and medication management). Attending an adult day program was one central (mandatory) concept of PACE to keep people in the community. Outcomes from the PACE programs have been positive including lower nursing home admissions, better self-reported health, lower mortality rates, and lower healthcare costs (than traditional Medicare fee-for-service). Also the participants have been more likely to be able to die at home if that was their wish. However, the criticisms of the PACE program are substantial and include that it is not easily affordable for middle income older adults, whereas it does help those who are eligible for Medicaid. Some have found the requirement of using adult day services and giving up their own primary care provider too restrictive. Finally, not only is there a lack of awareness, but also a lack of funding. At the onset, grant funding paid for the majority of PACE startup costs, but this is no longer available.[50] Nonetheless, innovation and creatively working together to improve healthcare outcomes do seem to be necessary if we are going to be able to manage the huge numbers of older adults who will need extensive care over time.

REHABILITATION   **Rehabilitation** is the process of helping someone regain the highest possible level of functioning after an injury or illness. Rehabilitation specialists, including **physiatrists** (who are physicians specializing in rehabilitation), nurses, and therapy practitioners in the fields of occupational therapy, physical therapy and speech-language pathology, work with patients or clients in the home, community, residential facility settings, and hospital. Rehabilitation services are provided at different levels of intensity. In an acute rehabilitation setting, where a patient can stay for days or a few weeks, the patients generally receive 3 or more hours of skilled therapy per day, at least 5 days per week. Through medical management and therapy, the patients are expected to make significant gains in a reasonable and expected period of time. Therapists, rehabilitation nurses, and physiatrists are experts in judging whether this is likely to occur given various factors and the patient's current condition.

For example, after a stroke, or cerebrovascular accident (CVA), patients often can make good progress in regaining their strength, balance, and motor control to do the tasks they want or need to do. If they make excellent and quick gains, they may return home directly from the rehabilitation hospital. However, if their gains are slower or not as significant, they may need alternative placement (e.g., assisted living or a nursing facility) prior to or instead of going home. Or if their level of endurance cannot withstand the intensity of the acute level of rehabilitation, they may receive a lower intensity of therapy services in a **skilled nursing facility** (SNF).

Through rehabilitation, which includes exercise, education, and training/retraining in ADLs, IADLs, mobility, communication, and other functional tasks as needed, many people have been able to return to their former level of independence and their former living situations. This is accomplished through the restoration of function and/or through the use of compensatory measures and environmental adaptations to make up for lost skills.

ADULT DAY SERVICES   **Adult day services** (ADS) are community-based group programs with specialized plans of care designed to meet the daytime needs of individuals with functional and/or cognitive impairments. Unfortunately, these programs are highly fragmented, because they are not currently regulated in the United States, at least at the federal level.[51] According to a U.S. industry market research report,[52] although the growth of ADS programs slowed in 2010–2011, growth increased again in 2012, and the need is expected to continue to increase as the older population continues to increase. There were approximately 3,400 adult day centers in the United States in 2002. This was fewer than half of the 8,500 that would have been considered adequate.[53] The average program size included 38 participants, with just over half of those attending having the diagnosis of dementia. Participants also included people with frailty (41%), mental retardation or developmental disabilities (24%), and chronic mental illness (14%).[53] ADS programs tend to follow one of the following models: the medical model (21%, in which rehabilitation and health services are offered), the social model (37%, these offer no medical services), or a combination of both medical and social (42%).[53]

Because they offer structured care in a protective setting (but are considered more than "babysitting"), these services can help people with disabilities live at home, while allowing caregivers time to work or rest. Participants usually have opportunities for social engagement, activities, and meals, in an environment that offers staff assistance when needed. Although some state programs, long-term care insurance policies, Medicaid, and Veterans' Affairs programs can help with funding, most adult services are paid for privately.[54] The nationwide average cost for adult day services was $70 per day in 2012. However, fees vary greatly from state to state, in part due to state regulations.[55]

More research needs to be conducted on the outcomes of day services, but to date, although little research has been conducted, ADS programs have shown initial promise for decreasing caregiver stress related to caregiver job requirements, family needs, and recreational constrictions. The caregivers are better able to deal with problem behaviors, perhaps due to spending time away from the person.[56] Another study found that the caregivers reported an improved ability to be adaptable and showed decreased signs of stress, anger, and depression. The caregivers also reported a decreased sense of subjective burden.[57] Finally, Zarit found that caregiver stress decreased significantly on days that their care recipient was in an ADS program, compared to other days (but only for caregivers who lived with the care recipient).[58] He also found that the care recipient had less disturbing "dementia" behavior and better sleep patterns.[58] Ultimately, effective ADS programs could help to delay institutionalization for those at risk by providing caregivers needed support so that they can extend the time they are able to undertake this vital role.

LONG-TERM RESIDENTIAL CARE   **Residential care facilities** can have multiple labels, including adult residential facilities, adult group homes, domiciliary homes, personal care homes, family care, adult foster care, rest homes, board and care homes, and assisted living facilities. All have the common theme of bridging the gap between independent living and 24-hour-per-day nursing care.[59] States have different definitions and degrees of licensing and regulation for the various types of facilities. The Assisted Living Federation of America defines **assisted living facility** as a long-term residence option that provides resident-centered care in a residential setting. It is designed for those who need extra help in their day-to-day lives but who do not require 24-hour-per-day skilled nursing care.[60] Residents rent rooms or apartments and receive needed assistance with ADLs and IADLs as part of their monthly rental fee. The amount of assistance available varies among facilities and regions. Most states regulate these facilities. This model of housing seeks to allow independent decision making, while promoting the safety of all residents. Most apartments are "homelike" and environmentally accessible. Residents are encouraged to bring personal furnishings and continue their community involvement.

Community or shared space is also a feature of assisted living facilities. Dining rooms, laundry areas, libraries, and activity/physical fitness areas are located to promote social interactions.[61] Although an initial move is necessary to establish themselves at an assisted living facility, many older people find relocating is well worth the consequent security it brings. Although residents are encouraged to maintain an optimal level of functioning, they also can trust that if health issues do arise, they will receive the needed care in their new home for as long as possible.

In 2009, there were approximately 36,000 assisted living residences in the United States, housing more than 1 million people.[62] Facility sizes vary greatly, as do fees charged and services provided. Residences typically provide 24-hour supervision, up to three meals per day in a group dining room, personal care, social activities, housekeeping, and arrangements for transportation. The most frequent resident needs included:[63]

- Help with medications (86%)
- Help with bathing (72%)
- Help with dressing (57%)
- Help with toileting (41%)

Some assisted living facilities offer specialized units for people with dementia to ensure both their safety and their engagement in meaningful activities. Other facilities may opt not to accept residents with significant cognitive impairments; for example, if the facility is not set up to accommodate safety concerns such as wandering. The typical assisted living resident is white, female, and over 85 years old. Generally the woman has at least one cognitive impairment (52%) and usually pays for her care privately. Only 11% of assisted living residents received Medicaid assistance for their assisted living costs.[63] The average cost for assisted living in 2012 was $3,550 per month, with the lowest cost in Arkansas ($2,355) and the price double or higher in parts of the northeast. The highest rate was in Washington, D.C. ($5,933).[55] It remains unclear why these costs vary so greatly, but it seems to fit with the notion that assisted living still is not financially accessible for a large segment of the older population of the United States.[64]

Board and care facilities are also considered to be in this residential care spectrum, but they differ from many assisted living centers in that they tend to be located in traditional, large single-family homes. These homes typically provide meals, transportation, other services, and "protective oversight" as needed. A board and care home generally has one to six beds, which may be located in either private or shared bedrooms.[65]

CONTINUING CARE RETIREMENT COMMUNITIES   Health care for life can be obtained at **continuing care retirement communities** (CCRCs), which have existed for more than a century, but which have just recently gained popularity in the United States. These facilities are specifically designed to provide lifetime care within one community (i.e., opportunities for aging in place), so residents often move there while still independent and then change residences within the community if medical and/or personal care services are needed.[65] To join, the person generally pays an entrance fee and a monthly fee, and in return gets a home and certain services (specific to that CCRC).[66] These homes are arranged in a community and may be free-standing houses, condominiums, or apartments and include residential treatment facilities. The services may be optional for the resident and may range from no outside services at all to comprehensive healthcare services as needed. Services available may include housecleaning, meals, recreational programs, transportation, grounds upkeep, laundry service, individual medication management, respite care, rehabilitation, nursing services, health promotion programs, recreational programs, assistance with personal care, and social services. Although CCRCs can be not-for-profit entities, they are still considered on the higher end of the housing payment spectrum, and therefore are not an option for all older adults.

HOSPICE CARE   Supportive comfort care provided to people at the end of life is part of the **hospice** movement. The focus is on pain relief and quality of life, rather than curative treatments. Although the concept of hospice care dates to ancient times, the first hospice in the United States was started in 1974. Medicare added a hospice benefit in 1983. Services may be provided in a client's home (including assisted living and nursing facilities), hospital, or a separate hospice facility. Services include medical, emotional, and spiritual care for terminally ill people and their families. Under the Medicare hospice benefit, eligibility includes a prognosis of 6 months or less, "if the disease runs its normal course." Beneficiaries receive a wider range of covered services and supports than would be available under traditional Medicare Part A.[67]

Hospice care is well known for those with cancer, but also can be appropriate for people with many other medical diagnoses, including end-stage cardiac or pulmonary issues, renal failure, dementia, and neurological degenerative conditions. Although it is available through the last expected 6 months of life (and beyond, if a person survives longer), many patients use the benefit less than a week, which may indicate a reluctance on the part of patients, families, or medical personnel to address a terminal prognosis.[67] Trends indicate that as more patients and families are educated about its possible benefits, hospice may become a more attractive alternative in the final months of life.[67]

NURSING FACILITIES   Nursing facilities house only a relatively small percentage (4.5%) of the total 65 and older population, but the percentage increases dramatically with age, ranging from 1.1% for persons 65–74 years to 4.7% for persons 75–84 years and 18.2% for persons 85 and older.[23] Nonetheless, an impression persists among some older adults and the general public that nursing home care is an inevitable, and undesirable, part of growing older. A 2007 survey of more than 800 older adults and adult children revealed that people were more fearful of losing their independence (26%) or moving into a nursing home (13%) than they were of dying (3%). Adult children's concerns about their parents' well-being if they had to leave their homes centered on the older adults' sadness at loss of independence (89%), fear of leaving their homes (70%), the risk of mistreatment (82%), and potential unhappiness in a facility (79%).[68]

Nursing facility care may be needed by those people who have disabilities interfering with their self-care skills. Because of their physical or cognitive impairments, others must assist them in completing their daily tasks. If the need for assistance is greater than what is available through family caregivers and/or professional providers in other settings, a move to a nursing facility may be the option of choice for safety and comfort. The average cost per year for nursing home care ranges from $81,030 for a semi-private room to $91,520 for a private room. Again the rates vary considerably by state, with the lowest rates in Texas and Oklahoma and the highest rates (nearly $700 per day) in Alaska.[55]

Nursing facilities provide around-the-clock care through the use of paid caregivers, primarily nurses and aides. In the past, people generally entered a nursing home to live out their final days. In recent years, the concept of nursing facility care has been changing, and the services provided are increasingly focused on rehabilitation. Older people are often admitted to the facility for a short stay to receive rehabilitation services and improve their functioning enough so that they are able to transfer to a less restrictive environment.

Oversight of long-term care is performed by a number of entities. Medicare audits and surveys providers who participate in the Medicare program to ensure that they are in compliance with all state and federal requirements. States also survey licensed facilities. Agencies and facilities opting for additional accreditation, such as those provided by The Joint Commission (TJC) or the Community Health Accreditation Program (CHAP), are subject to additional requirements related to care provided. The Long Term Care Ombudsman Program, which is part of the Administration on Aging, works with long-term care providers and consumers to improve quality and resolve issues.[69]

In spite of the need for long-term care facilities and the oversight provided, there still seems to be "widespread animosity toward nursing homes."[70] People do not eagerly anticipate becoming residents of long-term care facilities as they grow old. Therefore, many are rethinking the continuum of care to both improve the long-term care facilities that do already exist and to come up with better alternatives to 24/7 institutionalization unless

Table 10-1 Anticipated Trends in Housing for Older Adults (2010–2020)

1. Energy-efficient and environmentally friendly design

2. Universal design

3. Technology (including sensor technology, social and wellness connections, and interactive applications for health care)

4. Flexibility of amenities (to meet individual desires)

5. Services at home (where people want them)

6. Naturally occurring retirement communities (NORCs)

7. Continuing care retirement communities (CCRCs)

8. Housing that empowers residents

9. Increasing need for memory care (due to the increasing number of people with Alzheimer's disease)

10. New ways to finance housing needs (need for partnerships and creativity)

Adapted from Schubert, E. (2010). Ten Senior Housing Trends for the Next Decade. Retrieved April 29, 2013 from http://www.seniorhousingdevelopment.org/posts/view/75-10-Senior-Housing-Development-Trends-for-the-next-10-Years/

absolutely necessary. In addition, the Medicare system allows interested parties to compare nursing homes based on their ratings of health inspections, staffing, adherence to residents' rights, and pharmaceutical services. This website (www.medicare.gov/NursingHomeCompare /search.aspx) can be very helpful in determining which facilities provide the best care in any desired location.

Table 10-1 provides an overview of housing trends that may occur over the next few years. Several of these trends have been addressed throughout the chapter.

OLD AGE CARE IDEAS FROM AROUND THE WORLD

Around the world there is talk of a "silver tsunami" coming as the population everywhere is quickly heading into old age in unprecedented numbers. With limited resources, we will be challenged to find creative solutions to housing and care issues. Scandinavia has long been noted as providing the pinnacle of old age care. Although what they provide is not inexpensive, in general the care is less burdensome on the individual during old age (taxes being higher throughout life to ensure a secure old age).[71] A few of the ideas are worth sharing to stimulate thinking beyond our current constraints.

- In Europe, long-term care facilities seem to most often have private rooms including universal design features such as private bathrooms with standard walk-in showers (**Figure 10-5**). Access to the outdoors and walking paths is expected (**Figure 10-6**). In Norway and other Scandinavian countries, people pay a portion of their retirement income for long-term care housing (generally 75–80%) (H. Danielson, personal communication, March 20, 2012).

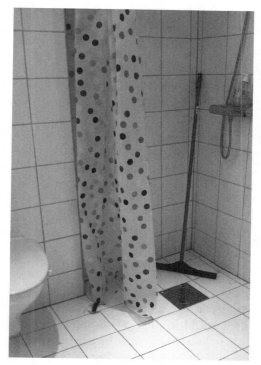

Figure 10-5   An accessible walk-in shower (universal design).

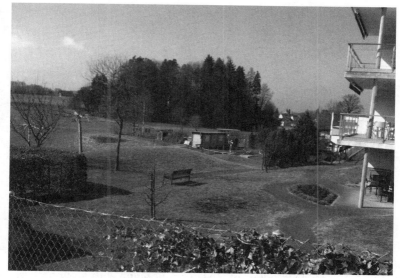

Figure 10-6   Opportunities to enjoy the outdoors.

- Many long-term care facilities abroad have cafés that are open and inviting to the public. When you walk into these facilities the smell of baked goods is pleasing, and therefore the cafés are frequented by local community members looking for light fare at a reasonable cost or a convenient place to meet friends. Perhaps the best outcome of this design is the seamless integration of the public into the facility.
- In Norway, among other Scandinavian countries, a comprehensive coordinated care plan is set into motion at age 75 (or earlier as needed), beginning with an in-depth home visit from a community nurse who becomes the person's case manager to arrange services and equipment as needed from then on (H. Danielson, personal communication, March 20, 2012). Community nurses and therapists have their offices in the state-run long-term care facilities so they get to know the residents well. Adaptive equipment is loaned out and then refurbished, at no direct cost to the recipient.
- In Scandinavian countries, people also value independent living and staying at home for as long as possible. Based on a professional assessment, people can obtain in-home assistance as needed, even if this need grows to several times per day (M. Lilja, personal communication, March 22, 2012).

Two specific examples of long-term care are also worth sharing. In the Netherlands, Hogeweg is a village specifically designed for those with severe dementia. People live in the village, just as they would in their own homes, doing whatever they like to do, but instead of being on their own they are constantly monitored for safety. The residents can shop, walk, visit, eat out, take care of their homes, or engage in whatever they would like to do (**Figure 10-7**). However, behind the bucolic scenes of community life are trained

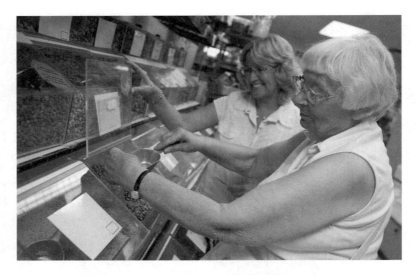

Figure 10-7   A possible resident of Hogeweg shopping with an unobtrusive helper.
© iStockphoto/Thinkstock

elder-care specialists, ready to redirect residents as needed. The Hogeweg idea is seen by some as truly inventive and creative, and by others as a *Truman Show* reality fraught with deception of the residents.[72]

The Lotte, in Copenhagen, may seem like an ordinary, albeit pleasantly appointed, long-term care facility located in an old brick home in the heart of the city (**Figure 10-8**). However, this home, started by a nurse, Thyra Banks, is certainly out of the ordinary in its day-to-day operations. The 23 residents, volunteers, and staff seem genuinely happy to be there and are eager to greet visitors. Based on the Eden Alternative, the residents have private rooms and are free to do what they like. There is no problem with wandering because if residents want to take a walk, someone simply goes with them. There are no strict rules; if people want to stay up late singing and dancing, they are welcome to do just that. Partying is encouraged, and sleeping pills simply are not necessary (A. Garvold, personal communication, March 17, 2012). Perhaps the most unusual and outstanding event that takes place is the annual vacation for the residents and staff to Spain or Greece. Nearly everyone goes, and family members are invited too. The vacation is largely paid for out of the staff sick-pay fund, which the Lotte is able to use because people so rarely call in sick.[73]

Throughout the world providers and policy makers are rethinking how to support people in their quest to age well. One approach mentioned as being used at the Lotte and currently gaining visibility is the **Eden Alternative**. This nonprofit organization

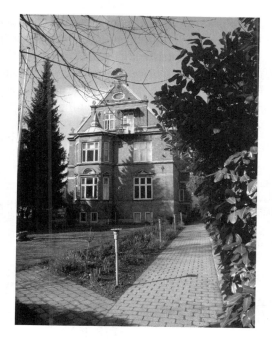

Figure 10-8 The Lotte in Copenhagen

provides education and resources to help long-term care organizations change their culture and environments from being facilities to warehouse the frail to being habitats to support living human beings. Their focus is on promoting meaning in life and a variety of activities in a friendly warm atmosphere. The philosophy includes encouraging resident autonomy; creating opportunities for meaningful activities, including caring for other living things (e.g., pets, plants, and engaging with children); and enhancing spontaneity and variety throughout the day.[74] To date, 300 long-term care homes in the United States, Canada, Europe, and Australia have registered to commit to using the Eden Alternative philosophy. Research is beginning to surface about the benefits of this model. For example, the West Midlands–based Accord Housing Association in the United Kingdom reported a precipitous decrease in the use of psychotropic drugs (from 47% to 2%) by adhering to the Eden Alternative and giving residents more choice and control.[75]

SUMMARY

A desired, or at the least, satisfactory living situation can provide the foundation for maintaining quality of life for older adults. Although safety is paramount, perhaps an equally important consideration is respecting choices made by competent older adults and supporting their quality of life in the environments of their choosing. Such a home, described by Garrett,[2] "fulfills many needs: it is a place of shelter and security, inspires a sense of belonging and mastery, and allows the person to be him- or herself, reinforcing (by the presence of significant personal items) their life and identity."

Older people have a variety of opportunities to live in such a home, whether it is a house, apartment, SRO, CCRC, assisted living facility, or nursing facility. The home, not just a space to reside, should be a place as pleasing, as affordable, and as accessible as possible to the individual. Along with safe and enjoyable surroundings, older people also need social support systems (provided by their families or beyond) and opportunities to participate in personally meaningful activities and contribute to their communities, for these are the ingredients needed to promote a healthy and fulfilling aging experience.

Review Questions

1. Most older people in the United States would prefer to live _____ if widowed.
   A. Alone
   B. With their children
   C. In their own home
   D. In an SRO

2. Universal design
   A. Supports aging in place
   B. Can be used only with new construction

    C. Requires single-story construction
    D. Is helpful only to people with disabilities

3. All the following characteristics describe SROs, *except*
    A. Private bathrooms
    B. One room
    C. Limited kitchen facilities
    D. Low cost

4. Which one of the following services is not available at CCRCs?
    A. A continuum of long-term care as long as needed
    B. Assistance with personal care
    C. Rehabilitation services
    D. Hospital services

5. _____ is/are an option for short-term rehabilitation care before moving to another setting.
    A. Single-room occupancies
    B. Skilled nursing facilities
    C. Subsidized housing
    D. Residential care facilities

Learning Activities

1. The seven principles of universal design are:[76]
   - Equitable use
   - Flexibility in use
   - Simple and intuitive use
   - Perceptible information
   - Tolerance for error
   - Low physical effort
   - Size and space for approach and use

   Discuss how these relate specifically to an aging population. Come up with specific examples. You may need to do some additional research online to relate these to concepts learned in this chapter.

2. Without referring back to the chapter, individually list the five most important things for you when considering your own environment when you are older. Compare your answers with the group. What can you learn from the answers of others?

3. Brainstorm about different ways that older people can improve their quality of life. Be creative. Remember, in brainstorming there are no wrong answers. How can a variety of healthcare professionals assist in the improvement process? Give specific examples from different professional perspectives.

4. Spend some time designing your future retirement community. You can list features or draw them out. Be specific. Share the designs among the group. Discuss the cost of the design elements and care you plan to provide. Will your community be suitable and affordable for the general population? Why or why not?

5. Do a little additional research on continuing care retirement communities (CCRCs). What are some advantages and disadvantages of this type of setting? How could these be made more accessible for older people?

REFERENCES

1. MacDonald, M, et al. Research considerations: The link between housing and health in the elderly. *Journal of Gerontological Nursing*, 1994;20:5–10.

2. Minkler, M. Community organizing among the elderly poor in the United States: A case study. *International Journal of Health Services*, 1992;22:303–316.

3. National Association of Triads. The Makeup of Triad. Retrieved July 2, 2008, from http://www.nationaltriad.org/tools/Triad-at-a-Glance.pdf

4. National Aging in Place Council. Aging in Place Glossary of Terms. Retrieved July 9, 2008, from http://www.naipc.org/AGuidetoAginginPlace/GlossaryofTerms/tabid/103/Default.aspx

5. Hood, A. Coming home for elders may take a village. *Aging Today,* 2011;32(4), 14.

6. Alley, D, Liebig, P, Pynoos, J, Banerjee, T, Choi, IH. Creating elder-friendly communities: Preparations for an aging society. *Journal of Gerontological Social Work,* 2007;49(1/2):1–18.

7. Kerschner, H, Pegues, JA. Productive aging: A quality of life agenda. *Journal of the American Dietetic Association*, 1998;98(12):1445–1448.

8. Terracciano, A, et al. Personality predictors of longevity: Activity, emotional stability, and conscientiousness. *Psychosomatic Medicine*, 2008; 70(6):621–627.

9. Phillips, EM, Davidoff, D. Normal and successful aging: What happens to function as we age. *Primary Psychiatry*, 2004;11(1):35–38, 47.

10. Hong, LK, Duff, RW. Widows in retirement communities: The social context of subjective well-being. *Gerontologist*, 1994;34:347.

11. Cox, J. It's a lifeline. *Elderly Care*, 1996;8:13–15.

12. National Alliance for Caregiving and AARP. *Caregiving in the US*. Bethesda, MD: National Alliance for Caregiving, 2004.

13. Yarry, S, Stevens, EK, McCallum, TJ. Cultural influences on spousal caregiving. *Generations, American Society on Aging*, 2007;31(3):24–30. Retrieved February 14, 2009, from http://www.asaging.org/publications/dbase/GEN/Gen.31_3.Yarry.pdf

14. Center for Universal Design, North Carolina State University. About Universal Design. Retrieved July 16, 2008, from http://www.design.ncsu.edu/cud/about_ud/about_ud.htm

15. Cannava, E. "Gerodesign": Safe and comfortable living spaces for older adults. *Geriatrics*, 1994;49:45–49.

16. Figueiro, MG. Lighting the Way: A Key to Independence. 2001. Retrieved April 15, 2013, from http://www.lrc.rpi.edu/programs/lightHealth/AARP/pdf/AARPbook1.pdf

17. Dethlefs, N, Martin, B. Japanese technology for aged care. *Science and Public Policy*, 2006;33(1): 47–57.

18. Saunders, P. Japan Proposes Robots to Help Elderly as Population Implodes. LifeNews.com (Tokyo). November 12, 2012. Retrieved May 10, 2013, from http://www.lifenews.com/2012/11/12/japan-proposes-robots-to-help-elderly-as-population-implodes/

19. Rantz, MJ, et al. Evaluation of aging in place model with home care services and registered nurse care coordination in senior housing. *Nursing Outlook*, 2012;59(1):37–46.

20. Houser, A. Long-Term Care Fact Sheet. AARP. 2007. Retrieved July 4, 2008, from http://www.aarp.org/research/longtermcare/trends/fs27r_ltc.html

21. Kassner, E. *Medicaid and Long-Term Services and Supports for Older People: Fact Sheet.* Washington, DC: AARP Public Policy Institute, 2005.

22. Garrett, G. But does it feel like home? Accommodation needs on later life. *Professional Nurse,* 1992;7:254–257.

23. Administration on Aging, U.S. Department of Health and Human Services. *A Profile of Older Americans: 2010.* Washington, DC: U.S. Department of Health and Human Services, 2010. Retrieved April 15, 2013, from http://www.aoa.gov/aoaroot/aging_statistics/Profile/2010/10.aspx

24. Coleman-Jensen, A, Nord, M, Andrews, M, Carlson, S. *Household Food Security in the United States in 2011.* Washington, DC: USDA ERS, 2012.

25. Ziliak, J, Gundersen, C. *Food Insecurity Among Older Adults.* A report submitted to the AARP Foundation, Aug. 2011.

26. Stucki, B. *Use Your Home to Stay at Home.* Washington, DC: National Council on the Aging, 2005.

27. National Reverse Mortgage Lenders Association. NRMLA. Retrieved April 15, 2013, from http://www.nrmlaonline.org/nrmla/default.aspx

28. Jewish Federation of North America. All About NORCs. Retrieved April 15, 2013 from http://www.norcs.org/page.aspx?id=119552

29. Enguidanos, S, Pynoos, J, Denton, A, Alexman, S, Diepenbrock, L. Comparison of barriers and facilitators in developing NORC programs: A tale of two communities. *Journal of Housing for the Elderly,* 2010;24(3/4):291–303.

30. Ormond, BA, et al. *Supportive Services Programs in Naturally Occurring Retirement Communities.* Washington, DC: U.S. Department of Health and Human Services, 2004.

31. Opp, A. Productively Aging: St. Louis's Naturally Occurring Retirement Community. American Occupational Therapy Association. Retrieved

July 10, 2008, from http://www.aota.org/news/centennial/40313/aging/40617.aspx

32. U.S. Census Bureau retrieved July 28, 2013, from http://www.insideeldercare.com/uncategorized/more-elderly-parents-living-with-adult-children/

33. U.S. Department of Housing and Urban Development. Single Room Occupancy Program (SRO). Retrieved July 28, 2013, from http://portal.hud.gov/hudportal/HUD?src=/program_offices/comm_planning/homeless/programs/sro

34. American Association of Homes and Services for the Aging. Aging Services: The Facts. Retrieved June 19, 2008, from http://www.aahsa.org/article.aspx?id=74

35. Cohousing Association of the United States. What Is Cohousing? Retrieved July 7, 2008, from http://www.cohousing.org/what_is_cohousing

36. U.S. Office of Personnel Management. *The Handbook of Elder Care Resources for the Federal Workplace.* Retrieved July 7, 2008, from http://www.opm.gov/Employment_and_Benefits/WorkLife/OfficialDocuments/Handbooks-Guides/ElderCareResources/index.asp

37. Rosenbeck, R, Bassuk, E, Salomon, A. Special Populations of Homeless Americans. Retrieved July 4, 2008, from http://aspe.hhs.gov/progsys/homeless/symposium/2-spclpop.htm

38. Genworth Financial. Compare Cost of Care Across the United States. 2013. Retrieved April 5, 2013, from https://www.genworth.com/corporate/about-genworth/industry-expertise/cost-of-care.html

39. Adams, PF, Kirzinger, WK, Martinez, ME. Summary health statistics for the US population: National Health Interview Survey, 2011. *Vital Health Statistics,* 2012;10(255):18. Retrieved April 16, 2013, from http://www.cdc.gov/nchs/data/series/sr_10/sr10_255.pdf

40. Agency for Healthcare Research and Quality. *Long-Term Care Users Range in Age and Most Do Not Live in Nursing Homes: Research Alert.* Rockville, MD: AHRQ, 2000.

41. Thompson, L. *Long-Term Care: Support for Family Caregivers.* Washington, DC: Long-Term Financing Project, Georgetown University Press, 2004.

42. U.S. Department of Health and Human Services, Assistant Secretary for Planning and

Evaluation. *The Future Supply of Long-Term Care Workers in Relation to the Aging Baby Boom Generation*. Report to Congress. Washington, DC: U.S. Department of Health and Human Services, 2003.

43. Kaiser Commission. The Medicaid Program at a Glance. 2013. Retrieved April 17, 2013, from http://www.kff.org/medicaid/upload/7235-02 .pdf

44. Ujvari, K. Long term care insurance: 2012 update. AARP Public Policy Institute Fact Sheet. Retrieved July 28, 2013, from http://www.aarp .org/content/dam/aarp/research/public_policy_ institute/ltc/2012/ltc-insurance-2012-update- AARP-ppi-ltc.pdf

45. Health, United States, 2011. National Health Expenditures. 2011 Highlights. Retrieved July 28, 2013, from http://www.cdc.gov/nchs/data /hus/hus11.pdf

46. National Association for Home Care and Hospice (NAHC). Home Page. Retrieved April 18, 2013, from http://www.nahc.org

47. Kinsella, A. About Home Telehealth. Retrieved April 18, 2013, from http://www.longtermcare- link.net/eldercare/home_telehealth.htm#patient

48. Winthrop University Hospital. Winthrop's Tele- health Monitoring Program: Making the Home the Preferred Place of Care. Retrieved April 18, 2013, from http://www.winthrop.org/news- room/publications/vol20_no1_2010/page6.cfm

49. The Joint Commission. Home—the Best Place for Health Care: A Positioning Statement from The Joint Commission on the State of the Home Care Industry. 2011. Retrieved April 19, 2013, from http://www.jointcommission.org/assets/1/18 /Home_Care_position_paper_4_5_11.pdf

50. Tanaz, P, Anderson, G. Program of All-Inclusive Care for the Elderly. Health Policy Monitor. April 2009. Retrieved April 18, 2013, from http://www.npaonline.org/website/download .asp?id=3034&title=PACE_-_HealthPolicy- Monitor_-_2009

51. MetLife Mature Market Institute. *Market Survey of Long Term Care Costs. The 2009 MetLife Market Survey of Nursing Home, Assisted Living, Adult Day Services, and Home Care Costs.* Westport, CT: MetLife, 2009. Retrieved April 19, 2013, from https://www.metlife.com/assets

/cao/mmi/publications/studies/mmi-market- survey-nursing-home-assisted-living.pdf

52. IBISWorld. Industry Report. Retrieved April 18, 2013, from http://www.ibisworld.com /industry/adult-day-care.html

53. Wake Forest University School of Medicine. Report: Shortage of Adult Day Services in Most U.S. Counties. 2002. Retrieved April 19, 2013, from http://www.rwjf.org/en/research-publica- tions/find-rwjf-research/2004/01/report--short- age-of-adult-day-services-in-most-u-s--coun- ties.html

54. Pandya, S. Adult Day Services. AARP. Retrieved July 4, 2008, from http://www.aarp.org /research/housing-mobility/homecare /aresearch-import-839.html

55. MetLife Mature Market Institute. *Market Survey of Long Term Care Costs. The 2012 Market Survey of Long Term Care Costs.* New York: MetLife, Nov. 2012. Retrieved May 9, 2013, from https://www.metlife.com/assets/cao/mmi /publications/studies/2012/studies/mmi- 2012-market-survey-long-term-care-costs.pdf

56. Schacke, C, Zank, SR. Measuring the effective- ness of adult day care as a facility to support family caregivers of dementia patients. *Journal of Applied Gerontology*, 2006;25(1):65–81.

57. Dabelko-Schoeny, H, King, S. In their own words: Participants' perceptions of the impact of adult day services. *Journal of Gerontological Social Work*, 2010;53(2):176–192.

58. Zarit, S H, Kim, K, Femia, EE, Almeida, DM, Savla, J, Molenaar, PCM. Effects of adult day care on daily stress of caregivers: A within-per- son approach. *Journals of Gerontology Series B: Psychological Sciences and Social Sciences*, 2011; 66B(5):538–546.

59. Golant, SM. *Housing America's Elderly: Many Possibilities/Few Choices*. Newbury Park, CA: Sage, 1992:229–246.

60. Assisted Living Federation of America. What Is Assisted Living? Retrieved July 4, 2008, from http://www.alfa.org

61. Just, G, et al. Assisted living: Challenges for nursing practice. *Geriatric Nursing*, 1995;16: 165–168.

62. National Center for Assisted Living. Assisted Living Facility Profile. Retrieved April 21, 2013,

from http://www.alfa.org/alfa/ALFA_Update.asp

63. Wright, B. Assisted Living in the United States. 2004. Retrieved July 6, 2013, from http://assets.aarp.org/rgcenter/post-import/fs62r_assisted.pdf

64. Cannuscio, C, Block, J, Kawachi, I. Social capital and successful aging: The role of senior housing. *Annals of Internal Medicine,* 2003; *139*(5 part 2, Suppl.):395–399.

65. Family Caregiver Alliance. Fact Sheet: Residential Care Options. Retrieved June 30, 2008, from http://www.caregiver.org/caregiver/jsp/content_node.jsp?nodeid=1742

66. AARP. About Continuing Care Retirement Communities. Retrieved July 8, 2008, from http://www.aarp.org/families/housing_choices/other_options/a2004-02-26-retirementcommunity.html

67. Hospice Association of America. Hospice Facts and Statistics. Retrieved July 4, 2008, from http://www.nahc.org/HAA/

68. Prince, D, Butler, D. *Final Report: Aging in Place in America.* Clarity and the EAR Foundation. Retrieved July 28, 2013, from http://www.slideshare.net/clarityproducts/clarity-2007-aginig-in-place-in-america-2836029

69. National Long Term Care Ombudsman Resource Center. What Does an Ombudsman Do? Retrieved July 28, 2013, from http://www.ltcombudsman.org/about-ombudsmen

70. Harmon, LC & Harmon, KM. We don't like nursing homes. Retrieved July 28, 2013, from http://www.alzheimersreadingroom.com/2010/03/we-dont-like-nursing-homes.html

71. Sørbye, LW, Hamran, T, Henriksen, N, Norberg, AA. Home care patients in four Nordic capitals. *Scandinavian Journal of Caring Sciences,* 2009;23:736–747.

72. Charter, D. For the Alzheimer Victims Lost in Time, a New Village of Care. March 31, 2012. Retrieved July 6, 2013, from http://www.thetimes.co.uk/tto/news/world/europe/article3370109.ece

73. Steed, J. Elderly thrive in Denmark. *The Star,* Nov. 9, 2008.

74. The Eden Alternative. Retrieved April 22, 2013, from http://www.edenalt.org

75. Dash. Housing Association Sees Dramatic Fall in Use of Psychotropic Drugs. 2011. Retrieved July 6, 2013, from http://www.24dash.com/news/housing/2011-07-07-Housing-association-sees-dramatic-fall-in-use-of-psychotropic-drugs

76. Centre for Excellence in Universal Design. The 7 Principles. Retrieved July 6, 2013, from http://universaldesign.ie/exploreampdiscover/the7principles

POLICY AND ETHICAL ISSUES FOR OLDER ADULTS

LANEY ANNE BRUNER-CANHOTO, PhD, MSW, MPH

It was once said that the moral test of government is how that government treats those who are in the dawn of life, the children; those who are in the twilight of life, the elderly; and those who are in the shadows of life—the sick, the needy and the handicapped [sic; today known as people with disabilities].

—Hubert Humphrey, 1977 speech*

Chapter Outline

Behavioral Objectives

Upon completion of this chapter, the reader will be able to:

1. List the eligibility criteria for Social Security, Medicare, and Medicaid.
2. Describe what is provided through Social Security.
3. Understand how Social Security, Medicare, and Medicaid are accessed.
4. Explain the differences among Social Security, private pension, and Supplemental Security Income.
5. Describe what is covered under Medicare and Medicaid.

---

* Congressional Record, November 4, 1977, Vol. 123, p. 37287.

6. Compare and contrast Medicare and Medicaid.
7. Explain the programs available through the Aging Network and their structures.
8. Describe how the Americans with Disabilities Act impacts health care.
9. Explain how long-term services and supports are funded in the United States.
10. Explain the limitations of a power of attorney for financial matters for older adults.
11. List the differences between a power of attorney and a conservatorship.
12. Compare and contrast a living will and a durable healthcare power of attorney.
13. List the ways in which healthcare decisions can be made on behalf of an individual.
14. Identify resources for cases of suspected elder abuse and neglect.

Key Terms

Advance directive	Long-term services and supports
Aging Network	Medicaid
Americans with Disabilities Act	Medicaid waivers
Area agencies on aging	Medicare
Competency (competent)	Medigap
Conservator	Older Americans Act (OAA)
Durable healthcare power of attorney	Power of attorney (POA)
Elder abuse and neglect	Social Security
Guardian	State units on aging
Living will	Supplemental Security Income (SSI)
Long-term care insurance (LTCI)	

Public policy issues and ethics affect everyone at all stages of life and in many different ways. Education policy requires certain behaviors of children and their parents. Transportation policy affects how people travel, whether on the interstate system that President Eisenhower began, on public transportation, or in environmentally friendly "green" vehicles. For older adults, specific policies have a real impact on their lives, including finances (Social Security) and health care (Medicare and Medicaid). Healthcare professionals need to know what these policies are, whom they cover, what services they provide, and how to access them to be able to fully help older clients and patients.

The specific policies covered in this chapter include income policies (Social Security and Supplemental Security Income, two distinct and separate policies) and healthcare policies (Medicare and Medicaid, also two distinct and separate policies). The specific federal policy for this population, the Older Americans Act, is discussed as an important foundation for services for older adults. A civil rights policy, the Americans with Disabilities Act, is also reviewed for its impact on elders who may have a disability.

Ethics also have an important place in the lives of older adults, especially related to decision making. All adults, including elders, are presumed to be autonomous and competent to make their own decisions. These decisions include financial, personal, and healthcare decisions. Healthcare professionals need to understand how decision-making processes and the legal mechanisms to assist decision making operate and can affect their elder clients and patients. Another ethical issue healthcare professionals may face is elder abuse and neglect. Knowing what abuse is and what resources are available, along with the decision-making resources and reporting laws, allows healthcare professionals to ensure that older patients and clients are able to live safely and as independently as possible.

This chapter is organized into three main sections. In the first, brief section, a high-level overview of the ever-evolving nature of policy and a historical perspective on elder policy is presented, with specific emphasis on current healthcare reform legislation under President Obama. In the second section, Policy Issues, specific policies related to older adults will be described including an overview, a brief history, a description of eligibility criteria, an explanation of benefits, and instructions on how to access the policy or program. The third section, Ethical Issues, concentrates on financial and healthcare decision making and then on elder abuse and neglect.

POLICY OVERVIEW

THE EVER-EVOLVING NATURE OF POLICY

Just as science and medical care have evolved over the years, so too have public policy and ethics. The issues described in this chapter are current as of 2013; however, they are ever-evolving. A prime example of this is the Patient Protection and Affordable Care Act (ACA) of 2010 (P.L. 111–148), President Obama's healthcare reform legislation. The ACA's individual mandate requires most individuals living in the United States to have health insurance through employer-based insurance, health insurance exchanges, or the optional expansion of state programs including Medicaid.[1] There are also some specific provisions that affect older adults. These provisions include drug rebates for Medicare beneficiaries and the eventual closing of the Part D "doughnut hole" (a prescription drug coverage gap in Medicare), the creation of a center to provide funds to states to implement programs for individuals who are dually eligible for Medicare and Medicaid, and the expansion of home- and community-based services benefits for Medicaid populations.[2]

If this chapter had been written right after the ACA was passed, one of the major benefits that would have been provided to future elders was the CLASS provision. The CLASS Act (Community Living Assistance Services and Supports) was to be a national voluntary home- and community-based services insurance program designed to provide a cash benefit, after an initial 5-year vesting period, to individuals who needed nonmedical services to remain in the community. The program was to be funded through payroll deductions. However, this provision was determined to be unsustainable through the proposed funding mechanism and was repealed.[3] Additionally, if the Supreme Court decision (which upheld much of the ACA) had struck down the entire law, this chapter might be focused less on Medicaid and more on private pay options for older adults.

Currently, the ACA has several specific and relevant points for older adults.[4] As mentioned, there are prescription drug discounts for certain medications covered through Medicare as well as the closing of the coverage gap for prescription drugs (the "doughnut hole"). Under Medicare, older adults receive an annual wellness visit and additional preventive screenings like mammograms and colonoscopies with no deductibles or copayments. With the ACA, Medicare and Medicaid fraud and abuse protections are expanded. The ACA seeks to enhance quality of care for all individuals, including older adults, through the implementation and evaluation of better coordination strategies and programs (like the accountable care organizations and dually eligible [Medicare and Medicaid] initiatives).

HISTORICAL PERSPECTIVES ON ELDER POLICY

Policies and programs for older adults in the United States are a relatively recent development. In the past, there were relatively few older adults, and the community, typically families, took care of aging individuals. Older adults without family were often relegated to poorhouses, subsisting on meager charity based on poor laws.[5]

With the passage of the Social Security Act in 1935, there was a dawning awareness of the need for policies and programs to assist individuals as they grew older. Much of the early policy focus for older adults was on finances and retirement, with amendments to Social Security expanding eligibility and eliminating limits in the 1950s and 1960s. Social Security has had a tremendous impact on the poverty rate of older adults, helping 14 million older adults out of poverty in 2011.[6,7]

During the 1960s, social service programs and funds, precursors to the current Aging Network of service providers, were also allocated for older adults. In 1961, the first White House Conference on Aging was held, followed by the establishment of the Commission on Aging in 1962. The Aging Network really took hold with the Older Americans Act of 1965, which created the Federal Administration on Aging and state units on aging.[8]

In fact, 1965 was an enormous year for both elder policy and healthcare policy affecting older adults. Medicare was established, creating federal healthcare insurance for older adults. Medicaid was also enacted, creating healthcare assistance programs at the state level for individuals with low income or resources (including older adults and people with disabilities).

In 1990, the Americans with Disabilities Act was enacted, calling for the integration of people with disabilities (including elders) into employment, services, and health care. Following the "independent living" philosophy, disability advocates who fought for the ADA are now influencing how services are provided to older adults.[9] All of these policies and programs exist today, though with amendments and specific changes dictated by current circumstances, politics, and demographics.

POLICY ISSUES

SOCIAL SECURITY

Social Security is the Old-Age, Survivors, and Disability Insurance (OASDI) program. It is funded through taxes on workers and employers. These taxes are paid into the Federal Old-Age and Survivors Insurance Trust Fund (better known as the Social Security Trust Fund). The current taxes pay for current benefits. Workers today are funding Social Security benefits for today's beneficiaries.

Much of the debate on Social Security revolves around whether Social Security will be able to pay out benefits to future generations of beneficiaries. This debate involves demographic and actuarial projections, which are uncertain. For example, life expectancy will play into the exact prediction of when the trust fund will be exhausted (that is, when expenses exceed the total trust fund income). The number of individuals in the workforce will be another factor. Even as baby boomers are retiring in greater numbers, if the relative good health they enjoy compared to past generations induces some baby boomers to delay retirement, then these individuals will continue to pay into the trust fund, rather than get "paid" from the trust fund.

History[10]   Franklin Roosevelt signed the Social Security Act in 1935; over the years, the act has been amended to evolve with the social, economic, and political tenor of the time. Social Security, at the federal level, was enacted to decrease the poverty rate among older adults, which was high during the Great Depression of the 1930s.

When it was enacted, Social Security covered all workers in commerce and industry (except for railroads). These categories excluded farm workers, domestic workers, and teachers, categories that were composed predominantly of women and minorities. The exclusions have been eliminated over time through amendments to the Social Security Act.

In addition, amendments in 1939 added spouses and children under the age of 18 years old for dependent benefits, in cases where the worker was still alive, and survivor benefits, when a worker experienced a premature death. Amendments in 1950 created cost of living allowances (COLAs), which increased Social Security amounts (which until then had been a static amount) by a certain percent increase. Further amendments allowed for additional COLAs, until legislation in 1972 created automatic COLAs.

In the 1980s, there was a concern about the financing of Social Security. This concern led to taxation of Social Security benefits and the slow increase in the retirement age from 65 to 67 in the 2000s. Other amendments have allowed older adults to remain in the workforce and still receive some Social Security benefits and, most recently, have excluded prisoners from receiving Social Security benefits.

Whom It Covers[11]   Although this is a chapter on policy issues for older adults, Social Security as a policy solution is not just for older adults or for retired workers. Nonelder beneficiaries of Social Security include workers with disabilities and dependents and survivors of workers who have participated in Social Security. Social Security covers workers who have earned enough credits through work. Typically, for people born in 1929 or later, they will need to have worked for at least 10 years to earn the 40 work credits needed to qualify for Social Security. Workers usually earn 4 credits for each year of work.

Individual workers can begin collecting Social Security benefits at age 62 (although workers with disabilities and dependents and survivors of workers may begin receiving Social Security benefits earlier). The benefit is greater for individual workers who wait until their full retirement age, which is based on their birth year. The benefit is reduced by 0.5% for each month Social Security benefits are begun before the worker reaches full retirement age. See **Table 11-1** to determine the full retirement age.

Workers need not stop working completely to receive Social Security; however, depending on how old the worker is and how much he or she makes, the monthly Social Security benefit amount may be reduced until the worker reaches the full retirement age. Workers can also delay the start of Social Security benefits until age 70, which will increase their benefits by a certain percentage, depending on year of birth (8% for people born in 1943 or later).[12]

Social Security also covers spouses and, in certain cases, former spouses of workers. Spouses may collect Social Security benefits based on their husband's or wife's work history or on their own, depending on which amount is higher. Former spouses may collect if they were married to the worker for 10 or more years and they have not remarried.

What It Provides[13]   Social Security was originally developed as a floor or foundation for workers' retirement income; it was not meant to be the only source of income. Currently, however, statistics show that Social Security provides the largest part of older adults' income: in 2010, 37% of income for individuals 65 or older was from Social Security, with earnings (30%), pensions (19%), and asset income (11%) rounding out the other main sources of

Table 11-1 Full Retirement Age

Year of Birth	Full Retirement Age
1943–1954	66
1955	66 and 2 months
1956	66 and 4 months
1957	66 and 6 months
1958	66 and 8 months
1959	66 and 10 months
1960 or later	67

Reproduced from Social Security Administration. *Understanding the Benefits* (SSA Publication No. 05-10024). Washington, DC: U.S. Government Printing Office, 2012: 9.

income.[13] For older adults with the lowest income, Social Security accounts for about 80% of their income. Benefits for Social Security depend on a worker's earnings, retirement age, working status, and relationship to the worker (in the case of spouses, dependents, and survivors).

How to Access[11]   Workers who are retiring should apply for Social Security benefits 3 months before they want to begin receiving benefits. Applications can be made online (www.socialsecurity.gov/applyforbenefits), on the telephone (1-800-772-1213, TTY 1-800-325-0778), or in person by making an appointment at the local Social Security office. Specific documentation is needed for the application process, and staff at the Social Security office can help to obtain the necessary documentation in the proper format.

Benefits are delivered electronically, either through direct deposit to a bank account or through a prepaid debit card program.

Supplemental Security Income[14]   The Social Security Administration also operates the **Supplemental Security Income (SSI)** program. The SSI program provides a monthly monetary payment for eligible individuals with little or no income and low resources. Eligibility criteria include individuals who are 65 years old or older, individuals who are legally blind, or individuals who are determined to be disabled. Many of these individuals may also receive Social Security benefits as noted previously, but an individual does not have to be receiving Social Security to receive SSI. Social Security and SSI are funded through different mechanisms. Whereas Social Security is funded through payroll taxes and eligibility is based on whether an individual or a member of his or her family paid into the system, SSI is financed through the U.S. Treasury's general funds.

Often individuals who receive SSI are eligible for Medicaid, although as shown later in this chapter, each state has different eligibility requirements for Medicaid. Also, most states supplement SSI benefits with an additional monetary payment each month. Furthermore, states can choose to have the federal government administer the entire benefit amount of federal SSI plus state supplement, have the federal government administer the entire benefit amount for some categories of recipients but not others (dual administration states), or administer the state supplement on its own. This arrangement matters to individuals when they need to contact someone about their benefit.

The amount of the SSI benefit (federal and state supplement) will be determined by an individual's income, resources, and living arrangement. For each of these categories, SSI has specific rules. Certain individuals are not allowed SSI benefits; these include fugitives from the law, individuals in prison or jail, individuals in publicly funded institutions, and individuals who only qualify for SSI because they gave away resources. SSI benefits also vary by who is paying for their room, board, and utilities.

Applications can be made on the telephone (1-800-772-1213, TTY 1-800-325-0778) or in person by making an appointment at the local Social Security office. No online SSI applications are available.

Pension/Retirement Income[15]   Many older adults have private pension or retirement income from a previous job(s), with about 50% of all private workers participating in some retirement plan/pension program. Retirement income typically comes in one of two forms: defined benefit or defined contribution programs. Initially, companies offered defined benefit programs. These pension programs were created such that individuals worked for a certain amount of time and then were guaranteed a specific amount (benefit) upon retirement as a lifetime annuity. Companies began moving away from those types of programs and now usually offer defined contribution programs like 401(k) accounts, where employees and employers set aside a specific amount into the program (defined contribution), which together with investment returns then determines the amount of the benefit upon retirement. Regular income of any pension type provides around 19% of the income for individuals 65 years or older. This, however, may not include income that is taken from other retirement accounts (like individual retirement accounts [IRAs]) because these amounts are often taken irregularly.

MEDICARE

Medicare is a social insurance program for older adults and certain other people. Social insurance is a government-sponsored program for which participation is generally mandatory for a defined population. A social insurance program's benefits and eligibility are defined by law and it is funded through taxes from or on behalf of participants. Medicare and Social Security are both examples of social insurance.[16]

History[17]   Medicare was created as the insurance program for elders in 1965 when President Lyndon B. Johnson signed H.R. 6675 (PL 89-97). Much of the early years of Medicare, through the 1970s, saw the expansion of eligible groups and covered services. For example, the Social Security Amendments of 1972 expanded Medicare to allow coverage for individuals with end-stage renal disease. In 1972, covered services also were expanded to include some chiropractic and rehabilitation therapy services.

In 1981, however, Congress became more concerned about slowing Medicare's growth and so put in place a variety of laws to limit Medicare spending. Laws were enacted that increased deductibles, instituted different payment methodologies for hospitals and physician services, and limited benefits such as home health and therapy services. For example, the Omnibus Budget Reconciliation Acts (OBRAs) of 1987, 1989, and 1993 modified payments to Medicare providers and changed physician billing. In 1988, the Medicare Catastrophic Coverage Act expanded coverage with a prescription drug benefit and caps on out-of-pocket expenses, and increased hospital and nursing facility benefits. However, by 1989, most of that act had been repealed. The Balanced Budget Act of 1997 continued the trend of implementing new payment methods for Medicare providers, including home health services and outpatient rehabilitation services. In 2003, with the Medicare Modernization Act, Medicare coverage was expanded to prescription drugs.

Current discussion revolves around the sustainability of Medicare and how it should be funded. Medicare is financed through payroll taxes kept in a trust fund, general revenues, premiums, and state payments (for certain benefits). Specifically, what people pay into the system is paying for the Medicare benefits of eligible individuals now. Debate centers on how long the Part A Hospital Insurance trust fund will remain solvent (insolvency will occur when the trust fund runs out of money to pay for Medicare benefits), with actuaries looking over a 70-year time horizon. The ACA enacted several provisions to slow Medicare spending and ensure the solvency of the trust fund, while improving benefits and the quality of care for beneficiaries. At present, the trust fund is expected to remain solvent through 2024.[18]

Whom It Covers[17]   Medicare covers people 65 years old and older, certain people under 65 years old with long-term disabilities, and adults with end-stage renal disease requiring dialysis or transplant. The inclusion of this specific disease category occurred in 1972 and was driven by Shep Glazer, who appeared before the House Ways and Means Committee while receiving dialysis. Since 2000, those with the diagnosis of another specific disease, amyotrophic lateral sclerosis (ALS), are also allowed to enroll in Medicare upon diagnosis instead of waiting the 24 months as other adults with disabilities do after a qualifying disability/disease.

What It Provides[18-20]   Medicare is composed of several different benefits or "parts," which provide specific help in covering certain healthcare services. Part A is also known as Hospital Insurance, and it covers inpatient hospital care, limited skilled nursing facility care (nursing homes), hospice, and home health care. Part B, also known as Medical Insurance, covers doctor/provider services, outpatient care, home health care, durable medical equipment, and some types of preventative services. Part C is Medicare Advantage plans, which include Part A and B services and are run by private insurance companies. Part D is the Medicare Prescription Drug Coverage, and is also run by private insurance companies.

Part A is financed through payroll taxes, paid by both employers and employees, and kept in the Hospital Insurance trust fund. In 2013 the payroll tax was 1.45% for employees and employers (total 2.9%) for all but higher-income taxpayers. Part A covers a semiprivate hospital room (unless a private room is medically necessary), meals, nursing services, and other medically necessary supplies and services. Part A accounted for 31% of Medicare spending in 2012. People with Medicare Part A are covered if there is an order from a doctor that the illness or injury requires inpatient hospital care, if the type of care can only be given in a hospital, if the hospital accepts Medicare, and if the hospital's utilization review process/entity approves of the hospital stay. Although Part A pays for the hospital stay, deductibles, coinsurance, and lifetime reserve days determine the amount that each Medicare hospital patient pays during a stay.

Part A also covers some skilled nursing facility care. Specifically, for up to 100 days, Medicare covers skilled nursing care, medications, supplies and equipment, medical social services, dietary counseling, physical therapy, occupational therapy, and speech-language pathology services, all as necessary to meet the patient's health/medical goals. To be covered, the Medicare recipient must have Part A with days left in the benefit period, a qualifying hospital stay, and a medical need for daily skilled care. A benefit period is how Medicare measures hospital and skilled nursing facility care. It begins on the first day a beneficiary received inpatient hospital or skilled nursing facility care and ends when the beneficiary has not had hospital or skilled nursing facility care for 60 days. There is no limit to the number of benefit periods. Similar to hospital stays, the person will be charged based on the number of days in a skilled facility.

Part A covers home health services including intermittent skilled nursing care, physical and occupational therapy, and speech-language pathology services. There are certain limitations to coverage for these services. To be covered, skilled nursing services must be only intermittent. Therapy services must be reasonable in amount and frequency, and specific, safe, and effective to treat the condition. In addition, the condition must be expected to improve with such treatment or else only a skilled therapist can safely create a maintenance program. Individuals receiving this benefit must have a doctor's order and the doctor must certify that the person is homebound (meaning they should not leave their house in their condition, they cannot leave home without help, and they cannot leave home without considerable and taxing effort). The benefit covers all costs for healthcare services; individuals must pay 20% of any durable medical equipment.

Part B or Medical Insurance covers medically necessary services (such as doctor visits) and supplies and services to prevent illness. Unlike Part A, Part B is funded through a premium system and general revenues. Part B accounted for 20% of Medicare spending in 2012.

Part B benefits include clinical research, ambulance services, durable medical equipment, mental health services, therapy services, and second opinions. Part B also provides an annual wellness visit, known as the "Welcome to Medicare" preventive visit, during the first 12 months of Part B coverage (under ACA provisions). Medicare beneficiaries who have had Part B coverage for longer than 12 months receive yearly wellness visits.[21] Additionally, tobacco cessation counseling and screenings are covered under Medicare Part B. Some services are never covered by Medicare Part A or B, including routine dental and vision care, hearing aid fitting, long-term nonskilled (custodial) nursing care, dentures, and regular foot care.

Part C (Medicare Advantage) consists of plans from private insurance companies that cover Part A and Part B benefits for individuals enrolled in the plans. Monthly premiums vary by plan. Part C accounted for 22% of Medicare spending in 2012, with over 13 million individuals enrolled in Medicare Advantage plans.

All Part C plans must cover emergency care as well as all of the services covered by Part A and B or "original Medicare." The only exception is hospice, which is covered by basic Medicare even if there is a Part C/Medicare Advantage plan in place. Part C plans do not have to cover any service that is not medically necessary; however, these plans may offer benefits that are not covered under original Medicare, like vision, hearing, or dental care.

Part D covers prescription drugs, and each private insurance plan has different lists of drugs that are covered. Similar to Part C/Medicare Advantage, Part D is funded through premiums that vary by plan. Part D accounted for 11% of Medicare spending in 2012. For some Part D plans, the lists (or formularies) are organized into tiers, with different tiers costing a beneficiary a different amount. Older adults and their healthcare providers should determine the formulary as well as the rules and limits for their specific Part D coverage (such as prior authorization requirements, quantity limits, and step therapy, in which a lower cost drug must be trialed before a higher cost medication is approved).

Most Part D plans have a coverage gap, called "the doughnut hole." This gap occurs when a beneficiary and his or her Part D plan have spent a certain amount of money on prescriptions. After that amount is reached, the beneficiary must pay for all prescriptions until a yearly limit on out-of-pocket costs is reached, and then the Part D plan again begins to help pay the prescription's cost. The ACA provides some relief for Medicare beneficiaries in the doughnut hole. First and foremost, the ACA closes the coverage gap by 2020. Second, if an individual reaches the coverage gap, there is an automatic 50% discount on covered brand-name drugs (although the full amount is counted toward the yearly limit), until the limit is reached. Third, beneficiaries in the coverage gap receive a 7% discount on generic prescriptions.[22]

Many older adults will purchase additional coverage to supplement their original Medicare (Parts A and B). This coverage is known as a **Medigap** insurance policy because it fills in certain gaps in original Medicare. These gaps are costs that original Medicare does not pay, including coinsurances, deductibles, and copayments. Other gaps in original Medicare, like services not covered (e.g., long-term nonskilled care, vision, etc.), are typically not covered with a Medigap policy. Medigap policies require premiums to be paid by the individual, which vary by plan. Medigap policies in the majority of states are standardized and identified by a letter, A–N, signifying exactly what the plan covers. (Exceptions to this standardization are in Massachusetts, Minnesota, and Wisconsin, which organize Medigap plans in a different way.)

For individuals with low incomes and little to no resources, states provide several programs to assist with paying for premiums. These programs include the Qualified Medicare Beneficiary (QMB) program, Specified Low-Income Medicare Beneficiary (SLMB) program, Qualifying Individual (QI) program, and Qualified Disabled and Working Individuals (QDWI) program. Each program has certain income and resource limits and pays for certain types of premiums and/or deductibles. Any individual who qualifies for one of these programs also qualifies for Extra Help, a Medicare program designed to assist with Medicare prescription drug coverage.

How to Access[19] For individuals already receiving Social Security, Social Security will contact them about 3 months before they turn 65 years old to make decisions about their Medicare coverage (discussed later in this chapter). A person can receive Medicare at 65 years old even if he or she is delaying the receipt of Social Security retirement benefits.

To apply for Medicare for older adults, a person needs to be 64 years and 9 months old. Individuals who have been determined to be disabled and are receiving Social Security disability benefits are eligible for Medicare 24 months after the disability determination is made. About 3 months before the 2-year period is completed, Social Security will contact them. As noted, ALS is a special case. Individuals with ALS may begin receiving Medicare upon the diagnosis, without waiting.

There are several decisions that need to be made. Individuals will need to decide if they want to receive original Medicare (Parts A and B) or receive their coverage through a Part C Medicare Advantage Plan (Parts A, B, and usually D). Then older adults will have to decide if they need to include prescription drug coverage (Part D). If they receive original Medicare, individuals need to determine if they want a Medicare supplemental insurance or Medigap policy. Individuals with a Medicare Advantage Plan are not eligible for a Medigap policy. The easiest time to purchase a Medigap policy is during the Medigap open enrollment period, which is the 6-month period that begins when an elder is 65 years old or older and enrolled in Part B. Medicare beneficiaries under 65 years old may not be able to purchase a Medigap policy, depending on the state.

For the Medicare Savings Programs (see QMB, SLMB, QI, and QDWI programs discussed previously), individuals with low income and low resources can contact their state Medicaid office for assistance with the application process and to determine eligibility.

MEDICAID

Medicaid is a public assistance program that provides health care to individuals of all ages with low incomes, including individuals with disabilities. Medicaid is a federal and state partnership, whereas Medicare is the responsibility of the federal government. Medicaid is a voluntary program for each state, although all 50 states currently participate. To participate, a state must agree to cover certain services (discussed further in this section) and follow Medicaid regulations.

History[17]   Medicaid was enacted at the same time as Medicare, in 1965. It is Title XIX of the Social Security Act. As a voluntary federal–state program, states chose whether or not to participate. It was only in 1982 that all states chose Medicaid, when Arizona created its Arizona Health Care Cost Containment System. In the years since Medicaid was created, coverage and eligibility requirements and options have expanded. Other changes have been enacted to allow states to better control costs (such as the Medicaid Drug Rebate Program created by the Omnibus Reconciliation Act of 1990) and to allow for additional flexibility in meeting the needs of residents (such as Medicaid waivers). Still other changes have made it easier for certain Medicaid beneficiaries with disabilities to work without losing all Medicare and Medicaid benefits (Ticket to Work and Work Incentives Improvement Act of 1999).

The federal government "matches" a percentage of the costs of the Medicaid program in each state. This percentage is known as the Federal Medical Assistance Percentage

(FMAP). The FMAP ranges from 50% (for wealthier states) to up to 83% (for poorer states). FMAPs are determined by financial criteria for each state and are in place for 3-year periods.[23]

Whom It Covers[24] Medicaid's eligibility requirements differ by state. There are mandatory eligibility groups that include children, elders, parents/caretaker relatives of children up to 18 years old, and those people with disabilities who meet specified minimum income levels. The ACA offers states the opportunity to expand eligibility to include all individuals meeting 133% of the federal poverty level. Some states are more expansive in their eligibility criteria than others because Medicaid law allows for flexibility in determining which groups are covered.[25]

Each state has specific income levels and resource amounts for qualification for Medicaid. There are limits to how much an individual may own and also limits to how much an individual can transfer to another person in the previous 5 years if he or she is trying to qualify for Medicaid (the 5-year look back for transfer of assets). These limits are in place to ensure that Medicaid benefits are given to individuals with lower incomes and few resources, not to individuals who are trying to appear to have lower incomes and few resources, but in fact, have access to such funds. Individuals can, however, spend down their resources and income through paying for health care to qualify for Medicaid. Spouses of individuals qualifying for Medicaid have protections, known as Spousal Impoverishment standards, to allow them to keep income, resources, and home equity.

What It Provides[24] Medicaid programs in each participating state must provide the following medically necessary services (medical necessity is determined by each state's requirements):

- Physician services
- Inpatient/outpatient hospital services
- Laboratory and x-ray services
- Early and periodic screening, diagnostic, and treatment services for people under the age of 21
- Federally qualified health center and rural health clinic services
- Family planning
- Nurse practitioner services
- Nurse midwife
- Nursing facilities for adults (age 21 and older)
- Home health care for nursing-facility–eligible individuals
- Medically necessary transportation

Each state may provide additional optional services (e.g., prescription drugs, personal care services, dental services, respiratory care, and intermediate care facility services for individuals with intellectual or developmental disabilities). The services that a state's Medicaid program covers are described in the State Medicaid Plan, a document that must

Table 11-2 State Medicaid Program Names (Examples)

State	Name of Medicaid Program
California	Medi-CAL
Massachusetts	MassHealth
Oklahoma	SoonerCare
Tennessee	TennCare

be approved by the Centers for Medicare and Medicaid Services (CMS). States can change what is in their State Medicaid Plan, at any time, through the State Plan Amendment (SPA) process. Amendments can be based on new data, changes in state or federal law, or a court order, and must be approved by CMS.[26]

How to Access   Each state operates its own Medicaid program. Each program has local eligibility offices where an older adult can apply. Information also is available online and can be viewed by searching for the state's Medical Assistance Office. State Medicaid programs may be known as Medicaid or another name (see **Table 11-2** for some examples).

To apply for Medicaid, an older adult will need to complete an application form and provide documentation about finances and functional level.

THE AGING NETWORK

The **Aging Network** is the name of the collaboration of the Administration on Aging (AoA), **state units on aging**, **area agencies on aging**, tribal and native organizations, service providers, and volunteers. On February 12, 2012, before the Senate Special Committee on Aging, the Assistant Secretary on Aging, Kathy Greenlee, testified:

> Last year [2011] the national aging services network served nearly 11 million seniors and their caregivers through home and community-based services. This was made possible by the Administration on Aging (AoA), 56 State and territorial units on aging, 629 area agencies on aging, 246 tribal and Native Hawaiian organizations, nearly 20,000 direct service providers, and hundreds of thousands of volunteers. These critical supports complement medical and health care systems, help to prevent hospital readmissions, provide transportation to doctor appointments, and support some of life's most basic functions, such as assistance to elders in preparing and delivering meals, or helping them with bathing. This assistance is especially critical for the nearly three million seniors who receive intensive in-home services, half a million of whom meet the disability criteria for nursing home admission but are able to remain in their homes, in part, due to these community supports.[27]

AoA, funded through the Older Americans Act, provides block grants for services through state and territorial units on aging, designated by the governor or legislature of each state/territory. These units then procure services through area agencies on aging and their network of service providers and volunteers.[5]

History[28] The **Older Americans Act** (OAA) was signed into law in 1965, following the first White House Conference on Aging in 1961. The Older Americans Act established the Administration on Aging (AoA). Originally, the OAA designated its population as anyone 65 years or older. However, in subsequent amendments and reauthorizations, the age was changed to 60 years and older to allow individuals approaching "elderhood" to benefit from information and referral resources as part of their preretirement planning.

In addition, as elder policies have evolved, Older Americans Act amendments have established the Aging Network framework through area agencies on aging (1974), added funding for senior centers (1974), created the Long-Term Care Ombudsman program for nursing facilities (1978) (and later board and care homes and other residential options in 1981), added services related to elder abuse (1992), and focused interventions on caregivers (1992, 2000). Some of the amendments and reauthorizations have emphasized the role of the Aging Network in providing supportive services for older adults in the community so that they remain at home (1984, 2006). Bearing this emphasis in mind, in 2012, the Department of Health and Human Services brought together the Administration on Aging, the Administration on Developmental Disabilities, and the Office on Disability to create the Administration for Community Living to further strengthen federal efforts to respond to the community living needs and preferences of people with disabilities of all ages, including older adults. Ongoing operations and management within these three agencies, including AoA, are not expected to change with this reorganization.[29]

Whom It Covers The Aging Network and the Older Americans Act define an older American as being 60 years old or older. Caregivers of older Americans are also covered.

What It Provides[5] The AoA provides funds to state units on aging and tribal organizations to provide specific services as mandated by the Older Americans Act. State units on aging then fund area agencies on aging to provide these services to local older adults through service providers. The specific services include nutritional services (Title IIIc of the Older Americans Act), which involves both congregate services (group dining) and home-delivered meals (Meals on Wheels); supportive services, which includes transportation, in-home care/personal care, adult day care, and information and referral; preventive health services; elder rights services, including the Long-Term Care Ombudsman program; and the National Family Caregiver Support Program, which offers counseling, training, and respite care to caregivers.

How to Access Area agencies on aging are the primary access point for the Aging Network. To find an area agency on aging or a specific service provider at the local level, an older adult, family member, or healthcare professional can contact the Eldercare Locator. This resource is maintained by the Administration on Aging and consists of a telephonic and web-based database of resources at the state and local level. To contact the Eldercare Locator, call 1-800-677-1116 or visit the website, www.eldercare.gov.

AMERICANS WITH DISABILITIES ACT

Thirty-seven percent of older adults report some type of disability in terms of hearing, vision, cognition, ambulation, self-care, or independent living.[30] This rate increases with age. Some elders have disabilities or functional limitations that prevent them from performing activities and fully integrating into community living. The **Americans with Disabilities Act** (ADA) is an important policy for all individuals with disabilities, including older people. The main aim of the ADA is to integrate individuals with disabilities into all aspects of living in the United States. The ADA prohibits discrimination of individuals with a disability in all areas of everyday life including employment, transportation, public facilities, health care, and telecommunications.[31]

History[32,33]   The Americans with Disabilities Act was signed into law by President George H.W. Bush in 1990. This law represented a culmination of decades of work by people with disabilities and other advocates to have official recognition of discrimination due to disability as a civil rights issue. Just as the civil rights movement demanded equal treatment under the law for people of all races, so did the ADA for people with disabilities.

According to the National Council on Disability, the ADA has provided tremendous gains in accessibility in many areas for individuals with disabilities. These gains occurred despite several Supreme Court decisions in the 1990s that limited the ADA. However, the ADA was amended in 2008 (Americans with Disabilities Act Amendments Act [ADAAA]). These amendments have sought to broaden and strengthen the ADA and its mandate of equal treatment regardless of disability.

Whom It Covers[31]   The ADA covers anyone who has a disability, which the ADA defines as "a physical or mental impairment that substantially limits a major life activity." The ADAAA further provided examples of life activities that include caring for one's self, eating, sleeping, walking, standing, and communicating. Thus, many older people with self-described disabilities are covered under the ADA.

What It Provides   Importantly, for older adults, the ADA provides for the accessibility of health care and healthcare facilities. For example, hospitals and doctor's offices must be physically accessible to individuals with disabilities. Accessibility comes in many forms and may involve architectural access as well as specific access to medical equipment. According to www.ada.gov, access also means that generally healthcare providers cannot examine individuals who come to their offices in wheelchairs because the providers are not giving equal medical services to people with disabilities.

How to Access   In general, the ADA is not a policy that individuals access; rather, it is a policy that provides access to individuals with disabilities. Individuals with disabilities can bring complaints and/or lawsuits under the ADA if they believe that an organization (e.g., doctor's office, provider, or hospital) is discriminating against them due to their disability. Healthcare professionals can access additional ADA information and training through their professional organization or www.ada.gov.

THE SPECIAL CASE OF LONG-TERM SERVICES AND SUPPORTS[34]

Long-term services and supports are those services that individuals, including older adults, need when their ability to take care of themselves is limited due to disability or chronic disease. As the name suggests, these services are often needed for long spans of time—years for older people and perhaps decades for individuals with disabilities. About half of all individuals who need long-term services and supports are 65 years old or older. These services may involve healthcare services, like skilled nursing, physical or occupational therapy services, which are required for the ongoing treatment of a condition or the maintenance of functioning, or more personal care services like bathing assistance or meal preparation. Long-term services and supports are available in both facility (e.g., nursing facilities or assisted living facilities) and community settings (for example, at home).

In 1999, a Supreme Court decision (*Olmstead v. L.C.*) impacted long-term services and supports in the United States. The *Olmstead* decision supported the belief that institutionalization was discrimination based on disability and was against the Americans with Disabilities Act. Under the *Olmstead* decision and the ADA, states were required to make modifications to programs to avoid institutionalization and provide services in the most community-integrated setting possible. It is within this policy background that current long-term services and supports are provided.[35]

Other trends have also impacted long-term service and support delivery for older adults and individuals with disabilities: independent living, self- or consumer-direction, and person- or family-centered care. Independent living is a philosophy and advocacy position of people with disabilities, who strongly support and demand that people with disabilities have the right to live independently and make their own decisions about their lives. "Nothing about us without us" is one mantra of this group, which advocates for long-term supports and services in the setting of one's choice (typically, home and community). Self- or consumer direction is about the organization and management of long-term services and supports that allow individuals receiving care or their chosen surrogates/representatives to plan and implement their own services through a variety of mechanisms. Self-direction may include the ability to hire and fire personal care workers, set the specific schedule of workers, buy equipment to take the place of workers, or buy different services chosen by the individual. Person- or family-centered care could include self-direction, but is more about how service providers are oriented to individuals needing care and their families.[36] These types of long-term services and supports take an individual's needs, preferences, goals, and desires into account as the organizing framework around which all care is to be provided. For older adults, often the term used is *family-centered care* to underscore the prominence of the family in caring for elders needing care.

In spite of the *Olmstead* decision and the ADA, there is still an institutional bias in many policies and programs. Policy makers, advocates, and other stakeholders have been working over the last two decades to balance long-term supports and services so that more services are provided in the community and fewer services are provided in facility settings. This is particularly true for Medicaid. Medicaid pays for a large part of long-term services and supports, both in facilities and in home- and community-based settings. In 2009, home- and community-based services accounted for almost 45% of all Medicaid long-term care spending. However, among services for older adults, home- and community-based spending accounted for 19% of Medicaid spending.[37]

Long-term services and supports can be quite expensive. In facilities, the cost of a semi-private room can average $75,000 a year or more. For personal care services in the community, costs in 2011 averaged $11,000 a year; home health services bill an average of $21 an hour. Depending on the types of services an individual needs, typically community-based care will be less expensive than facility-based care. In 2009, the total long-term services and supports expenses were $240 billion.

Medicare[34,38]   Many older people and their families mistakenly believe that Medicare covers long-term services and supports. It is true that Medicare funds some long-term services and supports, with about 24% of long-term services and supports paid for through Medicare. Specifically, Part A funds skilled nursing facility care, rehabilitation, and home health care; however, this coverage is limited and not intended for long-term stays or custodial care. Medicare can cover certain types of nursing facility stays, but only for 100 days and only if certain conditions are met. Personal care in the community is never covered through Medicare.

Medicaid[34,38]   The largest payer of long-term services and supports in the United States is Medicaid. This includes both nursing facility care and home- and community-based services. Over 40% of the $240 billion spent on long-term services and supports is paid for through Medicaid. In fact, nursing facility care is one of the mandatory services covered by Medicaid in all states. This institutional bias is being addressed, but at present, home- and community-based services are not mandated as Medicaid requirements. Community Medicaid services are provided through mandatory home health services, through any optional services that a state chooses to provide as part of its state plan (including but not limited to personal care attendant services), and through a specific regulatory device called a Medicaid waiver (see the following section). For all Medicaid services, individuals must meet the eligibility requirements for their state's Medicaid program to qualify for any long-term services and supports, even if they do need long-term assistance. Often, even if they do not initially qualify financially for Medicaid at the beginning of the need for long-term services, they soon use their resources and "spend down" their assets and income to the point where they then do qualify for Medicaid.

Medicaid HCBS Waivers and Special Programs[39,40]   Medicaid services that states provide must meet certain requirements. For example, states cannot limit or deny services because of specific conditions or diagnoses: the comparability requirement. States must fund services that are in effect throughout the state: the state-wideness requirement. However, because of certain amendments to the Medicaid Act, states can "waive" specific requirements and provide services in alternative ways. Notably, **Medicaid waivers** are available for states to provide home- and community-based services (long-term services and supports available in nonfacility settings). Many of these waivers are called either 1915(c) waivers, named after the section of the Social Security Act that authorizes them, or home- and community-based services (HCBS) waivers. These HCBS waivers allow states to provide services to Medicaid recipients who would otherwise be in a nursing facility.

Medicaid also funds the Money Follows the Person demonstration program currently active in 41 states and the District of Columbia. This program was expanded as part of the ACA. Money Follows the Person (MFP) programs have helped more than 19,000 people transition from facilities into the community since 2008. In each of these MFP states, enhanced Medicaid funding is available to the state (through a higher FMAP amount) for certain services designed to assist individuals with Medicaid currently residing in a nursing facility or other long-term care facility to transition into the community with a menu of services including state-specific State Plan services, Money Follows the Person demonstration services, and/or HCBS waiver services. With this enhanced funding, states are expected to strengthen the home- and community-based service system for these individuals transitioning out of facilities as well as individuals already in the community who require home- and community-based long-term services, to allow them to be diverted from an admission into a nursing facility. Each state's Money Follows the Person program is unique, with specific requirements and criteria approved by CMS.

In addition to MFP demonstration expansions, additional ACA benefits include a greater flexibility for states to offer home- and community-based services through a state plan amendment. Another program, the Balancing Incentive program, provides enhanced Medicaid funds to states that currently have less than half of their long-term services and supports spending in home- and community-based services to make these community services more accessible and understandable.

The Aging Network [34]   About 2% of long-term services and supports expenses are funded through other public funding, including Older Americans Act funding and the Aging Network. The Aging Network provides supportive services and nutritional services that can make up part of an older adult's long-term services and supports requirements. These services can include personal care and homemaker services, Meals on Wheels/dining options, transportation, and respite care. The Aging Network can also provide help through case management and information and referral programs. Benefits counseling, available through local Aging Network service providers, may also be of value for older adults needing long-term services and supports. In contrast to Medicaid, these services are available to all elders (individuals 60 years old or older) no matter their incomes, but are targeted to lower-income, minority, or rural older adults, or those with frailty or other disabilities.

Private Funding[34,41]   Some of the long-term services and supports that older adults need in the United States are provided either through private pay or by informal caregivers (family or friends). About 19% (or $1 out of every $5) of long-term services and support expenses are paid out of pocket. Older adults often have savings, income, or other resources to pay for services. As noted previously, some older adults will need to spend their savings and other resources before they can qualify for Medicaid long-term care. Families of older adults may also pay for services. A certified elder law attorney or financial planner can assist older adults and their families in determining the most appropriate long-term services and supports financing options. Benefits counseling through the Aging Network may also be of assistance.

Informal caregivers perform all types of caregiving activities including both activities of daily living and instrumental activities of daily living to the tune of an annual economic value of $450 billion, which dwarfs formal (i.e., paid) caregiving expenses. Activities of daily living (ADLs) include eating, toileting, transferring, dressing, and bathing activities. Instrumental activities of daily living (IADLs) include using the telephone, laundry, housekeeping, transportation, shopping, managing medications, and handling finances.

These caregivers are more likely to be women and typically spend about 18 hours per week providing unpaid care. One study found that most older adults who receive long-term services and supports in the home receive only informal care, with no publicly funded services.[42] These informal caregivers are often at risk for a decline in their own physical and emotional health, with resulting depressive symptoms, stress, anxiety, and other chronic conditions.

Long-Term Care Insurance   Some older adults may have **long-term care insurance**. There are about 8 million private long-term care policies in force.[43] Taken together, these policies currently fund about 7% of long-term services and supports expenditures in the United States.

Depending on the policy and its coverage, the policy may cover home- and community-based services (such as home health care, personal attendant services, assisted living, and adult day care) as well as nursing facility care. Each policy will have different eligibility criteria and service requirements. Typically, a policy holder will qualify for benefits when he or she requires help with ADLs. Policies can be expensive, and premiums usually rise with age.

ETHICAL ISSUES

For older people, many ethical issues revolve around decision making and potential harm. This section focuses on specific ethical situations that healthcare professionals may encounter: decision making, financial decision making, healthcare decision making, and elder abuse.

DECISION MAKING[44]

Adults (18 years of age or older) are assumed to be **competent** and able to make decisions on their own behalf unless a legal court has judged them to be incompetent. Competent individuals can make decisions about finances (to buy, give, or sell property or assets, for example) and health care (to accept or refuse a specific treatment or medical recommendation). For older adults, a number of different situations may affect their competency or capacity to make decisions. A health condition may leave them temporarily or permanently unable to make decisions. For example, an elder who has suffered a catastrophic stroke may be unable to speak or write, or pay his or her bills. Alzheimer's disease and related disorders could similarly and permanently affect an older adult's competency. Depending on the competency of an older adult, there are several legal issues to consider related to both financial and healthcare decision-making processes.

Financial Decision Making[45]   If an older adult is competent, he or she may designate a **power of attorney**, an individual who can make decisions on his or her behalf. Depending on the scope of the power, this agent, then, has the ability to handle financial and business matters. In the case of a "regular" power of attorney, the older individual still can make decisions on these same matters. If an older adult is incapacitated or is declared incompetent, a regular power of attorney is usually then not effective. However, a durable power of attorney, which specifically designates that the power endures in the event of incapacitation, remains effective in that case.

If an older adult is thought to be incompetent or unable to handle financial matters, then a concerned individual may petition the court to determine competency (a **conservatorship** hearing). If the court, through its evaluations, determines that an older person is no longer able to take care of his or her own financial matters, it appoints a conservator to perform those duties.

Healthcare Decision Making   Healthcare decision making is an equally important aspect of older adults' lives, given that their lives are often impacted by health concerns. There are several legal vehicles that elders and their caregivers can use to direct healthcare decision-making processes. **Advance directives** are documents that let an older adult take part in his or her health care even when too incapacitated to express preferences.

Durable Healthcare Power of Attorney[46]   A **durable healthcare power of attorney** (also called a durable power of attorney for health care) allows an individual to choose a person (agent) to represent that individual and make healthcare decisions on his or her behalf should the individual not be able to. It differs from a general power of attorney in that the general power of attorney only provides authority to the agent until the individual is unable to make decisions, whereas the durable healthcare power of attorney and the authority of the agent endure even after an individual is unable to make decisions.

To execute a durable healthcare power of attorney, the older adult needs to pick the agent (also known as a proxy or surrogate), notify the agent of the decision, complete the required form, and typically have the signature witnessed by two adults (who are not the agent). Each state's forms may differ, so contact the local area agency on aging or a lawyer for additional requirements.

Living Will[46]   A **living will** is a document that allows individuals to explain what kinds of health care they do and do not wish for themselves should they be unable to make decisions. Decisions can include whether to use ventilators (i.e., breathing machines), to resuscitate (or not; when there is a decision not to perform CPR if breathing or the heartbeat stops, it is often known as a DNR, Do Not Resuscitate, order), to feed and hydrate via feeding tubes or IVs, to treat pain, or to donate organs or body tissues. These are often very challenging and difficult decisions that families may have to make at the end of a relative's life. A living will can ensure that one's wishes are known. Some states do not have a specific law recognizing the living will as a binding document; in those states, it is more useful to have an executed durable healthcare power of attorney. However, the guidance that a living will can provide may be extremely useful to families making decisions. To complete a living will, the older adult decides on the specific healthcare activities that he or she wants and does not want, and completes the state's required form.

For both durable healthcare powers of attorney and living wills, it is important that the older adult ensures a few things. First, the elder should make sure that the agent he or she appoints to be the power of attorney is aware of the advance directive, agrees to perform these duties, has a copy of the required form (each state has a different form and specific requirements), and is aware of the older adult's wishes and preferences for health care. Similarly, the older adult should give copies of all advance directives to family members (not only the agent), primary care providers, and long-term services and support providers (like nursing facilities or assisted living facilities). Copies of advance directives should also be available in a safe and accessible location in the elder's home; one practice is to place a copy of the form(s) on the refrigerator door or in the medicine cabinet. States may also have online registries or cards for wallets noting the presence of an advance directive.

All 50 states and the District of Columbia recognize specific types of advance directives including living wills and durable healthcare powers of attorney. States differ in terms of their requirements and forms as well as whether they will recognize other states' advance directives. Federal law requires healthcare facilities that accept Medicare and Medicaid to inform individuals of their rights to complete advance directives. Many hospitals, upon admission, offer an incoming patient the opportunity to execute a living will and/or a durable healthcare power of attorney. Older adults may or may not be able to take advantage of the opportunity, depending on their biopsychosocial condition. Above and beyond the noted legalities, however, advance directives are a powerful method to initiate and allow for conversations about healthcare decision making by and on behalf of older adults.

Other Vehicles[45]   Advance directives are used when individuals are of sound mind and are legally competent to make healthcare decisions. Similar to the earlier financial decision-making discussion, there are cases when older people may become incapacitated and may not be able to make healthcare decisions. If no advance directives (especially a durable healthcare power of attorney) have been completed, then caregivers may need to initiate a formal legal proceeding, called a **guardianship** hearing, to evaluate an older adult's competency. If he or she is determined to be legally incapacitated, the court will appoint a guardian and determine over which decisions the guardian will have authority. States differ in terms of requirements, so an attorney should be consulted if guardianship proceedings are warranted.

ELDER ABUSE AND NEGLECT

According to the National Center on Elder Abuse, "**Elder abuse** is any knowing, intended or careless act that causes harm or serious risk of harm to an older person—physically, mentally, emotionally or financially."[47] There are many forms of elder abuse, including physical abuse, emotional abuse, sexual abuse, exploitation, neglect, abandonment, and self-neglect. Elder abuse can take place in an older adult's own home, in a healthcare facility, or in a long-term support provider location (e.g., senior center). Family members or professionals may be abusers.

There are different signs or symptoms depending on the type of abuse. For physical and emotional abuse, signs include unexplained bruises, burns, injuries with the outline of an object (hand, belt, etc.), poor skin condition, torn clothing, being withdrawn or frightened, or hesitating to talk freely. Sexual abuse may be seen as bruising around the breasts or genitals or unexplained sexually transmitted diseases. Exploitation or financial abuse is often typified by a change in finances, changes to wills, and checks or withdrawals for loans and gifts. Neglect (including self-neglect) may include signs such as poor hygiene, unexplained/untreated medical conditions, pressure ulcers, and malnourishment/dehydration.

Statistics[48]   Recent research indicates that only 1 in 14 elder abuse incidents are reported to the authorities, suggesting that current statistics severely underestimate the real prevalence of abuse.[49] Acierno et al. surveyed older adults and found that 11% of them (excluding those individuals with dementia or living in long-term care facilities) reported experiencing some type of abuse during the past year.[50]

Risk factors for elder abuse are myriad; it is important to remember that elder abuse can occur anywhere. Some research suggests that women and adults who are 80 years or older are more at risk. Dementia, mental health diagnoses, and substance abuse are other noted risk factors, as is social isolation.

Reporting   There is no federal law against elder abuse; however, all states have some form of law or laws against elder abuse. These laws also provide for the reporting of suspected elder abuse. Depending on the state law, healthcare professionals, including doctors, nurses, rehabilitation therapists, and social workers, are usually mandatory reporters.[51] It is vital that healthcare professionals assess for signs of abuse and report when there are signs because often older adults are reluctant to report the abuse themselves. The local adult protective service agency and local law enforcement agency are two places to report suspected elder abuse. Reporting will typically involve giving the name, contact information, and specific details of the elder suspected of being abused, and may include the reporter giving his or her own information. Some states allow for anonymous reporting, in which the states protect the confidentiality of reporters.

What to Do

Healthcare professionals usually have a mandate to report elder abuse, but there are other actions they should take to make sure that elder abuse is identified, treated, and prevented. The National Center on Elder Abuse recommends the following:[52]

- Keep in contact with older adults to decrease isolation and give them a chance to talk.
- Be aware of the possibility of abuse and look out for the signs and symptoms.
- Contact the local area agency on aging to identify potential resources, programs, and supports.
- Volunteer with agencies providing services and supports to older adults.
- Raise awareness of the issue by talking about elder abuse and participating in World Elder Abuse Awareness Day on June 15.

Raising public awareness is one strategy to address elder abuse at a societal level. Other strategies advocated by the National Center on Elder Abuse include enhancing and expanding services for individuals harmed by elder abuse, enhancing the system of adult protective services, providing law enforcement and mandated reporters with additional training and education, and conducting more research on aspects of elder abuse.

SUMMARY

Policy and ethical issues can affect every aspect of an older adult's life, from how much money he or she receives each month, to what health care he or she receives, to the types of medications he or she can afford, to whether or not he or she can continue to live in his or her own home, to how he or she makes healthcare decisions or has them made on his or her behalf. This chapter has presented several specific policies healthcare professionals working with older adults should understand to better assist older individuals with these aspects of life.

The policies and programs covered in this chapter include:

- Social Security, a policy impacting retired workers, spouses, dependents, and individuals with disabilities
- Supplemental Security Income, a program providing resources for lower income individuals including older adults and people with disabilities
- Medicare, health insurance for older adults and certain people with disabilities
- Medicaid, a program providing health care for people with lower incomes and few resources

- The Aging Network through the Older Americans Act, which provides social, nutritional, and supportive services to older adults and their caregivers
- The Americans with Disabilities Act, a law providing civil rights protection to people with disabilities including older adults

Each policy affects different aspects of life, with a variety of eligibility criteria and covered benefits or programs. Healthcare professionals and organizations can assist older adults in determining which policies or programs impact them and how to access specific benefits.

Healthcare professionals can also help older adults with decision-making processes to ensure that their decisions are followed and with potential abuse issues to ensure their safety. Advance directives and proxy vehicles such as powers of attorney can be useful tools for older adults that, together with the listed policies and program, can help older adults live the lives they wish.

Review Questions

1. Match the policy or program to the characteristic.

   1. Social Security
   2. Supplemental Security Income
   3. Medicare
   4. Medicaid
   5. Americans with Disabilities Act
   6. Older Americans Act

   a. Created the Aging Network
   b. Designed during the Great Depression
   c. Civil rights law
   d. Health insurance funded through payroll taxes
   e. Federal–state partnership providing health care
   f. Can be administered by the state or by the federal government

2. The "donut hole" of Part D of Medicare refers to the gap:
   A. In prescription drug coverage
   B. In coverage for emergency room visits
   C. In rehabilitation coverage after 30 days
   D. In coverage for nursing home care

3. If an older adult who has worked for 40 years wants to retire with full Social Security benefits, what is the most important factor to consider?
   A. Date of birth
   B. Length of work history after 40 years
   C. Marital status
   D. Availability of a 401(k)

4. What is the name of the federal agency that provides funding for aging services?
   A. Social Security Administration
   B. Centers for Medicare and Medicaid Services

C. White House Conference on Aging

D. Administration on Aging

5. _____ is the insurance program for older adults and certain younger people with disabilities.

A. Medicare

B. Medicaid

C. Medigap

D. Social Security

Learning Activities

1. Because the names are so similar, people often get Medicare and Medicaid confused. Compare and contrast Medicare and Medicaid in terms of eligibility, services, and funding. Develop a simple way to present this information (e.g., PowerPoint presentation, table, notes, or illustrations). Ask someone to review it for clarity.

2. An older adult client needs long-term services and supports and wants to stay in her home. She is on Medicare and Medicaid, and receives modest Social Security benefits. What resources would you pursue to assist her?

3. Think about a situation in which you might need elder resources (maybe a family member needs long-term services and supports or a friend is nearing retirement or someone close to you has to make a healthcare decision). Check out the websites listed under "Resources."

   a. Which websites or resources were the most helpful to you? Why? What kinds of information were available, accessible, and most interesting to you? Were you able to find out what you needed or wanted to know?

   b. Based on your experiences and knowledge, develop your own pamphlet or resource for older adults and their families/caregivers.

4. The year 1965 comes up several times in this chapter. What happened in 1965 related to elder policy issues? Why was 1965 such an important year for elder policy issues? Dig a little deeper. What was going on in the United States at that time? Talk to an older friend, client, or relative to find out what their perspective is.

5. Conduct a research project to determine how another country funds long-term services and supports. Compare and contrast that country to the United States in terms of public versus private funding, the balance between institutional and home- and community-based services, and informal caregiving.

CASE STUDY

Mrs. S., who is 80 years old, has a diagnosis of dementia and has been living with her younger sister (Ms. R., 68 years old) for 2 years since the death of Mrs. S.'s husband. Mrs. S.'s two children live 3 hours away and visit on holidays. She has few other visitors, and Ms. R. rarely takes her out of the house because they don't have a car. Ms. R. gets groceries delivered and uses local senior center transportation for Mrs. S.'s infrequent doctor's appointments. A neighbor is concerned because she saw Mrs. S. with some bruises on her arm when she came over to chat with Ms. R. Ms. R. said that Mrs. S. falls down and bumps up against the furniture. The neighbor reached out to you as a healthcare professional. You want to help.

Do you think that Mrs. S. is being abused? Why or why not?

If you are unable to make a decision, what other information do you need? If you do think she is being abused, what should you do?

If you don't think she's being abused, what should you do?

What resources could be helpful to you, Mrs. S., and Ms. R.?

With whom would you consult?

RESOURCES

Social Security	www.ssa.gov
SSI	www.ssa.gov/pgm/ssi.htm
Pensions	www.pensionrights.org/counseling-projects
Medicare	www.medicare.gov
Medicaid	www.medicaid.gov
Aging Network	www.eldercare.gov
	www.aoa.gov
	www.n4a.org
Americans with Disabilities Act	www.ada.gov
	www.ncd.gov
Decision making	www.caregiver.org/caregiver/jsp/home.jsp
	www.americanbar.org/groups/law_aging
	www.nsclc.org
Elder abuse and neglect	www.ncea.aoa.gov

REFERENCES

1. Henry J. Kaiser Family Foundation. Focus on Health Reform—Summary of New Health Reform Law (#8061). Retrieved December 31, 2012, from http://kff.org/health-reform/fact-sheet/summary-of-new-health-reform-law

2. U.S. Department of Health and Human Services. Key Features of the Affordable Care Act, By Year. Retrieved December 31, 2012, from http://www.hhs.gov/healthcare/facts/timeline/

3. O'Connor, M. HHS Halts Implementation of the CLASS Program. 2011. Retrieved February 1, 2013, from http://www.natlawreview.com/article/hhs-halts-implementation-class-program

4. The Five Things You Need to Know About the Affordable Care Act. Retrieved December 31, 2012, from http://www.healthcare.gov/seniors

5. Gelfand, DE. *The Aging Network: Programs and Services*. 6th ed. New York: Springer, 2006.

6. Center on Budget and Policy Priorities. Top Ten Facts about Social Security. Retrieved December 31, 2012, from http://www.cbpp.org/cms/?fa=view&id=3261

7. Center on Budget and Policy Priorities. Social Security Keeps 21 Million Americans Out of Poverty: A State-by-State Analysis. Retrieved April 21, 2013, from http://www.cbpp.org/cms/?fa=view&id=3851

8. Administration on Aging. Historical Evolution of Programs for Older Americans. Retrieved December 31, 2012, from http://www.aoa.gov/AoAroot/AoA_Programs/OAA/resources/History.aspx

9. Gibson, MJ. Beyond 50.03: A Report to the Nation on Independent Living and Disability. Retrieved January 30, 2013, from http://www.aarp.org/health/doctors-hospitals/info-11-2003/aresearch-import-753.html

10. Social Security Administration. Historical Background and Development of Social Security. Retrieved January 26, 2013, from http://www.ssa.gov/history/briefhistory3.html

11. Social Security Administration. *Understanding the Benefits* (SSA Publication No. 05-10024). Washington, DC: U.S. Government Printing Office, 2012.

12. Social Security Administration. *How Work Affects Your Benefits* (SSA Publication No. 05-10069). Washington, DC: U.S. Government Printing Office, 2013.

13. Federal Interagency Forum on Aging-Related Statistics. *Older Americans 2012: Key Indicators of Well-Being.* Washington, DC: U.S. Government Printing Office, June 2012.

14. Social Security Administration. *What You Need To Know When You Get Supplemental Security Income (SSI)* (SSA Publication No. 05-11011). Washington, DC: U.S. Government Printing Office; 2011.

15. Federal Interagency Forum on Aging-Related Statistics. *Older Americans 2012: Key Indicators of Well-Being.* Washington, DC: U.S. Government Printing Office, June 2012.

16. Committee on Social Insurance of the American Academy of Actuaries. *Social Insurance* (Doc. No. 062). Actuarial Standards Board, July 1998. Retrieved July 30, 2013, from http://www.actuarialstandardsboard.org/pdf/asops/asop032_062.pdf

17. Henry J. Kaiser Family Foundation. Medicare: A Timeline of Key Developments. Retrieved January 6, 2013, from http://kaiserfamilyfoundation.files.wordpress.com/2005/06/5-02-13-medicare-timeline.pdf

18. Talking about Medicare: Your Guide to Understanding the Program, 2012. Retrieved July 30, 2013, from http://kaiserfamilyfoundation.files.wordpress.com/2013/03/7067-02_medicare-at-a-glance.pdf

19. U.S. Department of Health and Human Services, Centers for Medicare and Medicaid Services. *Medicare Basics* (CMS Product No. 11034). Washington, DC: U.S. Government Printing Office, May 2011.

20. www.Medicare.gov. Accessed December 31, 2012.

21. Healthcare.gov. If I Have Medicare, Do I Need to Do Anything? Retrieved December 31, 2012, from http://www.healthcare.gov/law/features/65-older/medicare-preventive-services/index.html

22. Healthcare.gov. If I Have Medicare Do I Need to Do Anything? Retrieved December 31, 2012, from http://www.healthcare.gov/law/features/65-older/drug-discounts/index.html

23. U.S. Department of Health and Human Services. Federal Medical Assistance Percentages or Federal Financial Participation in State Assistance Expenditures FMAP. Retrieved January 31, 2013, from http://aspe.hhs.gov/health/fmap.htm

24. Kaiser Commission on Medicaid and the Uninsured. Medicaid: A Primer. Retrieved July 30, 2013, from http://kff.org/medicaid/issue-brief/medicaid-a-primer/

25. http://www.medicaid.gov/. Accessed December 31, 2012.

26. Medicaid.gov. Medicaid State Plan Amendments. Retrieved January 26, 2013, from http://www.medicaid.gov/State-Resource-Center/Medicaid-State-Plan-Amendments/Medicaid-State-Plan-Amendments.html

27. Kathy Greenlee. Testimony. Retrieved January 26, 2013, from http://www.aoa.gov/AoARoot/Press_Room/Speeches_Testimony/archive/2012/docs/WestVirginiaTestimony_022012.pdf

28. Administration on Aging. Historical Evolution of Programs for Older Americans. Retrieved December 31, 2012, from http://www.aoa.gov

/AoAroot/AoA_Programs/OAA/resources
/History.aspx

29. Administration on Community Living. About Us: Questions and Answers on the Establishment of the Administration for Community Living. Retrieved January 26, 2013, from http://www.hhs.gov/acl/about-us

30. Administration on Aging. Profile of Older Americans. 2011. Retrieved December 31, 2012, from http://www.aoa.gov/aoaroot/aging_statistics/Profile/index.aspx

31. Americans with Disabilities Act. Home Page. Retrieved January 20, 2013, from http://www.ada.gov

32. Frieden, L. *NCD and ADA 15 Years Later*. Washington, DC: National Council on Disability, 2005.

33. Frieden, L. *Righting ADA*. Washington, DC: National Council on Disability, 2004.

34. Howard, J. Long-Term Care. Retrieved December 31, 2012, from http://www.kaiseredu.org/Tutorials-and-Presentations/Long-Term-Care.aspx

35. Department of Justice. Olmstead: Community Integration for Everyone. Retrieved January 20, 2013, from http://www.ada.gov/olmstead/

36. Feinberg, L. *Moving Toward Person- and Family-Centered Care* (Insights on the Issues 60). Washington, DC: AARP Public Policy Institute, 2012.

37. Kaiser Commission on Medicaid and the Uninsured. Medicaid's Role in Meeting the Long-Term Care Needs of America's Seniors. Retrieved January 6, 2013, from http://kaiserfamily foundation.files.wordpress.com/2013/02/8403.pdf

38. NIH Senior Health. Paying for Long-Term Care. Retrieved January 6, 2013, from http://www.nihseniorhealth.gov/longtermcare/payingforlongtermcare/01.html

39. Department of Health and Human Services. *Understanding Medicaid Home and Community Services: A Primer*. Washington, DC: U.S. Department of Health and Human Services, Office of the Assistant Secretary for Planning and Evaluation, 2010.

40. Affordable Care Act Supports States in Strengthening Community Living. Retrieved July 30, 2013, from http://www.hhs.gov/news/press/2011pres/02/20110222b.html

41. Medicare.gov. Paying for Long-Term Care. Retrieved January 6, 2013, from http://www.medicare.gov/LongTermCare/Static/PayingOverview.asp

42. Thompson, L. *Long-Term Care: Support for Family Caregivers* [Issue Brief]. Washington, DC: Georgetown University, 2004.

43. Stevenson, D, et al. The complementarity of public and private long term care coverage. *Health Affairs*, 2010; 29:96 –101

44. AARP. Planning for Incapacity. Retrieved July 30, 2013, from http://www.aarp.org/relationships/caregiving-resource-center/info-11-2010/lfm_planning_for_incapacity.html

45. American Bar Association. Health and Financial Decision Making. Retrieved January 6, 2013, from http://www.abanet.org/aging

46. AARP. Advance Directives: Creating a Living Will and Healthcare Power of Attorney. Retrieved July 30, 2013, from http://www.aarp.org/relationships/caregiving-resource-center/info-11-2010/lfm_living_will_and_health_care_power_of_attorney.html

47. National Center on Elder Abuse. *15 Questions and Answers About Elder Abuse*. Washington, DC: NCEA, 2005.

48. National Center on Elder Abuse. *How to Answer Those Tough Questions About Elder Abuse*. Washington, DC: NCEA, n.d.

49. National Center on Elder Abuse. *National Elder Abuse Incidence Study*. Washington, DC: NCEA, 1998.

50. Acierno, R, et al. Prevalence and correlates of emotional, physical, sexual and financial abuse and potential neglect in the United States: The National Elder Mistreatment Study. *American Journal of Public Health*, 2010; 100:292–297.

51. Steigel, L, Klem, E. *Reporting Requirements: Provisions and Citations in Adult Protective Services Laws, By State*. American Bar Association Commission on Law and Aging. Retrieved May 4, 2013, from http://www.americanbar.org/content/dam/aba/migrated/aging/docs/Mandatory ReportingProvisionsChart.authcheckdam.pdf

52. National Center on Elder Abuse. *Why Should I Care About Elder Abuse?* Washington, DC: NCEA, 2010.

Chapter 12

HEALTH LITERACY AND CLEAR HEALTH COMMUNICATION: TEACHING AND WRITING SO OLDER ADULTS UNDERSTAND

SUE STABLEFORD, MPH, MSB

When you wish to instruct, be brief; that men's [people's] minds take in quickly what you say, learn its lesson, and retain it faithfully. Every word that is unnecessary only pours over the side of a brimming mind.

—Cicero, 106-43 BC

Chapter Outline

Behavioral Objectives

Upon completion of this chapter, the reader will be able to:

1. Compare the reading level of health materials with the reading abilities of the majority of older adults, and discuss the mismatch or gap between them.
2. Define the terms *literacy* and *health literacy*.
3. Describe the health literacy skills of older adults according to their performance on the 2003 National Assessment of Adult Literacy, as well as according to other research studies.

4. Describe the impact of older adults' limited health literacy skills on their health.
5. Describe the role of health system communication.
6. List six plain language standards for verbal patient teaching.
7. List 5 to 10 plain language standards for written information.
8. Discuss the impact that plain language and clear health communication could have if effectively implemented across healthcare delivery systems.

Key Terms

Chronic condition
Health literacy
Health Resources and Services
   Administration
The Joint Commission
Limited literacy skills
Literacy
Numeracy

Osteoarthritis
Plain language
Plain language standards
Reading levels
Sensory deficits
Shame-free environment
Teach-back

A PATIENT'S EXPERIENCE OF HEALTH COMMUNICATION

Meet Marjorie. She is 78 years old and lives independently in the same town as her daughter and grandchildren. She has **osteoarthritis**, which makes it a little hard for her to get around. At a recent medical visit, her doctor noticed that she was somewhat depressed and prescribed an antidepressant. When the office nurse called to see how she was doing, Marjorie was upset. Here is what she told the nurse:

> I don't know why the doctor thought I should take pills. I'm not crazy, you know. He asked me some questions about how I've been feeling and I told him. It's hard to get old and not be able to do all the things I used to be able to do. Sometimes I have trouble sleeping. And, I get lonely, especially when my daughter is too busy to come over and visit. The doctor said I'm depressed, but I don't understand how taking a pill will help. He gave me a pamphlet to read about it, but the print was so small and it was so complicated that I gave up.

PATIENT/CONSUMER COMMUNICATION: THE GAP BETWEEN HIGH LEVELS OF INFORMATION AND THE LIMITED LITERACY SKILLS OF AMERICAN ADULTS

Marjorie's experience is not unusual. Many, if not most, older adults have trouble understanding both verbal and written health communication. This may be due to **sensory deficits** such as decreased vision or hearing. Sometimes stress and anxiety are so high that it is impossible to listen or read with understanding. Many patients in our increasingly diverse society do not speak or read English well or at all, and need help from medical interpreters at clinical visits and materials that have been translated into other languages. And sometimes communication fails because health professionals communicate at high levels, both verbally and in writing—way beyond the abilities of most adults to understand.

Hundreds of research studies have documented the high **reading levels** of most health and medical information—typically high school and college level.[1] At the same time, researchers for the U.S. Department of Education have shown in two national adult **literacy** surveys (1992 and 2003) that most adults cannot read at these levels. On the most recent survey conducted in 2003, compared to other age groups, "Adults ages 65 and older had the lowest average prose, document, and quantitative literacy."[2]

On the **health literacy** section of that 2003 survey, older adults again scored the lowest of all age groups. About 60% had *below basic* or *basic* health literacy skills. But, they most likely need better skills to care for themselves effectively. One of the health literacy tasks labeled as *intermediate* was this: "Determine what time a person can take a prescription medication, based on information on the prescription drug label that relates the timing of medication to eating."[3] Essentially, this means that a majority of older adults, lacking an intermediate level of health literacy skills, cannot read, understand, and use this type of medication label. And remember, this age group takes the most medications!

In this electronic age, you might think that "print is dead" and that the Internet is the major source of health information. For working-age and younger adults, this can be true. According to the most recently available Pew Internet survey, about 81% of American adults go online and about 72% have searched for health information in the past year.[4] However, Pew Survey data also show that older adults are far less likely than younger adults to go online or look for health information on the web. Other studies show that web-based health information is usually at the same high reading level as print materials.[5]

Additionally, what happens when healthcare providers teach patients verbally? Patients again often struggle to understand, especially when time is rushed and a vast amount of information is shared quickly.

EXPANDING UNDERSTANDING: THE CONTEXT OF HEALTH LITERACY AND NUMERACY

Health literacy from a patient perspective means using literacy skills—reading, writing, speaking, listening, and computing (math)—in a health context. This context is, for many, like visiting a foreign country where they do not know the language or the customs.

Patient health literacy challenges include: (1) having the specialized vocabulary, knowledge, and skills to manage one's own health; (2) using multiple information formats in multiple locations to accomplish multiple tasks (e.g., reading food labels in the supermarket, medicine instructions at the pharmacy, safety regulations at work, consent forms in the hospital); (3) mastering the arcane U.S. health insurance and health delivery systems; and (4) simultaneously overcoming high levels of stress and anxiety associated with health decision making.

Viewed this way, it is likely that few adults have fully adequate health literacy skills. If an adult does not speak fluent English or does not know or accept the assumptions of Western medicine, understanding is further compromised.

Limited *numeracy* skills may also compromise patients' abilities to understand and act on health information. Although the term *health literacy* has traditionally included math skills (quantitative literacy), limited numeracy skills are increasingly being recognized as an independent cause for concern. On the 2003 National Assessment of Adult Literacy skills, more than 70% of adults age 65 and over had below basic or only basic quantitative literacy skills.[6] Limited numeracy skills impact a person's abilities to measure and time medicines, interpret food labels, read medical devices, assess risks, and so on.[7] Health literacy and numeracy challenge everyone, albeit in varying circumstances and to varying degrees. Older adults are an especially high-risk group for misunderstanding.

LITERACY AND HEALTH LITERACY SKILLS: MAJOR KEYS TO GOOD HEALTH

Research studies conducted over the past 20 years have highlighted the huge impact of **limited literacy skills** on health and health outcomes.[1] One study of more than 3,000 older adults enrolled in a Medicare managed care plan (Prudential) provides rich data regarding the literacy skills of older adults and the relationship of limited literacy to health. In a series of publications, study collaborators shared these conclusions:

- Older adults with inadequate health literacy often misread simple prescription instructions, information about the results of blood sugar tests, and other vital healthcare information.
- Literacy and health literacy skills decline with age.
- Inadequate health literacy is independently associated with greater risk of hospital admission, lower use of preventive health services such as flu and pneumonia shots, poorer physical and mental health, and higher all-cause mortality.[8-13]

THE IMPACT OF SYSTEMS ON HEALTH LITERACY: CONNECTING COMMUNICATION WITH PATIENT SAFETY AND PATIENT-CENTERED CARE

From a *system* perspective, health literacy means attending to the communication demands placed on patients (and their families) and how well or poorly the system accommodates their needs. The responsibilities of medical offices, clinics, and systems are well articulated in a recent Institute of Medicine report titled *Ten Attributes of Health Literate Health Care Organizations*.[14] This report makes it clear that most organizations place health literacy demands on patients that are significantly beyond the reading and numeracy abilities of most patients. This can result in serious consequences for systems as well as the patients and their families. Major national groups are speaking out about the problem.

The Joint Commission, which accredits hospitals around the country, points out in a report, "The typical informed consent form is unreadable for any level of reader."

Further, it notes that communication failures are the underlying root cause of 65% of *sentinel events*—instances of serious patient harm. The Commission urges hospitals to make effective communications a priority to protect patient safety.[15]

Further, the Joint Commission has issued new accreditation requirements to improve patient–provider communication. The Roadmap for Hospitals integrates health literacy with cultural competence, and requires hospitals to meet the oral and written communication needs of all patients, including those with speech, hearing, and other possible disorders that compromise their communication abilities.[16]

The American Medical Association has played a leading role in alerting physicians and other care providers about the health literacy problem and in supporting solutions. It is one of a growing number of health profession organizations to publish policy statements as well as reports and tools to address the issue.[17-19] In its *Safe Practices* report, the National Quality Forum recognizes clear communication as essential to patient safety.[20] The National Committee on Quality Assurance requires that all staff in patient-centered medical homes be trained in effective communication for all segments of the practice's population. Its standards and guidelines also embrace the need for cultural inclusion and multiple forms of communication in helping patients learn about and manage their health conditions.[21]

The federal government has also issued relevant policies requiring linguistic access, culturally competent care, and public information written in **plain language** and published tools to support professional skill development. Here is a sample of the tools available.

- The **Health Resources and Services Administration** (HRSA) offers a freely accessible online training program titled Addressing Health Literacy, Cultural Competency, and Limited English Proficiency, linking these closely related issues.[22]
- The Agency for Healthcare Research and Quality (AHRQ) has published the Health Literacy Universal Precautions Toolkit to help healthcare professionals and delivery systems learn how to address health literacy and related communication issues. This entire toolkit is freely accessible online.[23]
- The Office of Disease Prevention and Health Promotion of the U.S. Department of Health and Human Services has issued a National Action Plan to Improve Health Literacy. This plan outlines concrete action steps for all sectors of our society to address health literacy, including schools, workplaces, and healthcare systems.[24]

Beyond policies, tools, and exhortation lies a business case for attending to this issue. The Centers for Medicare and Medicaid Services (CMS) now use standardized patient satisfaction survey data to help determine hospital reimbursement rates for all Medicare patients. Surveys mailed to patients after hospital or physician office visits ask specifically whether they received information they could understand, verbally and in writing.[25]

Medicare has also implemented new 30-day readmission policies for specified conditions that financially penalize healthcare systems with excessive readmissions. This supports hospital systems using effective communication programs at all times, but perhaps especially during care transitions.[26] The need for action has never been more clear.

CLEAR HEALTH COMMUNICATION: AN OFTEN OVERLOOKED NECESSITY

Despite the research studies and recent policy advances, public health and healthcare organizations often treat communication as an afterthought. Other issues command higher priority. Or perhaps it is assumed that adults working in health disciplines know how to speak, teach, and write well enough to get their points across. As Marjorie's experience as well as research studies show, however, although clear communication is essential to good health outcomes, it does not happen automatically.

A large and only partially answered question is how to best communicate, both verbally and in writing, so that patients/consumers do understand critical health information. What works to motivate and enable care systems to systematically address communication challenges? What are the best solutions from both the patient and the system perspectives?

Researchers have some partial answers, although much remains to be learned. One major national research review, completed in 2004, notes that we still have more questions than answers.[27] An update of that review, published in 2011, confirmed and somewhat expanded results.[28] Research *has* shown that using specific patient teaching techniques such as "teach-back" and certain plain language writing techniques increases the likelihood that adults will be able to understand and use health information.[29-31]

The organizations that have drawn national attention to this problem—The Joint Commission, the American Medical Association, the federal government, and others—have proposed similar solutions. The Joint Commission report contains 35 specific recommendations for improving communication in hospitals and across the continuum of care. Major emphasis includes teaching and writing in plain language.[15] Similarly, the AMA report, *Help Patients Understand*, states: "Providers should use clear communication skills, techniques and practices for interpersonal communication with *all* patients, not just those with limited literacy."[19] And the federal government devotes multiple websites to teaching employees and others how to communicate effectively in plain language.[32]

WHAT IS PLAIN LANGUAGE? HOW WILL I KNOW IT IF I HEAR IT?

Here are the six verbal communication tips that the AMA recommends that all physicians adopt to improve patient understanding.[33] (The author provides additional comments.)

1. *Slow down.* This is especially important to help older adults who may have hearing loss and who do not mentally process information as rapidly as when they were younger.
2. *Use plain, nonmedical language.* Another way to say this is to use everyday language or conversational language. Pretend you are talking with a relative or neighbor. Our usual spoken language is far simpler than formal communication.
3. *Show or draw pictures.* This is helpful in written materials as well. We know from research that pictures help older adults learn and remember information.[34] Similarly, using models can increase patient understanding. For example, anatomical models

can help patients understand how their bodies work. Food models can demonstrate healthy food choices and appropriate portion sizes.

4. *Limit the amount of information and repeat it.* This means prioritizing information to the three to five most important points. Most adults can remember only three things from a healthcare visit.

5. *Use the **teach-back** technique.* Sometimes this is called the "show me" or "demonstrate back" or the "teach to goal" technique. This means, have patients state in their own words what they are to do or demonstrate how they will perform a certain action, such as use a medical device. So, a provider might say something such as: "Ms. Smith, how will you explain what we've discussed to your family when you get home?" Or, "Ms. Smith, I want to make sure I've given clear directions. Would you tell me in your own words the key steps to take when you get home?" This gives the provider a chance to learn what the patient understands and to fill in or repeat missing information. The essential element of this technique is for the provider to take responsibility for being clear, not to "grill" the patient as if it were a test with shame attached for failure.

6. *Create a **shame-free environment**: Encourage questions.* Some providers say: "*What* questions do you have?" instead of the more common "*Do* you have any questions?" By asking "What questions do you have?," it is assumed that the adult does have some questions and now will feel more comfortable asking them.

Three additional tips also help older adults learn more effectively from healthcare visits:

1. *Frame the conversation first.* This means, tell the adult what you will be talking about before launching into the discussion. This helps prepare him or her to listen and hear information with understanding. So, you might say: "Ms. Smith, I'd like to start you on a new medicine. Let me explain what it is, how to take it, and how it should help." Then go on with your teaching points.

2. *Encourage older adults to bring a friend or family member to the visit.* Another set of eyes and ears, or someone to actually take notes, can help the patient remember what was discussed during the visit. However, the provider still needs to address the client, not the friend or family member. Often older adult clients are ignored, especially when a younger person attends the visit with them.

3. *Give plain language written information that reminds the patient of what to do, how to do it, and why.* Most of us forget up to 50% of what we've heard as soon as we leave the exam room.[35] We all need reminders about actions and next steps. It also is helpful for many older adults to have written information to share with family members who have not been at the clinical visit but help care for them.

If some of these techniques were used with Marjorie, how might the result have been different? If the doctor had used teach-back, he would have learned that Marjorie did not understand the diagnosis (depression) and did not agree with the treatment plan (medication). They could possibly have arranged an alternative plan that suited Marjorie better. If she had brought her daughter or a friend to the visit, they could have talked about it together later, and further understanding could have occurred. If the doctor had given Marjorie plain language and easy-to-understand print information about depression, perhaps she would have gained a better understanding of the diagnosis and reconsidered her treatment choices. She could have become an engaged patient, sharing decisions with her doctor.

WHAT IS PLAIN LANGUAGE? HOW WILL I KNOW IT IF I SEE IT?

The patient, Marjorie, also had trouble reading the information about depression that her doctor gave her. This is not surprising, given the high reading levels of most health and medical information. Although plain language is not a total solution to a complex problem, it is a great starting point for creating more accessible print and web-based materials. Plain language principles also apply to designing information for other media, such as DVDs and social media applications. Many groups publish **plain language standards**, including the National Institute on Aging. Its publication, *Making Your Printed Health Materials Senior Friendly*, is available online and in print.[36] To view a website targeted to older adults that models standards for accessibility as well as appeal, check out www.NIHSeniorHealth.gov. You will see that it reflects the following guidelines, and also incorporates visual and navigational elements that make it easy to use.

Plain language guidelines accepted by multiple expert groups include the following:

- *Content*: Information is accurate, up-to-date, and limited. Focus is on behavior—what the reader needs to *do*. The average reader can use and remember no more than about five major points at one time. If a topic is complex, such as managing depression, break it up into smaller sections so that an adult can read small amounts at a time.
- *Structure/organization*: Structure and organize information from the user's perspective. This means putting the most important information first and creating small chunks with good headers or subtitles. Some readers read just the subtitles, so headings really need to convey key points. Health writers typically lead off with explanations about anatomy or descriptions about how many people have a certain problem. Plain language reverses this and begins with clear action messages. The background information comes later because it is less critical.
- *Writing style*: Talk directly to the reader in a positive, friendly tone as much as appropriate and possible. As noted earlier, most adults best understand everyday language. These are typically short words (one or two syllables) common in spoken language. When medical terms are used, such as the name of a condition, a pronunciation should be given and the term explained. Sentences should also be short, about 12–15 words on average. Use mostly active voice and explain general principles with concrete examples. For example, instead of writing about regular exercise, write about walking

most days of the week for at least one-half hour. To engage your readers even further, use testimonials or short example stories of older adults who share the reader's concerns or who have solved a common problem.

- *Appearance and appeal*: The first few seconds that an adult looks at a piece (or a website) create a lasting impression. So, we need to make sure our print materials and websites are attractive, inviting, and look easy to read. This almost always means plenty of white space, not a page crammed full of print or a home page with too many visual distractions. The size of the print needs to be large enough for reading ease (usually about 13- or 14-point typeface for older adults), and the print/paper contrast should be sharp with dark print and light paper. Limit the use of fancy typefaces, underlining, and other visual tricks. Use appropriate pictures to humanize materials and show adults how to do recommended action steps.

Many organizations publish plain language guides and checklists that are easy to access online. Try using them when you are creating easier-to-read information.[37-39] One of the best-kept secrets about plain language is that it takes practice to write simply and clearly. One key to success is planning what you want to write (or say) before you sit in front of the computer and start writing. You must know both your audience and your purpose well. Ask yourself over and over: Who will use this? What do they need to know to take the action I am recommending? How can I suggest this in a way that is appropriate and compelling to the intended audience?

Showing what you have written to prospective users before you make many copies of it is also important. Be brave and ask for feedback and ways to make your material more clear. You will be surprised at what your trial readers do not understand and the great ideas they will offer to improve your piece.

Learn more about checking your materials with potential users in the Toolkit for Making Written Material Clear and Effective from the Centers for Medicare and Medicaid Services. This online publication is a thorough and complete manual about how to plan, write, design, and test plain language information—from soup to nuts.[40]

CLEAR COMMUNICATION: A CALL TO ACTION

Will using plain language and other clear health communication techniques ensure that older adults can read, understand, and use the information? Will it help to address our major national concerns with patient safety, quality, and costs of care? There is no one solution to the complex problem of communicating effectively with diverse patients and audiences. We do know from research in the fields of health education, reading, social marketing, and psychology that well-planned and simply written information can make a big difference in level of understanding.

But simply knowing what to do is not the same thing as doing it, and many factors can interfere with adults taking actions beneficial to their health. Understanding, however, is almost always the first step, whether in getting preventive vaccines, managing a **chronic condition**, preparing for a medical test, or following discharge and medication instructions.

Healthcare providers have a challenge and an opportunity to enrich their practice and the lives of patients. Health professionals must take the lead in learning effective verbal and written communication techniques. Good health and health care are too complex, important, and costly for us to continue bumbling along with materials that are too hard to read and verbal teaching that patients cannot remember and use. You can use the online resources and training programs listed in the references and attend workshops to learn more.

Clear communication is not only the right thing to do, it is essential to thrive in this new era of "pay-for-performance" and "bundled care." As payment models continue to shift to reimbursing for episodes and results of care and measuring them more accurately, effective communication will play an increasingly important role. Only if patients engage in their care as partners with their providers, and understand what to do and how to do it, will we be able to bend the cost curve. Only healthcare delivery systems and healthcare professionals that adapt will survive and thrive.

Consider how Marjorie's life might have been enhanced if she had better understood her physician's concern for her mental well-being and they had been able to talk about how to improve her quality of life. Marjorie may have agreed to try medication, or perhaps she would have chosen other therapies first. She would have better understood that depression does not mean she is "crazy"; nor is it a normal part of aging. It is quite possible that untreated depression will worsen Marjorie's physical health in the coming months, especially because she also has osteoarthritis. Depression can worsen other chronic conditions.[41] There are millions of "Marjories"—millions of older adults managing health conditions who will benefit from the extra care we take with our communications. And the care systems in which we serve will benefit as well.

Review Questions

1. Each of the following can negatively affect an older person's ability to understand our communication, *except*
   A. Sensory decline in vision or hearing due to aging
   B. Professional use of medical terms
   C. Limited adult literacy skills
   D. Printed information written at the sixth-grade level

2. Which statement about older adults' literacy skills is true?
   A. Those over 65 scored the highest on the 2003 National Assessment of Adult Literacy.
   B. Literacy skills tend to increase with age because of practice.
   C. Limited literacy skills are associated with greater health risks.
   D. Literacy skills are not related to hospital admission rates.

3. Which of these national groups issued an important report implicating communication failures as the cause of the majority of serious harmful patient events?
   A. American Association of Allied Health Professionals
   B. American Surgical Nurses Association
   C. The Joint Commission
   D. The American Medical Association

4. Which of the following statements about written plain language is *true*?
   A. Plain language is too boring to be helpful in increasing understanding.
   B. Plain language is conversational, meaning that it is clear and simple.
   C. Plain language does not include paying attention to any elements beyond words.
   D. Plain language dumbs down important healthcare information and may not be 100% accurate.

5. _____ have been shown to increase the likelihood that adults will use vital healthcare information.
   A. Detailed written materials
   B. TV shows
   C. Medically based instructions
   D. Teach-back techniques

Learning Activities

1. View the American Medical Association video *Health Literacy and Patient Safety: Help Patients Understand*, and discuss it with your classmates. (The video is online here: www.ama-assn.org/ama/pub/about-ama/ama-foundation/our-programs/public-health/health-literacy-program.page.) This multimedia program is a great kick-off to start building knowledge about literacy facts and how limited literacy affects patients in medical situations.
2. Download the handouts from the Ask Me Three program (available at www.npsf.org/askme3). Discuss how the handouts might promote patient–provider interaction.
3. View web-based health programs for older adults at www.NIHSeniorHealth.gov. Experiment with the various "buttons" on the site to see how users can change settings to suit individual needs. Consider how this site meets guidelines for plain language and accommodates possible sensory deficits in users.
4. Complete a health literacy audit of a local healthcare facility, preferably a hospital. Use the audit tool designed by Dr. Rima Rudd, Assessing the Health Literacy Environment. (available at www.hsph.harvard.edu/healthliteracy). Or, choose selected elements from the tool and create a mini-audit tool that can be completed more easily. There are other audit tools in the Health Literacy Universal Precautions Toolkit (accessible at www.ahrq.gov/qual/literacy/).

5. Use the checklists in one of the audit tools or one noted in references 37–39 of this chapter to evaluate health and medical materials for plain language. How well do the materials meet plain language guidelines?

6. Read and evaluate a key national report about health literacy. The executive summary of the Institute of Medicine report *Health Literacy: A Prescription to End Confusion* can be found at www.nap.edu/catalog.php?record_id=10883.

7. Look for research articles that link health literacy and your health occupation. A search in major databases will reveal articles published in most health fields, including nursing, physical and occupational therapy, social work, nutrition, pharmacy, dentistry, and medicine.

8. Complete the online training program sponsored by the Health Resources and Services Administration (HRSA) (available at www.hrsa.gov/healthliteracy/). Look for the course titled "Unified Health Communication: Addressing Health Literacy, Cultural Competency, and Limited English Proficiency." You must register for the course (online), which is free, and you can complete one unit at a time and print out the course handouts.

9. Try writing a one-page, easy-to-read information piece related to a specific issue in your field. If you have a clinical practicum and access to patients, ask some of them for suggestions of what to include and for feedback about your first draft. Practice using your piece for patient teaching along with the teach-back method.

10. Look up the Cultural and Linguistic Access Standards (CLAS). You can find them at http://minorityhealth.hhs.gov/templates/browse.aspx?lvl=2&lvlID=15. Discuss how they pertain to healthcare organizations.

REFERENCES

1. Nielsen-Bohlman, L, Panzer, A, Kindig, D (Eds.). *Health Literacy: A Prescription to End Confusion.* Washington, DC: National Academies Press, 2004.

2. Kutner, M, Greenberg, E, Jin, Y, Boyle, B, Hsu, Y, Dunleavy, E. *Literacy in Everyday Life: Results from the 2003 National Assessment of Adult Literacy* (NCES 2007-480). U.S. Department of Education. Washington, DC: National Center for Education Statistics, April 2007: 27.

3. Kutner, M, Greenberg, E, Jin, Y, Paulsen, C. *The Health Literacy of America's Adults: Results from the 2003 National Assessment of Adult Literacy* (NCES 2006-483). U.S. Department of Education. Washington, DC: National Center for Education Statistics, 2006: 6.

4. Fox, S. Pew Internet: Health. 2013, Feb. 1. Retrieved February 11, 2013, from http://www.pewinternet.org/Commentary/2011/November/Pew-Internet-Health.aspx

5. Berland, GK, et al. Health information on the Internet: Accessibility, quality, and readability in English and Spanish. *Journal of the American Medical Association,* 2001;285(20):2612–2621.

6. Kutner, M, Greenberg, E, Jin, Y, Paulsen, C. *The Health Literacy of America's Adults: Results from the 2003 National Assessment of Adult Literacy* (NCES 2006-483). U.S. Department of Education. Washington, DC: National Center for Education Statistics, 2006:6.

7. Apter, A, et al. Numeracy and communication with patients: They are counting on us. *Journal*

of General Internal Medicine, 2008;(12)2: 2117–2124.

8. Gazmararian, J, et al. Health literacy among Medicare enrollees in a managed care organization. *Journal of the American Medical Association*, 1999;281(6):545–551.

9. Baker, D, Gazmararian, J, Sudano, J, Patterson, M. The association between age and health literacy among elderly persons. *Journals of Gerontology Series B: Psychological Sciences and Social Sciences*, 2000;55B(6):S368–S374.

10. Baker, D, et al. Functional health literacy and the risk of hospital admission among Medicare managed care enrollees. *American Journal of Public Health*, 2002;92(8):1278–1283.

11. Scott, T, Gazmararian, J, Williams, M, Baker, D. Health literacy and preventive health care use among Medicare enrollees in a managed care organization. *Medical Care*, 2002;40(5):395–404.

12. Wolf, M, Gazmararian, J, Baker, D. Health literacy and functional health status among older adults. *Archives of Internal Medicine*, 2005;165: 1946–1952.

13. Baker, D, et al. Health literacy and mortality among elderly persons. *Archives of Internal Medicine*, 2007;167(14):1503–1509.

14. Brach, C, et al. *Ten Attributes of Health Literate Health Care Organizations*. Washington, DC: Institute of Medicine of the National Academies, June 2012. Retrieved February 11, 2013, from http://iom.edu/~/media/Files/Perspectives-Files/2012/Discussion-Papers/BPH_Ten_HLit_Attributes.pdf

15. Joint Commission. "What Did the Doctor Say?" Improving Health Literacy to Protect Patient Safety. 2007. Retrieved February 14, 2013, from http://www.jointcommission.org/What_Did_the_Doctor_Say/

16. Joint Commission. *Advancing Effective Communication, Cultural Competence, and Patient- and Family-Centered Care: A Roadmap for Hospitals*. Oakbrook Terrace, IL: The Joint Commission, 2010. Retrieved February 8, 2013, from http://www.jointcommission.org/assets/1/6/ARoadmapforHospitalsfinalversion727.pdf

17. Ad Hoc Committee on Health Literacy for the Council on Scientific Affairs, American Medical Association. Health literacy: Report of the Council on Scientific Affairs. *Journal of the American Medical Association*, 1999;281(6):552–557.

18. American Medical Association. *Improving Communication—Improving Care. An Ethical Force Program Consensus Report*. Chicago: AMA Press, 2006: 114.

19. American Medical Association Foundation. *Health Literacy and Patient Safety: Help Patients Understand. Reducing the Risk by Designing a Safer, Shame-Free Health Care Environment*. Chicago: AMA Foundation, 2007: 13.

20. National Quality Forum (NQF). *Safe Practices for Better Healthcare—2010 Update: A Consensus Report*. Washington DC: NQF, 2010.

21. National Center for Quality Assurance. PCMH 2011. Retrieved February 8, 2013, from http://www.ncqa.org/Home/PatientCenteredMedicalHome2011.aspx

22. U.S. Department of Health and Human Services, Health Resources and Services Administration. United Health Communication 101: Addressing Health Literacy, Cultural Competency, and Limited English Proficiency. Retrieved February 8, 2013, from http://www.hrsa.gov/healthliteracy/training.htm

23. DeWalt, DA, et al. *Health Literacy Universal Precautions Toolkit* (AHRQ Publication No. 10-0046-EF). Rockville, MD: AHRQ, 2010. Retrieved February 8, 2013, from http://www.ahrq.gov/qual/literacy/

24. U.S. Department of Health and Human Services. *National Action Plan to Improve Health Literacy*. Washington, DC: Author, 2010. Retrieved February 8, 2013, from http://www.health.gov/communication/hlactionplan/pdf/Health_Literacy_Action_Plan.pdf

25. Agency for Healthcare Quality and Research. CAHPS. Retrieved February 8, 2013, from http://cahps.ahrq.gov

26. Jack, BW, et al. The reengineered hospital discharge program to decrease rehospitalization. *Annals of Internal Medicine*, 2009;150: 178–187.

27. RTI International, University of North Carolina Evidence-Based Practice Center. *Literacy and Health Outcomes: Evidence Report/Technology Assessment Number 87*. Rockville, MD: Agency for Healthcare Research and Quality,

U.S. Department of Health and Human Services, January 2004.

28. Berkman, ND, et al. Low health literacy and health outcomes: An updated systematic review. *Annals of Internal Medicine,* 2011;155:97–107. Retrieved February 8, 2013, from http://www.ahrq.gov/clinic/epcsums/litupsum.htm

29. Schillinger, D, et al. Closing the loop: Physician communication with diabetic patients who have low health literacy. *Archives of Internal Medicine,* 2003;163:83–90.

30. Davis, T, et al. Intervention to increase mammography utilization in a public hospital. *Journal of General Internal Medicine,* 1998;13: 230–233.

31. DeWalt, D, et al. A heart failure self-management program for patients of all literacy levels: A randomized, controlled trial. *BMC Health Services Research,* 2006;6(30).

32. U.S. Department of Health and Human Services, Office of Disease Prevention and Health Promotion. Health Communication, Health Literacy, and e-Health. Retrieved February 8, 2013, from http://www.health.gov/communication/

33. Weiss, B. *Health Literacy and Patient Safety: Help Patients Understand. Manual for Clinicians.* 2nd ed. Chicago: AMA Foundation, 2007:29.

34. Houts, P, Doak, C, Doak, L, Loscalzo, M. The role of pictures in improving health communication: A review of research on attention, comprehension, recall, and adherence. *Patient Education and Counseling,* 2006;61:173–190.

35. Kessels, RPC. Patients' memory for medical information. *Journal of the Royal Society of Medicine,* 2003;96(5):219–222.

36. National Institute on Aging. Making Your Printed Health Materials Senior Friendly. Retrieved February 8, 2013, from http://www.nia.nih.gov/health/publication/making-your-printed-health-materials-senior-friendly

37. Maximus, for Covering Kids and Families National Program Office. The Health Literacy Style Manual. 2005. Retrieved February 8, 2013, from http://coveringkidsandfamilies.org/resources/docs/stylemanual.pdf.

38. Centers for Disease Control and Prevention. *Simply Put: A Guide for Creating Easy to Understand Materials.* 3rd ed. Atlanta, GA: Centers for Disease Control and Prevention, April 2009. Retrieved February 8, 2013, from http://www.cdc.gov/healthliteracy/pdf/Simply_Put.pdf

39. Plain Language Association International. Website. Retrieved February 8, 2013, from http://www.plainlanguagenetwork.org

40. Centers for Medicare and Medicaid Services. Toolkit for Making Written Material Clear and Effective. Retrieved February 8, 2013, from http://www.cms.gov/Outreach-and-Education/Outreach/WrittenMaterialsToolkit/index.html

41. Simon, GE. Treating depression in patients with chronic disease. *Western Journal of Medicine,* 2001;175(5):292–293. Retrieved February 14, 2013, from http://www.ncbi.nlm.nih.gov/pmc/articles/PMC1071593/

chapter 13

FUTURE CONCERNS IN AN AGING SOCIETY

PAUL D. EWALD, PhD

Anyone who gives you firm prognostications about what is going to happen is either a liar or a fool, because the uncertainties over trends in life expectancy, health and disability, and retirement age are quite high.

—Richard Suzman, Director of the National Institute on Aging's Office of Demography on Aging

Chapter Outline

Behavioral Objectives

Upon completion of this chapter, the reader will be able to:

1. Identify three critical age-related issues facing the United States in the future.
2. Describe ways in which the future generations of older adults are different from the older adults of today.
3. Understand and describe the respective roles of the family, the public sector, and the private sector in caring for frail older adults.

4. Understand that populations around the world are aging at different rates and be able to explain some of the reasons for this and consequences of it.

5. Explain how societal responses to aging vary around the world because of differing rates of change as well as different social, political, and economic policies.

Key Terms

Age composition	Private sector
Demographics	Public sector
Generational equity	Volunteerism
Lifelong education	Work life
Old-age dependency ratio	Young-age dependency ratio

The aging of the U.S. population is not unlike a good news–bad news story. The good news is that more of us are living longer, often in better health, more independently, and with greater security. The bad news is that these advances carry considerable economic and social costs. The good news is that many of us have been, and will continue to be, the beneficiaries of technological and biomedical advances. The bad news is that we will be faced with increasingly difficult resource choices, ethical dilemmas, and political decisions. The good news is that there will be more opportunities for growth and personal enhancement in later life. The bad news is that there may be more years of dependency in later life.

Whether we attend to the good news or the bad news side of the story depends in large part on the social perceptions and attitudes we hold of old age, both individually and as a society. Do we think of it as a time of leisure, relaxation, reflection, and happiness? Or is it a time of greater dependency, illness, and loss? One can see elements of truth in both of these characterizations. Most of us hold dual stereotypes about the nature of old age because we can usually find validation for both the good and the bad in our day-to-day experiences: recalling our vibrant and wise grandparents one day; paying a visit to a nursing home the next.

As we come to terms with the realities of a society in which the number of older adults is increasing steadily, our perceptions and attitudes will undergo rapid change as well. Attitudes and perceptions, however, will not likely converge into a single way of understanding our elders. From the inception of gerontology as a field of study, researchers and observers have emphasized the diversity within the older population and the difficulty in drawing generalizations and conclusions. As the older population increases, it also is becoming more diverse, with multiple sources of variation.

Gerontologists have always been future-oriented. The engine that drives the enormous expansion of interest in the phenomenon of aging is **demographics**. Demographers have relentlessly drawn the attention of researchers, health care providers, and policy makers to the facts of a graying population. The basic facts are undisputed. The exact rates of growth and the consequences of this growth, however, are more speculative, and in some circles, hotly debated.

Demographers lay out their predictions of population growth and change on the basis of different assumptions. These assumptions most often concern fertility rates (adding new people into the population), mortality rates (subtracting people from the population), and migration (the addition and subtraction of people from the population). By examining trends over time, predictions about future growth and change can be made with a certain degree of confidence. But because the future can never be known with absolute certainty, demographers develop multiple series of projections based on assumptions of different rates. Which series to accept, of course, becomes critically important when faced with questions of healthcare planning or economic policy development. Beyond predicting basic rates of fertility, mortality, and migration, other factors quickly enter into discussions of the future of an aging population:

- Will healthcare costs continue to escalate at the present rates?
- How will family structures change as a result of divorce, separation, and an increasing number of people never getting married?
- How secure is the Social Security system?
- Will older adults continue to retire at relatively early ages?
- Will Americans' savings rates improve?
- Will the U.S. economy continue to expand?
- Will young adult and middle-aged women continue to enter the full-time workforce at current rates?
- How will the demand for other federal expenditures change over the next 50 years?

The answers to these questions are often a great deal more speculative than fertility and mortality statistics, and yet, each will have a profound effect on the quality of the lives of older Americans in the next century—and consequently, the quality of American life. Thus, the task of prediction becomes precarious, and the careers of predictors often short. The seriousness of the concerns identified in this chapter rests on assumptions and, to a degree, on speculation. They will change as answers to some of the questions just posed change or become known. They are based on (usually conservative) demographic predictions and should be thought of in an if/then sense. *If* things develop as we suspect they will, *then* it is likely that . . . and so forth. You are encouraged to consider the issues identified in this chapter critically and with skepticism. Consider how the concerns may or may not materialize depending on how we come to view our elders; on how future generations of Americans come to understand issues of obligation, dependency, and entitlement; on how we behave toward different age groups; and on how we vote and behave politically. Shifts in our collective behavior will assuredly influence these concerns for better or for worse.

From among the many concerns in a rapidly aging population, this chapter focuses on three main categories of issues. First, some differences between today's older adults and the older adults of the future are identified. It is this future population with which we are mostly concerned, and they are unlike their predecessors in several important respects. Second, concerns over generational equity and distribution of resources have been raised since the 1980s and are likely to become more pressing as the expected population trends unfold. Third are concerns around how the burden of economic support, and social and medical care, will be distributed. This last concern is discussed from the perspectives of several different nations.

Populations around the world are aging at different rates, allowing us to look at different levels of societal response to the problems and challenges of aging. It will become clear that these are all very complex issues, and the answers to many questions are not known. In many cases, the scope and dimensions of the problems and challenges are only partially understood. The goal in this chapter is to identify several of the major issues that have received the attention of planners, researchers, and the public and to try to provide some context for understanding and thinking about these issues. First, demographic shifts most important to an understanding of these concerns are reviewed.

SIGNIFICANT DEMOGRAPHIC SHIFTS

In 2010, there were 40.3 million Americans older than 65 years, and they constituted 13% of the population.[1] This group is expected to grow to more than 71 million by 2030, representing about 20% of the U.S. population.[2] Within today's older population, the proportion that is older than age 85 numbers approximately 5.3 million. By 2050, the over-85 age group will number nearly 21 million. Much of our interest in, and concern over, our aging society is with this group that is older than 85, whose growth is outpacing all others. This is a heterogeneous and complex age group to study. They are often characterized as frail older adults. Indeed, the likelihood of hospitalization or nursing home placement rises considerably with advanced age. Dementias and cognitive impairments that many of us have come to associate with advanced age do, in fact, increase dramatically in rate to a point among surviving older adults. Mobility is reduced; chronic conditions multiply; impoverishment and social isolation are greater risks. There is reason for concern as we see the unprecedented expansion of this age group. And yet, there is evidence to suggest that for a substantial proportion of those who survive into their 80s, there is a sort of mortality grace period that is marked by vitality and relatively good health.[3] And as suggested in the following sections, today's population of individuals older than 85 may not be the best guide to understanding future older adults.

Be cautious about generalizing circumstances found in the United States to other parts of the world. Societies throughout the world are aging at different rates as a result of different degrees of modernization, industrialization, and economic development. In general terms, developed nations have older populations. The countries of the developing world currently have relatively young populations, but over the next half century they will be experiencing population aging at a rate unprecedented in the developed nations. Countries like the United States have had the luxury, so to speak, of slower and steadier rates of aging throughout the 20th and 21st centuries, and with considerable foreknowledge. The dual challenges of poorer countries will be to deal with the pace of aging and, concomitantly, the problems associated with economic development.

Another statistic of interest to demographers and gerontologists is referred to as the dependency ratio. This ratio refers to those people in the population who are usually thought of as economically dependent to those who are economically productive, and can be calculated and considered in several different ways. The **old-age dependency ratio** refers to the number of people in the population older than 65 as compared with those between the ages of 18 and 64. Although all of those older than 65 are not necessarily retired or nonworking, and all of those between ages 18 and 64 are not necessarily working and economically productive, this ratio serves as a general indicator of the economic burden confronting the working segment of the population at any given time. The old-age dependency ratio increased throughout the 20th century and will continue to increase gradually through about 2020. After this date, not long after the baby boom generation begins to retire, the ratio begins to increase dramatically through 2030. Today, in crude terms, 100 workers contribute to the health and economic welfare of approximately 21 older adults. In 2020, 100 workers will contribute to the well-being of 27 or 28 older adults. The number of older adults per 100 workers grows to 35 by 2030 and then rises at a slower rate for the next few decades.[4] These ratios reflect the economic burden of an aging population.

Another type of dependency ratio is the **young-age dependency ratio**, or the ratio of those younger than 18 years to those between the ages of 18 and 64. Between 1970 and 1990, this ratio declined dramatically from about 61 young people to every 100 workers to 42 per 100. Since 1990 this ratio has remained relatively constant with minor fluctuations, and is expected to continue to remain constant well into the middle of the 21st century.[5]

The young-age and old-age dependency ratios can be combined for a total dependency ratio. This statistic shows that in 1990, there were about 62 young and old people to every 100 workers. This number is expected to increase to 67 by the year 2020.[5] Note, however, that the share of the total dependency ratio accounted for by children is declining, while the share accounted for by older adults is increasing. Consider also that the care of the young in the United States is considered to be primarily a private family responsibility, whereas the care of older adults carries with it more of a public responsibility (primarily through the Social Security tax and other taxes imposed on the working population). This issue and the ratios of economic dependency to productivity become significant in the discussion to follow concerning generational transfers and questions of equitable distribution of economic resources. But first, we consider what is known about the older population of today and the older adults of the future.

OLDER ADULTS TODAY

Data from the 2010 U.S. Census provide a portrait of today's older adults and a basis for understanding and predicting some of the population characteristics of future older adults. The educational attainment of the over-65 population is significantly below that of the total adult population. For example, college degree completion rates for all U.S. adults are currently about 25%, whereas just 16% of adults over 65 have 4-year college degrees or higher. A more dramatic contrast can be seen in those with less than a high school diploma. Among the oldest-old, over age 85, nearly half did not complete high school. That figure for the total U.S. adult population over age 25 stands at about one-fifth.[2] This is changing rapidly, however. For example, in 2006, men between the ages of 55 and 64 had levels of educational attainment comparable to men in the 25 to 34 age group.[6]

In 2000, 56% of older Americans were married, 28% were widowed, 7% were divorced, and 5% were never married. The number who are married declines with age. For example, two-thirds of those in the 65–74 age group were married compared to less than a third of the over-85 age group. This decline is explained largely by the difference in life expectancy for men and women, and the tendency for men to be slightly older than their wives. The 2010 U.S. Census reported a narrowing of the gap in life expectancy between men and women. In 1990 there were 82.7 men for every 100 women at age 65. By 2010 there were 90.5 men to every 100 women. These sex ratios have important implications for the availability of caregivers in the event of disability or impairment.[7] For the total over-65 population, in 2000, two-thirds lived in households with others, most often a spouse. Twenty-eight percent lived alone in a household. Women over 65 are still about three times more likely to live alone than are men.[2]

Since the early 1990s, labor force participation for men over 55 has increased. This reverses the prior trend toward earlier retirement decisions. This reversal has been attributed to changes in Social Security, the increased educational attainment referred to earlier, and significant shifts in employer pensions.[6] Briefly, Social Security eliminated its means test whereby a portion of benefits are withheld for workers earning more than specified amounts. Higher levels of educational attainment are associated with longer work lives, and men have made gains in education in recent years. Finally, over the last several decades employer-defined benefit pensions have declined and been replaced by 401(k) plans, which work like savings accounts and do not incentivize retirement at any particular age. These increased participation rates in the labor force have persisted through both the recessions of the past decade.[6]

For older age groups, disability becomes an important determinant of ability to work. The most common disabilities reported by older adults were physical in nature (27%), followed by difficulties with leaving the home (20%), and sensory difficulties such as blindness or hearing impairment (14%). All categories of disability increase significantly with age, with 47% of the over-85 population, for example, reporting difficulties leaving their homes.[2]

In sum, older Americans in 2000 had lower levels of educational attainment compared to the overall population, though the gap is gradually disappearing. They had high rates of home ownership and a modest level of financial security. Levels of disability, poor health, and living alone all rise with age, and women are more vulnerable than men because of their greater longevity. What is masked by this brief, stereotypical portrait is the considerable heterogeneity of the experience of aging and the variety of life circumstances found in late life. The future of aging in the United States is also changing as each successive cohort distinguishes itself from those that preceded them. The large baby boom generation began entering late life in 2011, and will surely experience this period of life differently from how their parents and grandparents did.

FUTURE OLDER ADULTS

The older population of the future, the baby boomers, will be characteristically different from their older predecessors of today. Notably, they have many more years of formal education. Higher levels of educational attainment are associated with lower mortality, better health, reduced poverty, and higher probability of being married, and hence less likelihood of being alone.[8] Family size of the older population has already begun to change and will continue to shrink in the coming decades. Until 2005, family size of older adults was increasing, with 35% of older adults having four or more children, and 46% having two or three children. Since 2005, however, only 11% have four or more children, and 55% have two or three. Family size has important implications for social and economic support for older adults. Some estimates are that as much as 80% of care for older adults is provided by family members, often by adult children. As family size shifts downward, the availability of family care declines commensurately. The proportion of older adults requiring formal assisted care may then increase.

The gap in life expectancy for men and women is narrowing. During the 1980s, women gained about 0.2 years in life expectancy and men 0.6.[8] Under today's mortality conditions, older Americans reaching the age of 65 can expect to live an additional 18.7 years on average. For those who reach the age of 85, women can expect another 7.2 years of life and men an additional 6.1 years.[2] This trend results in higher rates of marriage among older adults compared to previous generations. Women do not lose their husbands as soon because of death and thus spend fewer years alone. Beneficial consequences of this will probably include reduced rates of isolation and subsequently lower rates of depression and suicide, interdependency of intact couples, and less dependency of single older adults on societal and familial aid. Also, if the trends toward higher rates of divorce and separation among younger groups continue, combined with delayed childbirth and childrearing, available familial support is likely to decline even further than would be predicted by just the shrinking family size of older adults.

In the future, more women will retire from longer years of workforce participation. Participation in the workforce has increased among women over the last four decades. The largest increase has been among women ages 55–61, having gone from 44% working outside the home in 1963 to 64% in 2006.[2] For women older than 62, most of their increase in the workforce has occurred since the mid-1990s. This means that older women will be qualifying for their own pensions and Social Security benefits in larger numbers compared to years past.[8] This will have the effect of reducing poverty among older women and, combined with longer marriages, will increase the real income of older couples. Fewer are likely to need economic assistance. The paramount concern in this regard is how the Social Security system of revenue collection and benefits disbursement will be able to accommodate this larger cohort of beneficiaries with a reduced number of workers.

As the older population grows, so too grows the number of voters who are old. Inasmuch as older people vote more than younger people, and are more politically active generally, older adults are likely to become a more vocal and potent political force. In 1990, approximately 30% of federal expenditures were directed to the older population. Were this level of expenditures to be maintained through 2030, they could conceivably reach 60% of the federal budget.[8] Age-related voting behaviors and budget expenditures are both nearly impossible to predict for the short term, let alone over decades. If older adults vote in accordance with narrowly defined self-interests and maximize gains for older age groups, there will be fewer economic resources available for other purposes. If expenditures on defense and national security, for example, continue to increase as has been the case since 2001 to the present, pressure to reduce large federal budget items such as Social Security and other entitlements grows. Indeed, the pressure to restructure Social Security and other so-called entitlements was substantial during the 2012 election. There has been little evidence, until recently, that older adults vote with one mind on age-related issues, or any other issues for that matter. The 2010 elections revealed a greater tendency for elderly voters to vote as a bloc on age-related issues.[9] As pressure increases to reduce Social Security or Medicare benefits at the same time the older population expands, age politics are likely to become more pronounced. This will be unavoidable if income transfers across generations become greater. Questions about the equity of shifting more resources to older adults are exacerbated by the downward trends in the welfare and quality of life for children in the United States. This issue is examined in greater detail in the section on generational equity later in this chapter.

The difficulties in forecasting the future should be evident by now. Perhaps one of the greatest flaws in forecasting is in the assumption that today's notions about transitions from work to retirement will prevail in the future. The typical pattern of working from the completion of one's education in early adulthood to one's mid-60s, often for the same employer and in the same place, then abruptly leaving the workforce to pursue leisure and pleasure pursuits in retirement is not typical now—and for most Americans, never was. This is a pattern that fit middle- and upper-income white men for a relatively brief interval in our history. These are powerful stereotypes against which we must measure "the good life." The issues of generational equity and caring for frail older adults addressed in later sections are questions of resource availability and allocation. How we think about dependency, obligation, and the distribution of resources is influenced by whether we see others as needy, deserving, or a burden. In the United States, such determinations are made largely on the basis of what we believe one has earned through his or her own merit. Merit is awarded in our culture on the basis of education and training attained, work done, and contributions made. To what degree can we ascertain whether the future older adults will merit the benefits they reap? Are older adults cutting productive work lives unnecessarily short through early retirement? Could older adults stay on the productive side of the dependency ratio longer, thereby relieving some of the burden on younger generations?

WORK LIFE

Answers to these questions come from two very different directions that might be thought of as the supply and demand of work for older workers. As the absolute numbers of traditional-aged workers in the United States and other developed countries declines, employers are forced to rethink the attractiveness of older workers and modify work policies and practices. As life span, health, and opportunity extend, older Americans reconsider the balance of work, leisure, and social contribution in their lives.

Before the 1980s, retirement trends were quite clear. Women's participation in work outside the home stood at about half that of men. Most older workers retired as soon as they were able. The ability to retire was determined primarily on the basis of finances and health, factors working as incentives or disincentives depending on individual circumstances. By and large, the favorable balance of these two factors has provided great numbers of older male workers with sufficient incentive to take retirement at the earliest possible time. Labor force participation rates for older male workers declined steadily until the early 1990s. This decline was fueled by a reduction in the eligibility age for Social Security from 65 to 62 in the early 1960s. Older Americans had also accumulated greater amounts of lifetime wealth, allowing earlier retirement. Work participation for older workers leveled off in the mid-1980s for men. For men in the 65–69 age range, participation stood at 24% in 1985 but showed a gradual rise to 34% in 2006. Most of the increase in labor force participation for women older than 62 began in the mid-1990s.[1]

As the U.S. economy and the labor market shifted in the 1980s and 1990s, downsizing and reduction in the workforce became familiar terms to U.S. workers. Older workers were often targeted because of savings that would result from eliminating their higher salaries and the belief that their health insurance and benefits were more costly to employers. The Age Discrimination in Employment Act (ADEA) was introduced into law in 1967 to protect older workers from arbitrary and indiscriminate hiring and firing practices. The effect of downsizing is amply illustrated by the fact that between 1980 and 1987, one-fifth of all *Fortune* 500 companies' employees were eliminated.[10] In the early 1990s, an estimated 2 million people between the ages of 50 and 64 were able and wanting to return to work.[11] Workers in this age group often opt for "early retirement" after they have exhausted their work options. Those older than 65 years, generally in better health than previous generations, also show interest in continued employment, but more often in part-time or flexible employment opportunities.[11] These facts would suggest that the demand for work among older workers often exceeds the supply. Contrary to stereotypes, it appears that older workers are punctual, conscientious, sensitive to coworkers, and use fewer sick days than younger workers for acute problems. They are also loyal to employers and experienced.[12]

There is some evidence that older workers are losing their edge with regard to job security. Based on calculations of the U.S. Bureau of Labor Statistics' Displaced Worker Survey, displacement rate differentials for older and younger workers has disappeared. Two factors explain the decline in older worker's job security. First, following a decade of prevalent 401(k) plans, workers' average tenure in jobs shows a sharp decline since 401(k) plans offer little incentive to stay with the same employer. A second factor is the higher rate of displacement in the manufacturing sector. Even though this sector has been reduced since the mid-1980s, it has a displacement rate significantly higher than other employment sectors, and the likelihood of older employees working in manufacturing has declined.[6]

It is questionable whether extending the **work life** of older workers much beyond the gains already made over the last two decades is likely or realistic. The median age of retirement for men declined from 66 to 63 between the mid-1960s and the present. This was driven in large part by changes in Social Security allowing for partial benefit eligibility at age 62. As life expectancy continues to post gains, the ability to afford and sustain a comfortable or even reasonable postretirement lifestyle is becoming more challenging. Policy makers often search for ways to incentivize longer work lives, more savings, and reduced preretirement consumption. Some portion of the over-62 population, however, may simply be unable to work because of ill health or disability. Most older Americans are able to continue to work into their mid-60s, but it has been estimated that at least one-quarter of them may not be healthy enough to work beyond that. Other factors like the plateauing of educational attainment and the growing incidence of obesity may place real limits on people's ability to work.[13]

There also appears to be a mismatch between the needs and desires of older workers and the economics of employing older workers. Older workers report consistently that full-time work is less attractive and that they prefer part-time or flexible work opportunities, which are often unavailable. Recent proposals put forward by the Internal Revenue Service (IRS) may make phased retirement more feasible for older workers by reducing the extent of benefit coverage required by employers.[14,15]

Older workers tend to be the most expensive to employ. This can be balanced only by making them worth the cost to employers through, for example, ongoing educational, training, and professional development programs. Some industries, notably health care and higher education, have done well in this area by providing ongoing professional development, but by and large U.S. employers lag behind European and Japanese efforts in these areas.[16] In her comprehensive analysis, Munnell concludes that the only policy change likely to yield some significant extension of work life for older workers is to increase the earliest eligible retirement age from 62 to 64 or 65.[14] This both is politically challenging and would likely result in only marginal gains.

The pressure may come, however, from the other direction, that is, increased interest in and/or pressure to work among older adults themselves. People work either because they need to, they want to, or some combination of the two. The need to work, for some significant segment of the older population, may increase substantially, especially with the recent economic downturn. The crash of the stock market in 2008 resulted in a loss of about one-third of the value of 401(k) plans. Social Security in the future, for a variety of reasons, is not likely to cover as much of preretirement income as it now does. In 2006, the "average earner" who retired at age 65 received the equivalent of about 42% of previous earnings. After paying the automatically deducted Medicare premium, this drops to 38.7% of previous earnings. Current Social Security regulation is scheduled to reduce preretirement income replacement rates in the future through (1) the scheduled increases in the normal retirement age from 65 to 67, (2) increases in Medicare premiums, and (3) more taxation of Social Security resulting from exemption amounts not indexed to inflation.[14] Because Social Security provides the greatest source of aggregate income for older Americans, these changes are significant. In 2006, 37% of income for older Americans came from Social Security, 28% from earnings, 18% from pensions, and 15% from asset income.[14] Thus, the financial security of future older adults may be more tied to earnings than in the past. An AARP survey found two types of older workers, sustainers and providers, and estimated that about 61% of older workers work at least in part out of financial need. The proportion that needs to work may increase in the future, although the ability to work or the availability of jobs may not keep pace.[17] For this group, both income and health benefits, if available, are strong incentives to maintain employment.

For those who *want* to continue to work (estimated at 38% in the AARP survey) regardless of financial incentives, a number of powerful motives have been identified: maintenance of social networks, use of their knowledge, job autonomy, learning opportunities, involvement in decision making, supporting success in coworkers, job satisfaction, commitment to employers, a sense of responsibility, and making a contribution to society.[17] These motives are not very different from those identified by volunteers in a later section of this chapter.

It is important to note that powerful determinants of work and retirement patterns are the lifelong expectations we hold of each. As family structures change, as women participate in the paid workforce longer, as maternity and paternity leaves become more commonplace, and as education and retraining become more necessary, it is likely that older adults will become more accustomed to a mixed pattern of workforce entry, exit, and reentry. The expectation of a single sharp transition from work life to retirement will become less compelling. Combined with delayed benefit eligibility for Social Security, as well as general uncertainty about the stability of the Social Security system and the economy in general, adults will plan differently for retirement and alter their expectations of what is typical.

RETIREMENT AND FINANCES

How prepared are Americans for retirement? One measure of preparedness is derived from studies using the National Retirement Risk Index (NRRI).[18] The NRRI utilizes several measures to arrive at a risk estimate. First it projects an actual retirement income replacement rate based on preretirement income and wealth. The Index then constructs a target replacement rate that would allow households to maintain their preretirement standard of living in retirement. Finally, it calculates risk by estimating the gap between the projected and target rates. Using U.S. income and wealth data from the 2004 Survey of Consumer Finances, Munnell and her associates were able to identify the percentages of U.S. households that are ready to retire at any given age. The earliest age at which one becomes eligible for Social Security benefits is age 62. Estimates are that only 30% of households have the financial wherewithal to move seamlessly from work to retirement at this age. By age 66, when individuals are eligible for the full Social Security benefit and for Medicare, 55% of households are ready for retirement (including the 30% ready at 62). At age 70, about 86% of U.S. households are retirement-ready.[18] The average retirement age today is about age 63, suggesting a considerable gap between reality and need.

With the release of the 2010 Survey of Consumer Finances, Munnell et al. were able to estimate the impact of the recession on population retirement risk as measured by the NRRI.[19] For the overall elderly population, risk increased nine percentage points from 44% in 2007 to 53% in 2010, suggesting that many of today's workers face considerable challenges in adequately financing their retirements. This change was due to some of the worst investment returns in recent history along with the rise in Social Security's full retirement age, decline in housing values, and low interest rates (resulting in lower returns for annuitizing wealth). Further estimates that include explicit assumptions factoring in the escalating costs of health care put the at-risk percentage above 60% of households.[19]

Indeed, the cost of health care is a significant factor. In 2007, Medicare and Medicaid estimated the cost of out-of-pocket expenses for health care at $3,800 per year for an individual and $7,600 per year for a retired couple. For those requiring long-term care, the costs can be staggering. Private nursing home care is estimated to cost $90,520 per year.[20] These costs hit the elderly population differentially. Two-thirds of the elderly will require some form of long-term care; of this group, 40% will require 2 or more years of care. The need for long-term care is affected by race, ethnicity, education, living circumstances, and other variables.

Perhaps of greatest concern is that the levels of financial risk for the elderly are likely to increase with time. Late baby boomers will experience higher risk than the early baby boomers who are beginning their retirements now. In turn, Gen-Xers (those born between 1965 and 1974) will experience considerably higher risk than late baby boomers. Turning this state of affairs around must begin with greater knowledge of the challenges we face. Reduced risk will occur when we are able to better understand the financial resources necessary to live out our extended lifespans, are able to work sufficiently long to accumulate the resources we need, and can make significant improvements in our lifestyles to be healthy enough to extend our work lives sufficiently. Although this sounds like a tall order, we can look to other countries that have been successful in achieving these gains through policy initiatives. We return to this issue in the section on retirement practices in Japan.

LIFELONG EDUCATION

The growth of secondary and postsecondary education in the United States since World War II has been dramatic and impressive. Although the GI Bill created opportunities for returning veterans to obtain college credentials and marked the beginning of an educational expansion that continues today, not all segments of the population (those slightly older or women, for example) benefited equally or at the same time in their lives. In 1965, just 24% of the older population had completed high school and only 5% had college degrees. In 2009, the number of high school graduates among older adults increased to 77%, and 20% had completed a 4-year college degree.[21] The rates of high school completion for older men and women in 2007 were about equal, but the rates of bachelor degree completion differed, with 25% of men having completed but only 15% of women. Bachelor's degree attainment may have plateaued for older men, whereas gains for women are still likely.[13] Racial differences are more pronounced. In 2007, 81% of whites over age 65 had completed high school compared to 58% of African Americans and 42% of Hispanics. The bachelor's degree completion rates for whites, blacks, and Hispanics are currently 21%, 10%, and 9%, respectively.[2]

Later adult education takes many forms and, compared with the lock-step model of traditional early life education, is much more fluid and open-ended and can be considered **lifelong education**. Road Scholar (formerly Elderhostel) has become a well-known national and international program offering thousands of short-term courses of study each year. Geared to the college level and cultural enrichment, Road Scholar does not offer college credit and tends to appeal to those who are already well educated. Also, at least one-quarter of community colleges target older adults for particular kinds of course offerings. Those most commonly enrolled tend to be in the areas of financial planning and management, health and cultural enrichment, and contemporary civic issues.[22]

Increased enrollments of older adults in college and university courses were a boon to institutions that had been bracing themselves for declining enrollments during the 1980s. At that time, there was a decline in the pool of graduating high school seniors on the order of 25%. Yet, college enrollments went from 12 million to 13.4 million during 1 year as a result of older learners returning to school.[13] Among the adult college population, there are now more women than men, whites dominate on the order of 90%, and 85% of older students work, mostly full time. In order of frequency, the most common reasons given for returning to school are life transitions, learning as a satisfying activity, an opportunity to meet people, and a way to fill up free time. The kinds of life transitions precipitating a return to the classroom differ for older and younger adults. Those between 25 and 64 years cite career transitions. Those older than 65 more often cite leisure transitions and family transitions than do younger adults.[23]

It has been observed that adult education increases during periods of rapid social change. Changes in the economy, the age composition of society, technology, the family, and the roles of minorities and women all would appear to call for an increase in both traditional and less traditional forms of educational participation among older adults for some time to come.

VOLUNTEERISM

Wilson defines **volunteerism** as "engagement in proactive activities that involve commitment and whose benefits extend beyond the individual volunteers."[24] Similarly, Harootyan defines volunteering as "any activity intended to help others that is provided without obligation for which the volunteer does not receive pay or other material compensation."[25] Volunteering can be either formal or informal. According to the Current Population Survey of September 2005, 28.8% of the U.S. population engaged in formal volunteer work.[26] Older age groups participated somewhat less on average, with about 1 in 4 persons over age 65 engaged as volunteers.[26] Overall volunteer activity in the United States declined from about 80 million in 1987 to 63.4 million in 2010.[27] In a 2003 AARP study, the concept of volunteerism was broadened to include informal activity such as helping someone in the community. Among those older than age 70, 40% reported formal volunteer activity and another 40% reported informal assistance to someone in the community.[26]

Reasons given for volunteerism are multiple and include attaining higher levels of mastery, life satisfaction, and energy[26]; to make a contribution to society; to meet others[28]; to gain career-related experience; to enhance self-esteem; to reduce negative feelings; to strengthen social relationships; to learn more about the world; and to act on important values.[29]

Despite the significant contributions of older adults as volunteers, they are still considered to be an underutilized resource, and one that is growing in size. In addition to those who volunteer, there are a good many more who do not but say they would if asked.[30] Baby boomers who, relative to previous generations, are characterized by better health, higher levels of education, and greater financial security, report in high numbers (51%) that they intend to volunteer. Volunteer programs exist for most skill levels and interest areas. For example, the Older Volunteer Program of the ACTION Agency is an umbrella organization that includes the Retired Senior Volunteer Program (RSVP), Foster Grandparents, and Senior Companion Program. RSVP volunteers tend to be geared toward human services such as refugee services, literacy programs, long-term care, and youth counseling. Foster Grandparents and Senior Companions are targeted for low-income volunteers and provide small hourly stipends. RSVP allows for expense reimbursement. These programs are funded mostly with federal dollars, with some state and local contributions.[31,32]

AARP, formerly the American Association of Retired Persons, operates a Volunteer Talent Bank (VTB) for the purpose of matching volunteer interests and skills with agency and community needs. Set up originally to provide staffing for AARP volunteer needs, VTB now makes referrals to many outside agencies including the American Red Cross, the U.S. Fish and Wildlife Service, and the Peace Corps.[31]

The Service Corps of Retired Executives (SCORE) provides consulting and presents workshops for small business management assistance. By the early 1990s, after 30 years of volunteer service, SCORE had 13,000 volunteers providing voluntary assistance at 750 locations. In 1996, SCORE added online services and to date they have served more than 8.5 million clients. Consulting services are free of charge to client businesses and managers, and a small fee is charged for workshops to cover expenses.[31]

The organization Cross-Cultural Solutions offers an example of expansion of volunteer activity to international venues. Opportunities exist for adults over 50 in Asia, Latin America, and Africa to work with children, the elderly, the disabled, or in health care.[33]

In October 2006, the Older Americans Act (OAA) was reauthorized. The reauthorization included several steps to increase opportunities for volunteerism and civic engagement such as the availability of grants to organizations that engage older adults in services to meet community needs.[34] The OAA further asks area agencies on aging to participate in planning to support older Americans in civic engagement. Some proposals for policy makers include incorporating many of the structures of successful programs currently in place for younger age groups such as VISTA, the White House Fellows program, Troops to Teachers, and the Caro Fellows program. These proposals provide entry points, training, orientation, and structure to postcareer volunteer experiences.[34]

THE QUESTION OF GENERATIONAL EQUITY

Substantial gains have been made among the older segment of the population in terms of income and living conditions. In 1959, older Americans had the highest rates of poverty of any age group, with 35% living below the federally defined poverty line. Children under 18 were the second most poverty-stricken group then, with 27% below the federally defined poverty level, followed by working-age groups at 17%. By 1993, the poverty rate for older adults had dropped to 12.4%. Children did not make comparable progress. Following significant gains in the 1960s, poverty rates among children climbed in the early 1980s and again in the early 1990s when it reached 22.7% in 1993,[2,34] making children the largest poverty-stricken age group in the United States.

Fluctuations in poverty rates took unpredictable twists and turns following the 2008 recession. Between 2008 and 2009, poverty rates increased for every age group in the United States except those over 65, for whom it decreased by 0.8%. The greatest increase in poverty rate, 2.3%, was for the 18- to 24-year age group, with the under 18 and 25–34 age groups each increasing by 1.7%. The reduction of poverty for the elderly age group was due to adjustments to Social Security. For those over 65 who are in the lowest third of the income distribution, Social Security constitutes 84% of income. The cost-of-living adjustment in Social Security is designed to maintain purchasing power by indexing benefits to changes in the economy. These adjustments are calculated every October based on a comparison of third-quarter data of the Consumer Price Index with the previous year's numbers. Adjustments are made the following January. The 2009 January adjustment amounted to a 5.8% increase, the highest since 1982. In addition, the economic stimulus package of 2009 added one-time payments to Social Security beneficiaries. These two sources of additional income moved many elders at or below the poverty level to just above it.[35]

Given children's dependency on the adults around them for survival and well-being, childhood poverty is alarming and, some would argue, should be a source of national shame in a country as wealthy as the United States. These opposing trends have become the basis for the charge that older adults have become an overbenefited group at the expense of the young. There is concern that as the older population grows it will draw even more of our national resources away from an increasingly needy younger population. A way to remedy this circumstance and reverse the trend would be to recognize the importance of investing in young people, for example, by setting limits on expenditures and investments in the older population and redirecting those resources toward America's youth.

At first glance, this argument is a powerful one. It is indeed alarming to observe these opposing trends. It has been my experience that when even the most sympathetic students of gerontology become aware of these facts they quickly condemn the system that takes from children to benefit the old. The observation that the country's oldest adults seem to be enjoying an increasingly comfortable standard of living while the most dependent and vulnerable segment of the population is at greater risk carries with it images of selfishness, disregard for the future, and moral culpability. There are reasons to be cautious of these charges, however, and a need to examine the situation much more carefully. Researchers and gerontologists have argued that these impressions are misleading when taken out of context. Minkler summarized many of these contextual considerations and counterarguments at about the time when the disparity in age group poverty rates was reaching its peak.[36]

The way in which poverty is measured is sometimes different for the young and the old owing to estimated adjustments in living costs. Minkler argues that if the same definitions are used for the two groups, the poverty rate for older adults climbs about three percentage points. By any standard, income levels used to distinguish those in poverty from those not in poverty are artificial and set very low. When, for example, we consider 150% of poverty level as true poverty, sometimes described as poor and near poor, the poverty rate for older adults nearly doubles. In other words, although it is true that many of the old are no longer living below the poverty line as defined by the various government agencies, at least one-third of them are still living in extremely modest circumstances and would be considered by many to be poor. All of this is to suggest that poverty is more subjective and more complex than a magic cut-off number, and taken out of context these statistics can be misleading.[36]

More important is that the generational inequity argument strongly implies that monies are being taken away from the young and given to the old. In fact, the causes of childhood poverty and the causes of improved living standards for the old are quite independent and unrelated to one another. At the risk of oversimplification, the rise in poverty rates among children during the 1980s was attributable in large part to market forces. There was a decline in real wages among workers in the 1980s, an increase in substandard wage work, and loss of high-paying jobs in such areas as manufacturing, unfavorable employment trends for many, and an increase in single-parent, female-headed households. In other words, children are poor because young adults have declining opportunities in obtaining well-paying jobs and maintaining families. The declining poverty level among the old was primarily the result of changes in government policy in the 1970s. In 1972, Social Security payments were increased 20% and tied to annual rises in the Consumer Price Index to protect against inflation. If Social Security were reduced to its pre-1972 levels, this would both increase real poverty among the old and do nothing to alter the changes in markets and family structure that affected the young during this time with such devastating consequences.[36]

Much of the cost burden of supporting an aging population is directly related to the costs of increased demand for medical care and healthcare resources. Those who argue for greater **generational equity** imply that the cost is inflated because of the demands for high-technology medical care among older adults. In fact, much of the crisis in health care is a result not of high technology, but of the failure to control the costs of health care generally, costs that affect all ages. The costs of hospital care, for example, grew from $14 billion in 1965 to $167 billion in 1985. Healthcare costs increased at roughly twice that of the Consumer Price Index in this timeframe.[36]

Another flaw in the generational inequity argument is the suggestion that the distribution and redistribution of resources is a zero-sum game. This is not true of the political process generally, and there is no reason to believe that it should be true as the needs and demands of society change in a dynamic and fluid manner. The population is getting older. That calls for more resources of a particular kind. The Cold War ended over two decades ago, reducing the need for economic resources for defense, and national security has consumed substantial resources since September 2001. As needs change and as the composition of society changes, so too do the rules of resource acquisition and allocation change. This is evident in changes in tax laws, in retirement rules and benefits, in proposals for flextime for workers, and in uses of volunteer resources and energy. Corporate tax rates, for example, declined from 4.2% of the gross national product (GNP) in the early 1960s to 1.6% of GNP in the early 1980s. Although politically unpopular, perhaps we can no longer afford to forgo these sources of government revenues. Economic challenges, and the solutions identified to address them, must be understood as fluid and changeable.[36]

This section so far has considered inequities and imbalances between older adults and children. By the year 2000, the disparity in poverty levels between the young and old had narrowed to single digits, and by 2006 poverty rates stood at 9% and 17% for the old and for children under 18, respectively.[2] Today the debate is more often likely to focus on the equity of burden and benefit between the generations of working adults and retired adults. As the demographic shifts continue to move the United States toward an older age structure, and as grim economic forecasts predict insolvency in the Social Security system, age politics may take on a sharper edge. In 2006, Blackburn characterized the opposing camps in this debate on generational equity as the "generational accounting" supporters and the "generational solidarity" supporters.[37] The position held by the generational accountants, advanced in various forms since at least the late 1980s, is that taxing younger workers to finance the pensions of retirees is inherently unfair. This position amounts to a direct attack on the viability and equity of the Social Security program. Such accounting calculates the total contributions and the total eventual benefits for a given generation and necessarily takes cohort or generational size into account. When combined with a portrayal of a bankrupt Social Security system, generational accountants advance an emotionally packed economic argument with clear generational winners (larger cohorts) and generational losers (smaller cohorts). Variations derived from this basic position include policies that advance health savings accounts, voluntary personal retirement accounts, and various Social Security privatization schemes.[38] When age cohorts vary substantially in size, questions of fairness, equity, and generational justice present formidable challenges.

Those who support a position of "generational solidarity" argue, no less emotionally, that there is a social bond between generations of parents and children that transcends precise accounting (**Figure 13-1**). Those who advance this position favor a pay-as-you-go system of generational transfers and consider claims of the imminent collapse of the Social Security system and the crisis of an aging population as alarmist propaganda. In contrast, generational accountants argue that each generation should pay its own way and that risk pooling within generations is preferable to risk pooling between them.[37]

Blackburn, in his review of these positions, favors the reasoning of generational solidarity supporters but suggests that it too is flawed. He points to the duties and obligations of each generation toward the other but maintains that these obligations are not without limit. The economic alarmism of the generational accountants, Blackburn maintains, is

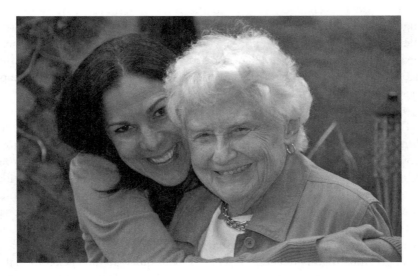

Figure 13-1   There is often a social bond between generations of parents and children that transcends precise accounting.
Courtesy of Paul Ewald.

based on arbitrary assumptions and distant time horizons that, when combined, point to massive, and likely erroneous, shortfalls in the system.[37]

The nation's stand on generational equity will be put to the test again soon, and often thereafter. An impact of the 2008 recession was to again raise longstanding concerns about the solvency of Social Security. The 2012 Social Security Trustees Report advanced the projected date of trust fund exhaustion from 2036 to 2033, based on its intermediate set of assumptions. Program finances were directly impacted by the recession due to the reductions in the payroll tax and the increase in benefit claims. The costs of the program began to exceed outlays in 2010, and this will continue. That means that Social Security is tapping the interest in the trust fund sooner than anticipated. By 2021, taxes and interest will fall short of projected outlays and the program will have to begin drawing on the trust fund assets. After trust fund exhaustion, projected for 2033, taxes will be the only revenue funding Social Security, and it will run deficits.[39]

Since the onset of the recession in 2008, government spending, deficit reduction, and taxes have dominated political discourse in the United States. The "sequestration" implemented on March 1, 2013, was the result of government gridlock and failure to come to terms with the balance of spending and revenue required to address the nation's economic situation. It is estimated that we could address the Social Security Trust Fund shortfall with a payroll tax increase of 2.68%—1.34% each for employers and employees. If such a tax increase was implemented immediately, the Social Security Trust Fund's solvency would be extended for 75 years. Each year of delay raises this number. As noted previously, Social Security accounts for 84% of total income for older Americans in the bottom third of the income distribution. In addition, elderly Americans are at greater and greater risk of financial shortfalls in retirement with each passing generation. (See "Retirement and Finances" earlier in this chapter.)

As has been stated repeatedly, increasing the tax burden on a shrinking cohort of workers is not an attractive option for many. What alternatives does this leave if we are to retain a viable and equitable pension system for America's older adults? One approach that has been advanced in Sweden (discussed later in this chapter), and that is under consideration in other developed countries, indexes retiree public pension benefits to the actual size of the current working age cohort. Another approach altogether would be to focus reform efforts less on publicly funded pension support like Social Security and more on employer-sponsored defined benefit pensions. These private pensions were more the norm from post–World War II until about the mid-1970s and resulted in considerably more retirement savings,[37,38] though at a higher cost to employers.

Related to the generational equity debate, and a large area of study in its own right, is whether age is being scapegoated when, in fact, there are sources of inequity within age groups that are greater than the inequities between age groups. It is important not to lose sight of the fact that older adults are certainly the most diverse age group in the population and that the aging experience varies enormously by race, sex, and class. To a lesser degree, this can be said of children as well. The likelihood of growing up in poverty, for example, is many times greater for an African American child in the United States than for a white child. The best predictor of poverty in old age is poverty throughout life. The study of aging from a life course perspective underscores the fact that economic resources and assets in old age result directly from continuous progressive employment throughout adulthood that has been the predominant traditional life pattern in U.S. society only for white males.[40]

PROVIDING FOR OLDER ADULTS

An analysis of the future of an aging society results in the recognition that the older population is growing at a rapid rate, and the segment of that population that is most frail and in need of greatest support (i.e., those 85 and older) is growing at an even faster rate than the rest. In response to that growing need, we can look to essentially three sources of resources and support—the family, the public government sector, and the private business sector. A brief review of the current system of resource provision and support in the United States follows. The U.S. system is then contrasted with the systems currently in place in Sweden and Japan.

Sweden is selected for two reasons. It has one of the oldest populations in the world and, in that sense, offers a glimpse of the future. It also has among the most elaborate public sector support systems for older adults in place anywhere. For that reason, it does not offer a probable glimpse of the future in the United States, inasmuch as few would suggest that the United States would or should adopt so extensive a social welfare arrangement.

Japan offers a startling demographic contrast to the United States. Compared to the over-65 cohort making up 13% of the U.S. population, Japan today has an older population that accounts for more than 20% of its citizens. Other contrasts exist in older labor force participation, cost and availability of health care, healthcare service utilization patterns, and societal attitudes toward older adults. Japan, because of the accelerated rate at which it achieved an older age structure, has had to consider and adopt many economic and health-care policies the United States and other developed countries are just now considering.

Finally, general conditions in the developing world are described. These conditions differ enormously from those in the developed countries of western Europe and North America. Like Japan, though for very different reasons, these countries will experience a period of explosive old-age population growth in a relatively brief time.

Based on these sketches, we see several different scenarios for the future of the older population. The United States is in a state of flux right now, and the aging of its population is a political football. It is unlikely that younger generations can sustain substantially more of the burden of care for its elders both in terms of familial care and through tax support. Growth in the **private sector** is probable, but there is reason to be skeptical of the quality and sustainability of private sector options for the general older population. **Public sector** support involves a long-standing social contract that minimally must be sustained at near current levels and, some would argue, should be strengthened in certain areas.

In contrast, Sweden's system is impressive, but at a cost that would not be palatable to most Americans. In the future, the need will continue to expand in Sweden, although at a slower rate than in recent decades. As the need expands, it is unlikely that the Swedish public sector will expand any further. The difference is more likely to be made up by families and growth in the private sector.

Japan's greatest challenge is in the continued growth in its oldest population. The oldest-old is the fastest growing age group in the society. With increased disability and ambivalence about family care in younger age groups, providing high-quality care for this cohort will be challenging.

The developing world, by far, faces the greatest challenges. Most countries are ill equipped to cope with the growth in the older population. Governments in developing nations assume, out of necessity, that the traditional family structures will absorb the care of their older family members. Traditional family structures in the developing world, however, are undergoing significant changes as a result of urbanization and shifting labor markets, leaving families unable to provide the kind of support they might have in stable social systems or on the scale anticipated. In some countries the public sector recognizes this and is responding accordingly with the initiation of a variety of public economic programs. A more detailed picture is sketched later.

Some of the care for the very old involves what is described as long-term care. This is a level of care usually needed for chronic and ongoing conditions that are more prevalent in the oldest-old. These chronic and ongoing conditions often limit mobility, functioning, and self-care. In many respects it is medically low-technology care, including social care and supervision. As disease conditions progress, the level of care intensifies, and some may require around-the-clock care and supervision as well as more intensive medical care. Long-term care may be provided in homes or in institutions, primarily nursing homes.

THE UNITED STATES

In the United States, funding for older Americans' health care comes from a combination of individual resources (or out-of-pocket payment), public health insurance, and a welfare approach. All Social Security recipients are eligible for basic Medicare coverage. Medicare is a public health insurance program for older adults and covers about half of the total healthcare costs for older Americans. Medicare beneficiaries have some allowances for long-term care but only on a short-term basis.

The major source of coverage for long-term care (LTC), including home-based care, nursing homes, and community-based care, is Medicaid, which in 2008 covered 38.7% of total costs. Medicare covered 25.8% of LTC costs in 2008. Private insurance covered approximately 11% of costs, and recipients paid 21.4% of costs out-of-pocket.[41] Medicaid eligibility is income-based and provides payment for health care for those eligible, regardless of age, who do not have the private resources to pay for medical care. Medicaid was never intended to be the primary source of funding for long-term care for older adults, yet nearly half of nursing home revenues come from public funds, most of this from Medicaid.[2,5] Established in 1966 along with Medicare, Medicaid is jointly funded through state and federal funds, and by the 1980s it had become the biggest item in many state budgets, precipitating more stringent cost-containment measures.[42]

Because 61% of the nursing homes in the United States are proprietary and operated on a for-profit basis, the United States has the circumstance of having private sector nursing homes heavily subsidized with public funds.[43] Critics have argued that this has created a two-tiered class system of care.[42] Because government funding sources are income-based and favor institutional care, institutions end up providing for an inordinate number of poor or impoverished older adults. Many of these individuals require more social than medical care, but have neither the family nor other social support or financial resources to elect any option other than nursing home care.

Noninstitutional alternatives to nursing home care, which have increased in use in recent years, fall into either formal or informal service categories. *Informal care* refers to that which is provided by immediate family members or other relatives. According to the Family Caregiver Alliance, 43.5 million family caregivers in the United States currently provide care for someone over age 50.[44] Among these care providers, about half provided care for 8 hours or less per week, while 17% provided 40 or more hours of care per week. Women make up 61% of care providers of people over age 50, are somewhat less likely than male providers to work full time, and report more often that they had no choice in providing care. The combination of absence of choice and level of burden is the strongest predictor of physical and emotional strain and of experiencing financial burden. The average age of recipients of care is 75 years. Caregivers are most often taking care of a parent (44%) or a grandmother (11%). One-quarter of caregivers are assisting individuals with Alzheimer's disease, dementia, or other forms of mental confusion. Unpaid caregiving is estimated to provide services valued at about $257 billion per year.[45]

Formal support services pick up where family care leaves off or is unavailable. The availability and array of noninstitutional services vary considerably by community, but may include in-home assistance with meals, homemaker services, home health aides, transportation, telephone monitoring, respite for family members, daycare, and legal services. These services have been designed largely to complement or aid family caregivers and less to replace them or sustain completely independent living conditions for older adults. Older people may first recognize the need for some form of long-term care during or after a hospitalization. Older people require hospitalization at about four times the rate of younger people. Approximately 20% of all older people use inpatient facilities in a given year.[5] What distinguishes the institutionalized from the noninstitutionalized older adults is often the availability of family help. Where family help is limited or unavailable, formal in-home and community services are intended to fill the gap and forestall institutional placement. Restricted availability, lack of awareness of and use of community services, fragmentation, and cost-containment measures, however, may all reduce the effectiveness of institutional alternatives. Findings from studies of demonstration projects comparing the costs of community care and institutional care have been mixed. They have not provided clear evidence that home-based care is more cost effective. There is considerable consensus, however, that it is preferred, more humane, and less dehumanizing.[46-49]

A longstanding criticism of formal in-home and community services has been the fragmented nature of the service delivery system. This fragmentation is largely a function of the financing mechanisms in place. Eligibility is usually income based, with the major funding sources being Medicare, Medicaid, Social Services (Title XX of the Social Security Act), Supplemental Security Income (Title XVI of the Social Security Act), Administration on Aging, Veterans Administration, and Housing and Urban Development.[5] In addition to low-income requirements, many of the services are limited in volume per year or over the lifetime of the client. Other criticisms include limited access to services and a workforce providing care that is unskilled, untrained, underpaid, and overworked.[50]

In her review of care provision in the United States, Olson argues that the public sector falls short in providing for the eldest and neediest members of society.[43] Access to in-home and community-based services is limited and fragmented. With its emphasis on individualism and self-reliance, the United States places the primary financial obligation for care squarely on older adults themselves. When care providers are needed, family members take on the large majority of the responsibility. The public sector takes over when there are no resources or no family.

Since 1985 there has been a steady decrease in nursing home residence rates. The age-adjusted rate in 1985 was 54 people per 1,000 over the age of 65. This rate declined to 35 per 1,000 by 2004.[2] The sharpest declines were among the over-85 age groups. The decrease in rate of nursing home use is being replaced commensurately with more in-home alternatives and other forms of residential care and assisted living arrangements. Healthcare costs among residents of long-term care facilities averaged $52,958 annually in 2004, compared to $10,448 among community residents.[2] Even though there has been a decline in rate of use, the absolute number of occupied nursing home beds has increased as a result of the expansive growth of the older population.

The highest expenditures, naturally, occur among the oldest-old. Additional variability in health and healthcare costs, however, can be seen in demographic breakdowns of the population beyond age. For example, African Americans have higher costs than either whites or Hispanics. Low-income individuals and those with chronic conditions incur higher healthcare costs.[2]

The rising costs of prescription drugs have contributed significantly to the healthcare costs of older Americans. In 1992, prescription drugs constituted 8% of total healthcare costs for the older population. By 2004, they had reached 15%.[2] During this same period there were declines in both hospital stays and nursing home use that were offset by increases in outpatient hospital services and physician visits.[2]

In the aggregate, 53% of all healthcare services for older adults were covered by Medicare in 2004. Older Americans paid 19% of costs out of pocket, and another 19% was covered by other payers. Medicaid covered 9% of costs for all services.[2] The shift in the past decade to more community-based, noninstitutional care and services would seem to be a very positive one that adds to the quality of life for many older Americans. We have seen far less success in containing the costs of services and care, which continue to outpace nearly all other segments of the economy.

The coming decades will no doubt involve more political positioning and renegotiation of the social contract between society, older adults, and family support. Action has already been taken to prolong the work life, and thus reduce the dependency, of the next generations of older adults. Cutbacks in Social Security benefits are being discussed seriously. Shifts in the dependency ratio make it unlikely that any expansion in public sector financing and services will take place. More and more, one hears arguments for increasing family responsibility for care of older family members, but this ignores demographic trends that predict a reduction in the availability of care to the family, to say nothing of the economic, emotional, and psychological costs associated with prolonged caregiving. We are likely to see significant growth in the private sector. How well a free-market approach to elder care would meet the needs of older adults and the medical and human goals of an aging society remains to be seen.

Still early in its implementation, the Affordable Care Act signed into law in March 2010 is not yet well understood. Some of the law's probable benefits to seniors include free preventive health services, prescription drug discounts, and expansion of employer health insurance coverage for early retirees between 55 and 65 years of age. In addition, states may elect to expand Medicaid coverage to low-income individuals and be eligible for matching federal funds, and small businesses may qualify for tax credits.[51]

JAPAN

Japan has the most rapidly aging population in history and consequently faces challenges unlike any other developed country. Japan's older population stood at 12% in 1990, and is approaching 22% today. By 2020, the over-65 population of Japan will constitute about 28% of the population. By contrast, the U.S. over-65 population is projected to reach 19.6% of the total population in 2030.[52] Most of the projected increase in Japan will be among the oldest-old. This growth in the older population will be accompanied by declines in the working-age population as well as the young age groups that would give birth to children. Fertility decline, however, is more linked to forgone and delayed marriage than absolute declines in birth-eligible women. Concomitant changes in attitudes toward child rearing, expectations to rely on one's children in old age, and toward older adults themselves are also evident in this rapidly changing society.[54]

Favorable post–World War II fertility and mortality conditions helped transform Japan into an economic superpower in the course of a few decades. These demographic conditions also contributed to relatively high savings rates. Both government and personal savings are expected to decline in the near term, which will in turn, of course, affect public pensions and healthcare funding.[53]

Population aging also slows labor force growth, a decline that has already begun. Participation in the labor force among older adults in Japan is actually considerably higher than it is in other developed nations; among men more than double that in the United

States, for example. It is unlikely, therefore, that policies directed at lengthening life span workforce participation will yield further gains. Changes in marginal and social security tax rates could increase women's participation, though there is little evidence of movement in that direction.[53]

Japan's higher labor force participation rate merits a closer look to better understand U.S. circumstances. In the United States in 2005, 25.6% of Americans over 60 were in the labor force, compared to 30.1% in Japan. Women in the two populations had approximately equal labor force participation rates at about 21%; however, men in Japan participated at a rate of 40.5% compared to U.S. male counterparts at 30.4%.[54] This difference is attributable to multiple variables including public policy, cultural value differences, and health. In Japan, employers can establish mandatory retirement ages, and most do at age 60. Japan has a dual retirement pension program that combined amount to about 60% of salary replacement. However, workers don't get the full benefit until age 65, resulting in an income gap between the ages of 60 and 65 and in economic need if they wish to maintain the same standard of living. Continued employment is assisted by the government through the passage of the Law Concerning Stabilization of Employment of Older Workers in 1971, and subsequent amendments that provide outreach to older Japanese, subsidy programs for employers, and community-based employment opportunities for older workers. In addition to economic need, Japanese culture places greater value on prolonged productivity versus leisure, as well as an expectation that elderly Japanese will contribute to the economic well-being of children and grandchildren. Finally, studies by the World Health Organization that estimate disability-free life expectancy in industrialized nations rank Japan first, with a healthy life expectancy of 75 years. The United States ranks seventh at 69.3 years.[54]

Japan has a publicly financed social insurance healthcare system. About 80% of health care in Japan is provided in the private sector, with costs heavily controlled by the government. The entire population is served through five main medical plans. Premiums amount to 8% of a worker's earnings, equally divided between employers and employees. Premiums are not sufficient to cover total costs, and the government has subsidized health care since 1972. Costs are paid directly to doctors and hospitals, with patients making copayments of between 10% and 30%. Healthcare costs for older adults rose from 14% of total healthcare costs in 1975 to 31% in 1995 and will reach 50% within the next decade. By international standards Japanese health care is relatively cheap at 7% of gross domestic product (GDP), as compared to 14% in the United States. This is mostly because of cost containment and does not represent full actual costs. Among the disadvantages reported by MacKellar and Horlacher are unavailability of cost-effective treatments such as joint replacements and longer average hospital stays compared to other developed nations.[53]

Reforms in Japanese healthcare provision for older adults date to 1990 with the introduction of the "Golden Plan." This plan was directed toward increasing the number of nursing home beds and providing home-based services, short-term stay facilities, and elder daycare centers. These services are provided at low or no cost to older adults and their families, though there is some evidence that they have been underutilized. One explanation for this low use rate has been provided by Asai and Kameoka, who invoke the cultural concept of *Sekentei*.[55] *Sekentei* translates as "social appearance," and is an important concept that reflects Japanese social values. The ideal of filial piety and care of one's elders commonly invoked in discussion of Asian cultures represents a set of social values that has undergone considerable change over the last several generations. The value of familial piety common to Confucian philosophy is considerably less relevant to younger generations of Japanese. Japanese scholars have challenged the concept for some time, arguing that older adults are no longer inordinately respected by family members or generally in Japanese society.[56,57] The suicide rate among older Japanese is the second highest in the world and is higher among older adults living with children than those living alone.[55] Other studies have found that Americans report higher levels of perceived parental care obligations compared to Japanese.[58,59] The concept of *Sekentei*, as used by Asai and Kameka, also translated as social pressure, results in a conflicted sense of shame in the use of nonfamily support services and thus may result in underutilization.

The Japanese pension system began as a fully funded arrangement but has gradually shifted to a pay-as-you-go system. It is a multitiered system consisting of a national flat beneficiary rate for all residents older than age 60, and a second tier employee pension that covers about 32 million private sector employees. There are also private corporation pension funds covering about 12 million workers. The beneficiary-to-worker ratio (or dependency ratio) within each of these systems is increasing markedly. Everyone between the ages of 20 and 59 contributes to the National Pension System. Pension reforms occurred in 1973, 1986, and 1994 and have variously increased pension levels, increased contribution rates, required mandatory coverage of employees' spouses, and imposed a minimum number of years of contribution for eligibility. Benefit formulas have been revised to discourage early retirement. The 1994 reforms raised the minimum eligibility age for the National Pension System from 60 to 65 to ensure that there would be sufficient reserves at the time of peak population aging.[53]

Additional reforms have been proposed and are under consideration including linking benefits to life expectancy, indexing pensions to real wages, linking the real incomes of beneficiaries to the real income of contributors (similar to Swedish proposals), and further raising eligibility to 67 years of age.

At the present time, pension payments account for about 70% of the income of older households, and about 50% of older Japanese rely exclusively on the public pension system. In the current arrangement, younger Japanese (born after 1950), unlike their parents, will contribute more to the pension system than they will receive in benefits, likely adding pressure to reform efforts.[53]

SWEDEN

In many respects, it is not possible to fairly compare Sweden with the United States. With 8.5 million people and a land mass equivalent to a midsized U.S. state, Sweden offers a very different model of elder care based on very different social and political philosophies. Sweden, therefore, is being offered in contrast to the United States to present an alternative approach. Whether it is one that the United States can or should emulate is a question that goes beyond the purpose of this chapter. The other feature that makes Sweden a fascinating example is that, like Japan, it is ahead of the United States, as well as most of the rest of the world, in the aging of its population. Almost 20% of Sweden's population is older than 65, compared with about 13% in the United States.

Sweden has one of the highest life expectancies in the world, and like other developed countries, its old-old population is the fastest growing segment. Much of Sweden's policy covering older adults is not age specific. In 1982, Sweden passed its Social Services Act, which provided municipal social services to all persons who needed them regardless of age. In the passage of this act, access to social services was established as a right of all Swedish citizens. The explicit goals of the act were to sustain self-determination and normalization by allowing for maximum choice and supporting the individual in remaining in his or her normal environment. The Health and Medical Services Act was passed in 1983 and provides health care and services to all members of society. Like social services, medical care and services are nearly all in the public sector. These publicly supported services available to all are supported through a tax system at the rate of about one-half of a working person's income. Approximately one-third of public expenditures goes to social insurance and social welfare programs. Of this expenditure, approximately 40% is used for various forms of old age support and care, mostly pensions and housing. There is widespread public opinion support for these policies in Sweden.[60]

Despite this generous public sector support directed toward independent living, Sweden does not differ from the United States in the proportion of its older adults who are institutionalized. It stands at about 5–6% of those older than 65 at any given time, with lifelong chances of being institutionalized being about 25–30%. The pattern of institutionalization for older adults, however, does differ somewhat. Generally, the older person is more likely to have a short-term stay in an institution and return home, possibly going back and forth several times. Trends are also for these stays to occur among the very old, near the end of life, and for shorter periods of time. The official policy goal is to keep people in their own homes to as great an extent as possible. The result has been that more are spending their final days in institutions but for a shorter time and at older ages. Also, as in the United States, Swedes' chances of spending time in an old-age home or nursing home are greater if they have no family.[60]

Sweden has one of the highest proportions of older adults who live independently. Estimates are that about 46% of Swedes older than 70 live alone. In Stockholm, 7 of 10 women older than 80 live alone. These rates are among the highest in the world. About 15% of older adults receives regular "home help" services. The trend in recent years has been toward more services being provided to fewer clients among the old-old. These services include cleaning, cooking, washing, and personal hygiene. The client pays a copayment of 5–10%, with the balance publicly subsidized.[60] The services are need-based, and the overall effect has been to reduce differences in use across classes. Studies have demonstrated that when health is controlled for, class differences in use disappear.[60]

Subsidized community-based services not subject to needs assessments include municipal transport services, food services, home-delivered meals, hairdressing, snow cleaning services, and district daycare centers. Most of these services are used by less than 10% of the elderly population.[60]

Studies of the Nordic countries generally find a ratio of formal caregivers to family caregivers of between 1:4 and 1:3. In Sweden, it is estimated that family and friends provide about two-thirds of all care.[60] Sweden's population is continuing to age and need will grow. It is unlikely that the public sector will expand any further. Sundstrom and Thorslund anticipate that the increased need will be met by a combination of increased family support and growth in private sector alternatives that, up until now, have not been common in Sweden.[60]

The Swedish pension system offers an intriguing model for other developed nations to consider. Pension contributions are made by the central government at a rate of 18.5% (in some cases based on pension credits awarded for such things as years spent on child care, national service, or studies), employers at a rate of 10.21%, and employees or the insured at a rate of 7%. Pension contributions are recorded on an ongoing basis in the bank books of the insured, but withdrawals are blocked until the age of retirement at 61. Savings accumulate with interest. Once retired, payment is reversed and disbursed to the insured for the remainder of their lives. Another feature of the system is that payment balances are affected by the survival rates of the cohort. That is, the pension balances of deceased members of the cohort, based on life expectancies, are added to the balances of surviving members of the cohort, increasing payments. Pensions, therefore, are based on pension credits, accumulated interest, and these so-called inheritance gains. Annually, Swedish citizens receive a statement allowing them to track growth year to year.[61]

The Swedish pension system was designed to be self-sustaining and self-correcting. It is influenced directly by employment growth and stock market fluctuations that result in payments into the system. These enter into asset-to-liability ratios that can trigger automatic adjustments to both payroll contributions and benefit levels. Costs and benefits may fluctuate down in response to drops in the employment levels and the stock market, or up (when there are surpluses), but balance out over the long-term. In 2008, the dramatic drops in financial markets tested the system's elasticity. The net effects of the recession and slow job growth would have resulted in a decline in benefits of 4.5% that would have taken effect in January 2010. Projected decreases in job growth in 2010 and 2011 put further stress on the system, which would have further decreased benefits by another 3.5% in 2011. Changes in benefits would not turn positive again until 2012. These circumstances forced a rethinking of the pension system, and policy makers responded by smoothing the impact of these dramatic shifts by using 3-year averages to value the funds. In this way, smaller decreases took effect over a 3-year period rather than all at once. This approach reduces the accuracy of the system's actual financial stability but also reduces hardship on beneficiaries. This represents a more dynamic system than in the United

States, where payroll deductions and benefits are more fixed. The U.S. Social Security program does utilize cost of living adjustments (COLAs), but in ways that affect benefits rather than maintenance of the trust fund.[62]

THE DEVELOPING WORLD

The expansion of the older population is a worldwide phenomenon, and the greatest increases by far will be in the developing world. The challenges this represents to societies in the developing world are compounded by the short time frame in which these changes will take place. For example, Guatemala, Singapore, Mexico, the Philippines, and Indonesia will all experience a tripling in the proportion of their older populations between the years 1985 and 2025. By comparison, growth in the United States in those years is estimated at 105%; in Canada, 135%; and in Sweden, only 21%.[61] In the next century, China will age faster than any other country. Official policy in China has led to sharp reductions in birth rates, which, if continued into the next century, could result in a population that is 40% elderly.[63]

So, although the entire world is experiencing a shift in the **age composition** of its population, this is happening at very uneven rates. Currently, Western Europe and developed countries in other parts of the world are the oldest countries with respect to age composition and will be aging at a relatively slow rate in the years to come. Developing countries are not only aging more rapidly than the developed world but are doing so at a pace the developed countries never experienced. The United States, for example, doubled its over-65 population from 7 to 14% over a period spanning 69 years (from 1944 to 2013). It will take South Korea only 18 years to experience the same proportional doubling (2000 to 2018). The developing world overall is therefore comparatively very young. Sub-Saharan Africa, for example, has one-fifth the proportion of older people today as Western Europe. In addition to the rapid rate of increase, developing countries will face the challenges of aging while still dealing with all of the attendant problems of economic, social, and political development. The rapid aging apparent in these countries is, in fact, a result of past successes in the areas of nutrition, vaccinations, and sanitation.[64] The world population of persons older than 65 increases by 870,000 each month. In 2008 the global population over age 65 was 506 million people. By 2040 it will be 1.3 billion people. Much of this increase will be in the developing world.[64]

It is not clear how the old will be provided for in many countries. Old-age pensions are not common in the developing world. In China, for example, only 10% of the workforce have pensions; in India, only 8%.[64] As economic development accelerates, traditional family patterns of care are likely to be disrupted. With urbanization, younger people move to the cities, often leaving older adults alone in villages and rural areas and without support.

In the developing world, healthcare provisions and expenditures are a fraction of those in the developed countries. According to World Bank figures, the U.S. per capita spending on health in 1990 was $2,763. By comparison, in Latin America, it averaged $105. In the world's poorest countries the average was $16.[64] As the populations of developing countries age, they will experience what demographers have referred to as the "epidemiologic transition" to the kinds of diseases and chronic conditions common to older age groups. This will occur while these countries are still grappling with infectious disease patterns common in younger age groups and developing countries. Hospitals, already available to only a fraction of the populations in these countries, may be overwhelmed with admissions, or demand for admissions, for cancers and cardiopulmonary diseases. Competition for resources could result in sharp class differences and age-based inequities.

Some of the wealthier countries in the developing world are initiating economic programs to reduce some of these problems. Taiwan, for example, has initiated a national health insurance system. Some Asian and Latin American countries have begun to look at mandatory pensions and savings plans.[64] But these sorts of reforms are still the exceptions rather than the rule. The more likely immediate solutions will be family and community based and emphasize low-tech, low-cost efforts to as great an extent as possible.

SUMMARY

Much has been said in this chapter about the way we might find the future as we grow older. Few of these claims are certainties. What is certain is that there will be many more older members of our society in the coming years, and the future cohorts of older adults will differ in significant ways from today's older adults. There are still gains to be made, although slight, in life expectancy, particularly among men. We can expect better overall health and greater independence. In the United States, the older adults of the future will be better educated as a group and, perhaps to an unprecedented extent, actively engaged in ongoing educational pursuits and community activities through both paid and unpaid work for longer periods of time. Despite this generally optimistic portrayal, the United States cannot afford to lose sight of the fact of heterogeneity in old age. This includes both a healthy diversity and a concern that aging is a very different experience for historically marginalized subgroups within the population. The aging population often magnifies the cumulative effects of inequality and inequity that have spanned lifetimes.

The major challenges facing our aging population in the future are the perennial concerns of today: care for those who cannot care for themselves, and the resources necessary for all persons to live their lives with dignity. These concerns will grow commensurate with the growth in the older population. To address these problems effectively, it is essential that they be reframed as shared national concerns, not as the problems of older adults. Younger generations, who must share the burden of growing costs and care, must be convinced that older adults merit their concern and their support and be assured that the same support systems and mechanisms will be there for them when they are old. This attitude toward the older adults of our society and confidence in the future are undermined by the divisive pitting of generations against one another in a falsely constructed zero-sum game. Such constructions must be rejected by an educated voting populace.

In terms of both age composition and ability to address the problems of aging, the United States finds itself on a middle ground relative to other nations of the world. Sweden was discussed as an example of an advanced and comprehensive system of care provision for one of the oldest populations in the world. Sweden's solutions, however, are not necessarily a good fit for the United States. Japan, as a result of the continuing rapid growth among older adults, is on a shorter timeline for solutions than is either Sweden or the United States. Issues of healthcare financing, pension reform, and public policy will continue to be acute in Japan for some time to come. Yet Japan leads the world in health indicators and workforce participation among older adults. In the upcoming years, the United States will be confronted with political and economic challenges in this arena that are unprecedented here. Effective policy formation and decision making will test our economic and political systems in unexpected ways. Solutions will call for creativity and probably the willingness to break with past patterns and expectations. Patterns of work, leisure, caregiving, and collective actions may all take forms not commonly practiced today. The uneven rates of change throughout the world will be one more strand in the complex web that draws us further into a global economy and worldwide network of associations. Just as the United Nations Children's Fund (UNICEF) was a global response to the needs of the world's children, there may also be the need for global responses to the concerns and problems of rapidly aging populations at a high risk for dependency.

Despite the uncertainties, the opportunity to live long, productive, and fully engaged lives in the United States is probably greater now than ever before. As aging becomes a more visible national phenomenon and more central to the national fabric, older adults will more often come to be seen as involved in all important aspects of public and private life. Attitudes among younger generations may well become more age-blind. We may become more adept at determining when and where age itself is or should be the significant criteria for sorting people into categories. What are age-related problems versus simply problems with living? When are age-based solutions called for versus need-based solutions? In what ways are the old and young alike rather than different? What do we share in common? These questions have not been prominent in the discussion thus far. They could mark a productive starting point for confronting some of the challenges that face us.

Review Questions

1. For future older Americans, family caregivers will
   A. Be more available to assist with care than they are today
   B. Be less available than they are today because of decreasing family size
   C. Be less available than they are today because of a declining willingness to help
   D. Be more inclined to provide financial support but not actual care

2. The number one reason older adults give for obtaining additional education is
   A. Boredom
   B. To socialize with younger people
   C. Life transitions
   D. Low cost

3. Older adults are most likely to do volunteer work in order to
   A. Fill time
   B. Avoid loneliness
   C. Prepare for paid employment
   D. Enhance self-esteem

4. Recent trends suggest that older workers and retired persons are
   A. More interested in continued work than in the past
   B. Less interested in continued work than in the past
   C. More likely than younger workers to be absent from work as a result of illness
   D. Less collegial and cooperative than younger workers

5. Childhood poverty in the United States
   A. Was eliminated in the 1990s
   B. Has increased because of the growing older population
   C. Is restricted to rural areas
   D. Is caused primarily by market forces and the problems of young adults

Learning Activities

1. Discuss ways in which corporations could design work schedules to better serve their older employees. Discuss possible contributions older workers can offer their employers.
2. Describe potential models for work-to-retirement transition in the 21st century.
3. Develop a curriculum for an elder college. In addition to possible course offerings and student services, design a physical environment suitable for these older students.
4. Describe challenges faced by developing countries in caring for growing older populations.
5. Discuss ways to achieve intergenerational harmony. What can the young offer the old and vice versa?
6. Interview three middle-aged individuals about what future concerns they have as they become older adults in an ever-aging society.

REFERENCES

1. U.S. Census Bureau. Age and Sex Composition: 2010. Retrieved August 2, 2013, from http://www.census.gov/prod/cen2010/briefs/c2010br-03.pdf
2. Federal Interagency Forum on Aging–Related Statistics. *Older Americans 2008: Key Indicators of Well-Being. Federal Interagency Forum on Aging-Related Statistics.* Washington, DC: U.S. Government Printing Office, March 2008.
3. Perls, TT. The oldest old. *Scientific American,* 1995;10:70.
4. U.S. Census Bureau. Aging Boomers Will Increase Dependency Ratio, Census Bureau Projects. Retrieved July 7, 2013, from http://

www.census.gov/newsroom/releases/archives/aging_population/cb10-72.html

5. Kart, CS. *The Realities of Aging: An Introduction to Gerontology*. 5th ed. Boston: Allyn & Bacon, 1997: 53.

6. Munnell, AH, Muldoon, D, Sass, SA. *Recessions and Older Workers*. Chestnut Hill, MA: Center for Retirement Research at Boston College, January 2009.

7. U.S. Census Bureau. Marital Status: 2010. Retrieved July 8, 2013, from http://www.census.gov/prod/2003pubs/c2kbr-30.pdf

8. Spencer, G. *What Are the Demographic Implications of an Aging US Population from 1990 to 2030?* Washington, DC: American Association of Retired Persons and Resources for the Future, 1993:8.

9. Binstock, RH. Older voters and the 2010 U.S. election: Implications for 2012 and beyond? *Gerontologist*, 2011;52(3):408–417.

10. Rupert, P. Contingent work options: Promise or peril for older workers. In *Resourceful Aging: Today and Tomorrow, Conference Proceedings*, 1991;4:51.

11. Patten, CW. Second careers: New challenges, new opportunities. In *Resourceful Aging: Today and Tomorrow, Conference Proceedings*, 1991;4:47.

12. Gamse, DN. Work and second careers: Executive summary and commentary. In *Resourceful Aging: Today and Tomorrow, Conference Proceedings*, 1991;IV: 9.

13. Munnell, AH, Soto, M, Golub-Sass, A. *Are Older Men Healthy Enough to Work?* Chestnut Hill, MA: Center for Retirement Research at Boston College, October 2008.

14. Munnell, AH. *Policies to Promote Labor Force Participation in Older People*. Chestnut Hill, MA: Center for Retirement Research at Boston University, January 2006.

15. Munnell, AH, Sass, S. *Working Longer: The Solution to the Retirement Income Challenge*. Washington, DC: Brookings Institute Press, 2008.

16. Taylor, P. Older workers and the labor market: Lessons from abroad. *Generations*, 2007; 31(1):96–101.

17. Roper, ASW. *Baby Boomers Envision Retirement II—Key Findings*. Washington, DC: AARP, 2004. Retrieved February 13, 2008, from

http://assets.aarp.org/rgcenter/econ/boomers_envision_1.pdf

18. Munnell, AH, Webb, A, Delorme, L, Golub-Sass, F. *National Retirement Risk Index: How Much Longer Do We Need to Work?* Chestnut Hill, MA: Center for Retirement Research at Boston College, June 2012.

19. Munnell, AH, Webb, A, Golub-Sass, F. *The National Retirement Risk Index: An Update*. Chestnut Hill, MA: Center for Retirement Research at Boston College, October 2012.

20. Metlife Mature Market Institute, Market Survey of Long-term Care Costs: The 2012 Metlife Market Survey of Nursing Home, Assisted Living, Adult Day Services, and Home Care Costs. Retrieved September 16, 2013, from https://www.metlife.com/mmi/research/2012-market-survey-long-term-care-costs.html?WT.ac=PRO_Pro3_PopularContent_5-18491_T4297-MM-mmi&oc_id=PRO_Pro3_PopularContent_5-18491_T4297-MM-mmi#keyfindings

21. U.S. Census Bureau. Older Americans Month: May 2011. Retrieved July 8, 2013, from https://www.census.gov/newsroom/releases/archives/facts_for_features_special_editions/cb11-ff08.html

22. Feldman, NS. Lifelong education: The challenge of change. In *Resourceful Aging; Today and Tomorrow, Conference Proceedings*, 1991;4:17.

23. Aslanian, CB. Adult learning and life transitions. In *Resourceful Aging: Today and Tomorrow, Conference Proceedings*, 1991;5:45.

24. Wilson, J. Volunteering. *Annual Review of Sociology*, 2000;26:215–240.

25. Harootyan, RA. Volunteer activity by older adults. In JE Birren (Ed.), *Encyclopedia of Gerontology: Age, Aging, and the Aged*. Vol. 2. San Diego, CA: Academic Press, 2006: 613–620.

26. Rozario, PA. Volunteering among current cohorts of older adults and baby boomers. *Generations*, 2007;30(4)31–36.

27. Wei, Y, Naveen, D, Bernhardt, KL. Volunteerism of older adults in the United States. *International Review of Public Non-profit Marketing*, 2012;9:1–18.

28. Warburton, J, Terry, D, Rosenman, L, Shapira, M. Difference between older volunteers and

non-volunteers: Attitudinal, normative, and control beliefs. *Research on Aging,* 2001;23: 586–605.

29. Clary, EG, Snyder, M. The motivations to volunteer: Theoretical and practical considerations. *Current Directions in Psychological Science,* 1999;8:156–159.

30. Okun, MA, Schultz, A. Age and motives for volunteering: Testing hypotheses derived from socioemotional selectivity theory. *Psychology and Aging,* 2003;18(2):231–239.

31. Costello, CB. Resourceful aging: Mobilizing older citizens for volunteer service. In *Resourceful Aging: Today and Tomorrow, Conference Proceedings,* 1991;2:15.

32. Thompson, E, Wilson, L. The potential of older volunteers in long-term care. *Generations,* 2001;25(1): 58–63.

33. Cross-Cultural Solutions. Volunteering Abroad Over 50: Retired Volunteer Abroad Programs. Retrieved August 2, 2013, from http://www.crossculturalsolutions.org/retired-volunteer-abroad-programs/?siteID=Google_Grants_retired_volunteers&gclid=CLbbgav-8rUCFe4-MgoduVUAsg

34. Gomperts, JS. Toward a bold new policy agenda: Five ideas to advance civic engagement opportunities for older Americans. *Generations,* 2007;30(4):85–89.

35. Munnell, AH, Wu, A, Hurwitz, J. *Why Did Poverty Drop for the Elderly?* Chestnut Hill, MA: Center for Retirement Research at Boston College, September 2010.

36. Minkler, M. Generational equity and the public policy debate: Quagmire or opportunity? In P Homer, M Holstein (Eds.), *A Good Old Age.* New York: Simon and Schuster, 1990: 222.

37. Blackburn, R. *Age shock: How finance is failing us.* Brooklyn, NY: Verso, 2006: 236–242.

38. Anrig, G. *The Conservatives Have No Clothes: Why Right-Wing Ideas Keep Failing.* New York: John Wiley and Sons, 2007: 206–229.

39. Munnell, A. *Social Security's Financial Outlook: The 2012 Update in Perspective.* Chestnut Hill, MA: Center for Retirement Research at Boston College, April 2012.

40. Stoller, EP, Gibson, RC. Advantages of using the life course perspective. In EP Stoller, RC Gibson (Eds.), *Worlds of Difference: Inequality in the Aging Experience.* Thousand Oaks, CA: Forge Press, 1994: 3.

41. *2009 Annual Reports of the Boards of Trustees of the Federal Hospital Insurance and Federal Supplementary Medical Trust Funds.* Washington, DC: U.S. Department of Health and Human Services. Retrieved September 16, 2013, from http://www.cms.gov/Research-Statistics-Data-and-Systems/Statistics-Trends-and-Reports/ReportsTrustFunds/downloads/tr2009.pdf

42. Olson, LK. Public policy and privatization: Long-term care in the United States. In LK Olson (Ed.), *The Graying of the World: Who Will Care for the Frail Elderly?* New York: Haworth Press, 1994: 25.

43. Centers for Disease Control and Prevention, National Center for Health Statistics. Nursing Home Facilities. 2006. Retrieved August 2, 2013, from http://www.cdc.gov/nchs/data/nnhsd/nursinghomefacilities2006.pdf

44. Family Caregiver Alliance. *Fact Sheet: Selected Caregiver Statistics.* 2012. Retrieved August 2, 2013, from http://www.caregiver.org/caregiver/jsp/content_node.jsp?nodeid=439

45. National Alliance for Caregiving and AARP. *Caregiving in the U.S.* New York: MetLife Foundation, April 2004.

46. Caro, FG. Relieving informal caregiver burden through organized services. In KA Pillemer, RS Wolf (Eds.), *Elder Abuse: Conflicts in the Family.* Dover, MA: Auburn House, 1986: 283.

47. Edelman, P, Hughes, S. The impact of community care on homebound elderly persons. *Gerontology,* 1990;2:570.

48. Pepper Commission, U.S. Bipartisan Commission on Comprehensive Health Care. *A Call for Action: Final Report.* Washington, DC: U.S. Government Printing Office, 1990.

49. Stephens, SA, Christian, TB. *Informal Care of the Elderly.* Lexington, MA: Lexington Books, 1986.

50. Cantor, MH. Family and community: Changing roles in an aging society. *Gerontologist,* 1991;31:337.

51. Munnell, AH, Hurwitz, J. *What Is "CLASS" and Will It Work?* Chestnut Hill, MA: Center for Retirement Research at Boston College, February 2011.

52. U.S. Census Bureau. *U.S. Interim Projection by Age, Sex, Race, and Hispanic Origin: 2000–2050.* Washington, DC: Author, 2004.

53. MacKellar, L, Horlacher, D. Population ageing in Japan: A brief survey. *Innovation,* 2000;13(4):413–430.

54. Williamson, JB, Higo, M. *Older Workers: Lessons from Japan.* Chestnut Hill, MA: Center for Retirement Research at Boston College, June 2007.

55. Asai, MO, Kameoka, VA. The influence of *sekentei* on family caregiving and underutilization of social services among Japanese caregivers. *Social Work,* 2005;50(2):111–118.

56. Hirayama, H. Public policies and services for the aged in Japan. In R Dobrof (Ed.), *Ethnicity and Gerontological Social Work.* New York: Haworth Press, 1987: 39–51.

57. Kumagai, F. *Unmasking Japan Today: The Impact of Traditional Values on Modern Japanese Society.* Westport, CT: Praeger, 1996.

58. Maeda, D, Sussman, MB. Young adults' perceptions of the elderly and responsibility of caring for the aged parents. *Shakai Ronen Gaku,* 1980;12:29–40.

59. Hashizume, Y. Salient factors that influence the meaning of family caregiving for frail elderly parents in Japan from a historical perspective. *Scholarly Inquiry for Nursing Practice: An International Journal,* 1995;12:123–134.

60. Sundstrom, G, Thorslund, M. Caring for the frail elderly in Sweden. In JK Olson (Ed.), *The Graying of the World: Who Will Care for the Frail Elderly?* New York: Haworth Press, 1994: 59.

61. Swedish Social Insurance Agency (SSIA). *Orange Report: Annual Report of the Swedish Pension System, 2006.* Stockholm: SSIA, 2006.

62. Sunden, A. *The Swedish Pension System and the Economic Crisis.* Chestnut Hill, MA: Center for Retirement Research at Boston College, December 2009.

63. Cockerham, WC. *This Aging Society.* Englewood Cliffs, NJ: Prentice Hall, 1991: 35.

64. Holden, C. New populations of old add to poor nations' burden. *Science,* 1996;273:46.

PATIENT[1] ADVOCACY FOR OLDER ADULTS

ELLEN MENARD, MBA, BSN, RN, and
REGULA ROBNETT, PhD, OTR/L

Culturally competent care and a high degree of knowledge in aging issues are central to the high performance expectations for today's healthcare professional. Innovations in care can be mind-boggling, especially to your aging patients. They will be counting on you to help them understand and navigate the healthcare maze. They will need you to advocate for them and, if possible, help them to advocate for themselves as they cope with rapid and complex systemic and personal change. As an excellent care provider, you want to rise to this challenge. Most patients and/or their families or caregivers will struggle mightily to navigate today's convoluted healthcare network. It is a space where already highly stressed people, who are often very sick as well, are bombarded with foreign-sounding medical and technological words, sterile equipment, distressing smells, odd sounds and sights, and even scarily masked healthcare professionals. The poking, prodding, and questioning that take place can be intimidating, humiliating, and even dehumanizing. These patients need help. Here are some of the key ingredients for successful patient advocacy.

---

[1] The term *patient* is used here because of its prevalence in the healthcare literature, but those healthcare professionals who work with clients can use the term *client* interchangeably with *patient* throughout.

TEAMWORK

Teamwork is an essential key ingredient to enhance patient advocacy. Complexities in care requirements have increased the need for information sharing and collaboration. It is a given that in order to thrive in today's milieu, patients require a coherent and cohesive care team approach. Interprofessional practice puts the patient's goals at the center of concern, and all work together in partnership to make the healthcare experience the best it can be. We owe it to our patients to be knowledgeable about other care professionals, to confer and join forces with each other, and to refer to one another, as needed. Care team members must be on the "side" of their patients. In practice, they must give their patients a voice, or sometimes be their patients' voices. When they voice the patient's concerns, they will have become their patient's advocate.

An emerging field of professionally trained patient advocates is helping to fill what at times can be a health literacy, communication, and healthcare vacuum. Enlightened hospitals, physician practice groups, insurance companies, and even patients/families themselves may employ these professionals to participate in and guide an individual's care or treatment plan. The role of patient advocate has been listed by *U.S. News and World Report* (Nemco, 2007) as a rewarding and necessary new healthcare career for "persuasive, persistent," and caring individuals. With or without a professional patient advocate on board, however, the entire healthcare team is still "on point" and fully responsible for their patient's care and safety.

PLAIN LANGUAGE

The use of *plain language* and being aware of appropriate health literacy is another key ingredient to ensure patients get the services and information they need. One might think that any health literacy deficits are a thing of the past, but the reverse actually is true. Consider the degree to which information has become available on the Internet and through social media, along with radio, television, libraries, and other nearly instantaneous ways to retrieve data. The amount of information out there is excessive. Envision already stressed patients and their families/caregivers accessing information that is often confusing and perhaps contradictory to other sources, including their own doctors. Information quests often can lead to more questions, uncertainty, anxiety, and frustration.

The Joint Commission estimates that medical miscommunication accounts for approximately 80% of serious medical errors (FierceHealthCare, 2010). Think of how easy it is to miscommunicate or misunderstand. One has only to imagine the children's game of "telephone" to understand the importance of clear and direct written and spoken language. In addition to speaking concisely in lay terms, paying close attention to the patient's responses and noting the nuances of tone and body language are also crucial.

For example, the healthcare professional might say: "Your case is terminal and we need to bring in the hospice people." The patient wonders what terminal means (or where the terminal is) and why hostile people need to be brought in. This may be an extreme example, but we should not assume that patients understand medical jargon and that they are hearing exactly what we are trying to say.

An interesting note is that patients may not even be aware of their lack of comprehension. In a study of emergency room patients and their level of understanding of the care they received and discharge instructions, the majority of patients (78%) demonstrated a deficiency in understanding, especially in the domain of discharge instructions, yet only 20% of the 140 English-speaking patients studied reported being aware of their lack of understanding (Engle et al., 2009). This is just more evidence to support the need for clear communication. We must refrain from assuming that just because patients are told what to do, they actually comprehend the information and can follow through.

LISTENING

Perhaps it is self-evident (although it is not as widespread as we might expect or hope) that another key to effective patient advocacy is *listening*. Too often we listen with biased ears, thus tuning out crucial information that does not fit with our assumptions of what we expect to hear. We cannot be successful as patient advocates unless we open our minds to truly hear what the person has to say. A technique that is helpful for ensuring understanding is to paraphrase what we have just heard and to ask patients if we are on the right track and thus understanding them correctly. Connect with patients, sit down at their level, get to know them, and listen to what they have to say (as well as what they [purposefully] do not say). All of us could listen harder.

Collaborating with and being on the patient's side does not necessarily mean always agreeing with or doing what patients want. Doing so would not serve either the patient or the healthcare team member well. The concept of patient advocacy means that patients (or others who care for and about them) act as their own advocates, and are informed and comfortable enough to have a voice and interact productively with the healthcare team, thereby optimizing patient quality and safety outcomes. When the interprofessional team operates within this contemporary frame of reference, optimal health care with improved patient outcomes occur routinely. Patients have better healthcare experiences. It helps to prevent errors. It saves lives.

Although misunderstandings occur among patients of all ages, older patients with potentially decreased sensory or cognitive functioning have unique care needs and are likely to be the most vulnerable population with whom you will work. You owe it to yourself and your profession to be fluent in the language of health care and to partner and collaborate with your fellow team members and patients—actively, proactively, and constructively.

SUMMARY

Patient advocacy is not about having all the answers. It is about establishing partnerships with colleagues and with care recipients. It is about staying current in your field, asking the right questions, listening, and engaging in clear two-way communications. Moreover, as a team member, an "insider," you will know the right resources to access and make the best referrals for best practice. Your involvement will go a long way to help your patients and families with the "when" and "how" to effectively engage their appropriate care provider, whether that provider is a nurse, surgeon, therapist, or any other healthcare professional.

Any person or organization with a stake in a patient's health and wellness is, by definition, a patient advocate. Innovations and advances in healthcare delivery will add to the intricate nature of the healthcare system. Not only will the layers of complexity continue to increase, but also medical specialization will likely be the norm, and care delivery may become more complicated and less seamless before the situation begins to turn around. Despite the best of intentions, training, and preparation, opportunities for mistakes, errors, or accidents will happen. In fact, in a study of premier hospitals in the United States, after a 10-year period, adverse events had increased and occurred in approximately one-third of all hospital admissions (Classen et al., 2011). These adverse medical events have contributed to as many as 180,000 deaths per year (*Lancet*, 2011). As a professional care provider, this should shock and dismay you. Patients and their families or caregivers need your help and constant vigilance. You can do *something*. You can begin by embracing your patient advocacy role in collaborating with the healthcare team to help your patients stay far away from the precipice—the danger zone—where they are most vulnerable. Quality and safety must be daily mantras. Being a dedicated and competent patient advocate is a laudable and necessary goal.

REFERENCES

Classen, DC, et al. "Global trigger tool" shows that adverse events in hospitals may be ten times greater than previously measured. *Health Affairs,* 2011; 30(4):581–589.

Engle, KG, Heisler, M, Smith, DM, Robinson, DH, Forman, SH, Ubel, PA. Patient comprehension of emergency department care and instructions: Are patients aware of when they do not understand? *Annals of Emergency Medicine,* 2009;53(4): 454–461.

FierceHealthcare. Joint Commission Center for Transforming Healthcare Tackles Miscommunication Among Caregivers. Oct. 21, 2010. Retrieved May 2, 2013, from http://www.fiercehealthcare.com /press-releases/joint-commission-center-transforming-healthcare-tackles-miscommunication-among-caregi#ixzz2SHiKnYPv

Lancet. Medical errors in the USA: Human or systemic? [Editorial] 2011;377(9774):1289.

Nemco, M. Patient advocate: Ahead of the curve. *US News and World Report.* Dec. 17, 2007. Retrieved May 2, 2013, from http://money.usnews.com /money/careers/articles/2007/12/19/ahead-of-the-curve-careers

AN OLDER PATIENT'S TRUE STORY

Paulette, a single, trim 79-year-old with thick eyeglasses and hearing aids is alone and sitting at the edge of her hospital bed, with a look on her very pale face like a restrained animal. She came into the hospital for simple colitis surgery 12 days ago and wound up with a serious and debilitating upper respiratory infection (URI). A deep rattling cough is evident but, at her insistence, the doctor has just signed the discharge order for her to go home, where she lives alone with her 60-pound dog. Even though she wore her doctor down and got her way about leaving, she appears to be in a foul mood. A beautiful suit, upscale shoes, and a handbag are on a nearby chair. She wants out! You walk into her room and assess your about-to-be-discharged patient.

Whatever role you play as part of the healthcare team, there are certain patient advocacy actions that should jump out at you as you contemplate the needs of this older woman. In collaboration with your patient and fellow team members, some questions must be asked and resolved *before* she leaves, or she will present a high risk for readmission. What are the clues or cues? What questions need to be raised?

CLUES AND CUES

Elderly
Lives alone
Mood and affect
Pale
Trim with nice clothing
Upper respiratory infection/productive cough
Discharge instructions

QUESTIONS TO ASK:

1. Are any family/support persons expected? When?
2. Will she have someone stay at her house, or will she be alone? Will home care be required?
3. Does she need a referral for rehabilitation? What rehab services might she need?
4. Will her eyesight require an enlarged font on the discharge instructions? (How will her eyesight impact her ability to live at home?)
5. Is she safe ambulating without assistance? Does she need a device? How are her transfers to sitting, standing, getting into and out of the shower, and so on?
6. Considering her visual and hearing impairments and distracted by her own mood, would she comprehend discharge instructions?
7. What is going on with her mood? Is this a change? If so, what is at the bottom of it?
8. Is she in pain or discomfort? Is she fearful? (of what?) Is she too proud (or private) a person to offer up this information?

9. What is her medical status due to her upper respiratory infection? Her surgery? Her cough?
10. What about her dog? Will she be able to handle the 60-pound dog and walk it daily?
11. What about her psychosocial needs? Loneliness?
12. If her affect today is not the norm for her, what is going on here? Is she depressed?
13. Has her care been compromised during this hospitalization? Has anyone explored and communicated the positives and negatives of her patient experience directly with her? Would she recommend this hospital to others? Why or why not? How does she feel about her doctor? The care team?

Considering the patient's entire story, including medical indications, is Paulette ready to be discharged, or is she at a safety risk and vulnerable to readmission? What do you think? If you think she's not ready, yet she's already been discharged by her doctor, what can you do about it now?

Create your own best-case-scenario solution for "Paulette."

CASE ANALYSIS

Unfortunately, this case presents an all-too-common situation, fraught with peril for the patient. Ideally, these typically busy care team members would have been consulted before the patient was discharged. In this case, the team conferred and ultimately decided Paulette was not ready to go home. They based their determination on the following evidence: The patient was demonstrating a completely different affect than in previous days. Because she had become very ill with her URI in the past week, Paulette had likely become dehydrated and was confused. The look on the patient's face expressed fear and confusion. The patient finally admitted she did not feel well enough to go home. Her independent streak was a deeply embedded personal trait. She was terribly worried about her dog. When priorities, including getting patients home into their own familiar environments or decreasing hospital days and costs appear to compete, staying on the side of the patient will always serve. For example, readmission of the patient or a preventable fall at home serves neither the patient nor the hospital.

CONCLUSION

The decision the care team (including the patient's doctor) made, in this case without the patient's immediate concurrence, was to seek a skilled nursing facility (SNF) short-term stay for Paulette. There, she would be helped to get back on her feet, follow her special colon diet safely, get rehabilitation services, and rehydrate. In short, she would be cared for, especially because she was still very ill from her URI and was still so early in recovering from her colon surgery. Taken all together, as a full picture, the patient presented ongoing care needs. Still protesting until she was settled into a local SNF, she did very well and was transferred home within 10 days.

CASE SUMMARY

As this case illustrates, the care team's good work serves not just the patient, but ultimately also the hospital. But, think of how proactive collaboration may have reduced the stress of this patient, or saved work that had already been started. What if everyone on the team was just too "busy," as is the norm? How would that have served the patient? What if she suffered a fall at home, breaking a hip or worse? Patient safety practices mandate vigilance. Besides, being on the same side as the patient saves the organization money, upholds its reputation, and decreases the risks of malpractice, readmission, and excess care charges. What if the team had not revisited the discharge order with Paulette's doctor? "What?," you say, "challenge a doctor's order?" Wrong frame, entirely. The correct frame is: We are *all* on the same side—the patient's side.

If you were not the patient's nurse in this story, you would have taken the team's concerns to the patient's primary nurse. Any concerns from your own health sciences vector, supported by the context supplied by the answers to the questions, would be fodder for the team's discussion. The patient's nurse would confer with the hospital's discharge coordinator or social worker, or go directly to the attending physician. Were you the patient's respiratory therapist? You would likely have had an excellent grasp of the patient's progress throughout her stay, her developing infection, and current cough. Were you another team member? How would your professional role fit into this scenario? Think of this situation as neither challenging the patient's wishes nor the doctor's discharge order. Many a patient, patient's family, doctor, and healthcare organization have ultimately been grateful for the collaborative work of the care team and their astute patient advocacy roles.

About the Contributing Author   Ellen Menard, MBA, BSN, RN, is a nationally recognized patient advocacy expert, speaker, and the author of *The Not So Patient Advocate: How to Get the Care You Want Without Fear or Frustration*. Her *New York Times*–recommended and multi-award-winning book is now in its fourth year of publication, continuing its wide reach to both healthcare practitioners and lay audiences. Besides serving in clinical and managerial roles in hospitals, Menard has gained 20 years of hospital administrator and corporate senior healthcare executive experience, and most recently was Senior Vice President, Organizational Effectiveness for Inova Health System.

ANSWERS TO REVIEW QUESTIONS

Chapter 1
1. B
2. E
3. B
4. B
5. D

Chapter 2
1. C
2. A
3. A
4. B
5. C

Chapter 3
1. C
2. B, A, D, C, E
3. A
4. C
5. D

Chapter 4
1. A
2. C
3. B
4. B
5. D

Chapter 5
1. B
2. D
3. C
4. A
5. C

Chapter 6
1. A
2. D
3. C
4. C
5. B

Chapter 7
1. A
2. D
3. A
4. A
5. C

Chapter 8
1. D
2. B
3. A
4. C
5. D

Chapter 9
1. D
2. B
3. A
4. C
5. A

Chapter 10
1. C
2. A
3. A
4. D
5. B

Chapter 11
1. 1. B; 2. F; 3. D; 4. E; 5. C; 6. A
2. A
3. A
4. D
5. A

Chapter 12
1. D
2. C
3. C
4. B
5. D

Chapter 13
1. B
2. C
3. D
4. A
5. D

GLOSSARY

A

AARP: An advocacy group for older adults, formerly known as the American Association of Retired Persons.

Activities of daily living (ADLs): Normal everyday activities such as eating, sleeping, bathing, and toileting.

Adaptation: Making accommodations to adjust to one's environment.

Adherence: A therapeutic alliance or agreement between the patient and prescriber; currently preferred over the now outdated term *compliance,* which suggests the passive following of the prescriber's orders.

Adult day services: Community-based group programs with specialized plans of care designed to meet the daytime needs of individuals with functional and/or cognitive impairments.

Advance directives: In *advance* of something happening to the individual, he or she signs a written *directive* stating who should make decisions for him or her in the event of incapacity.

Adverse drug reaction: An undesirable response associated with use of a drug that either compromises therapeutic efficacy, enhances toxicity, or both.

Age composition: Refers to the percentage of different age groups (e.g., younger or older) in a given population.

Age-associated memory impairment (AAMI): The most common age-related cognitive decline that is associated with mild forgetfulness.

Age cohort: A group or generation of elderly persons.

Ageism: Based on stereotypes, myths about aging, and language that conjures up negative images of older adults.

Agency on Aging: A community resource to help older adults connect with various services.

Aging in place: The ability to continue to live in one's home safely, as independently as possible, and comfortably, regardless of age, income, or ability level. It means living in a familiar environment and being able to participate in family and other community activities.

Aging network: The name of the collaboration of the Administration on Aging, state units on aging, area agencies on aging, tribal and native organizations, service providers, and volunteers.

Agnosia: A decrease in perceptual skills, such as not understanding what common objects are used for.

Alveoli: Thin-walled air sacs covered by capillaries that are the major site of gas exchange between air and the bloodstream.

Alzheimer's disease (AD): A degenerative brain disease that is the most common form of dementia.

Americans with Disabilities Act: An important policy for all individuals with disabilities, including older people. The main aim of the ADA is to integrate individuals with disabilities into all aspects of living in the United States.

Anemia: A decrease in hemoglobin level, causing a lower than normal oxygen-carrying capacity of the blood.

Aneurysm: Destruction of the inner layers of an artery's wall that can cause a saclike enlargement that can weaken the arterial wall.

Anhedonia: Difficulty experiencing pleasure doing formerly enjoyable activities.

Anorexia: A physiological change, often associated with aging, that can result in decreased appetite.

Anosmia: A complete loss of smell.

Apraxia: The inability to perform coordinated movements without muscular or sensory impairment.

Area agencies on aging: The primary access point for the Aging Network.

Assisted living facility: Long-term residence option that provides resident-centered care in a residential setting. It is designed for those who need extra help in their day-to-day lives but who do not require 24-hour skilled nursing care.

Atherosclerosis: The development of fatty plaques and the proliferation of connective tissue in the walls of arteries.

Attention: Being able to focus or concentrate.

Attrition: The wearing away of the tooth surface.

Autoimmune diseases: Marked by the mistaken immunological destruction of the body's own cells. In such diseases, the body loses the ability to distinguish "self" from "non-self."

Average life expectancy: Mean length of life, usually differentiated by country.

B

Baby boom generation: Those Americans born between 1946 and 1964.

Beers criteria: Criteria that look for potentially inappropriate medication (PIM) use in older adults.

Benign prostatic hypertrophy (BPH): A benign enlargement of the prostate.

Bereavement: A feeling of anguish at the death of a loved one.

Biopsychosocial: Biological, psychological, and sociological factors associated with old age and aging.

C

Cachexia: A wasting syndrome involving loss of weight, muscle atrophy, fatigue, weakness, and significant loss of appetite.

Calcium: A major mineral in the human body, needed for movement and to maintain strong bones. Derived from many foods such as dairy products.

Carbohydrates: Made up of one or more sugar molecules. They include bread, rice, grains, potatoes, sugar, and other like substances. Carbohydrates are classified as simple carbohydrates, which are made of fewer than three sugar molecules, and complex carbohydrates, which are made up of three or more sugar molecules.

Cardiovascular disease: Disease affecting the heart or blood vessels. It can include arteriosclerosis, coronary artery disease, heart failure, hypertension, and various other cardiovascular disorders.

Caregiver: One who provides care for another. This usually involves caring for a family member.

Cataract: An occurrence in which the eye becomes more opaque as its proteins become increasingly oxidized, glycosylated, and cross-linked.

Celiac disease: A digestive and autoimmune disorder that can damage the lining of the small intestine.

Cerebrovascular accident (CVA, or stroke): Infarction in the brain as a result of stenosis or occlusion of a blood vessel.

Cholesterol: A waxy substance found in animal products but not plant products. It is made by the human body and is necessary in making cell membranes, is a building block of some hormones, and is involved in the digestion of fats via bile.

Chronic bronchitis: Common in older adults, especially in those with a long history of cigarette smoking. It is clinically defined as a chronic cough ("smoker's cough") productive of sputum, occurring on most days for at least 3 months' duration over at least 2 consecutive years.

Chronic condition: A condition of long duration showing little or no improvement.

Chronic obstructive pulmonary disease (COPD): Emphysema and/or chronic bronchitis.

Cognition: Involves thinking, learning, and memory.

Cognitive behavior therapy (CBT): A behavioral psychotherapy that emphasizes the importance of thinking about what we do and how we perceive ourselves.

Cohousing: A type of collaborative housing in which residents actively participate in the design and operation of their own neighborhoods.

Competency: A measure of an individual's mental processes.

Congregate housing: Encompasses a multitude of different options, including independent living units, adult congregate living facilities, rental retirement housing, and senior retirement centers.

Conservatorship: When a person is appointed to make financial, investment, and property decisions for another.

Continuing care retirement community (CCRC): An established community that facilitates aging in place by meeting each resident's unique healthcare needs.

Contracture: A condition generally caused by joint immobilization that results in decreased range of motion, stiffening and subsequent structural changes, and pain on movement at one or more joints.

Convoy of support: A personal social network moving with the individual through life challenges and transitions.

Crystallized intelligence: Intelligence that tends to remain strong in those who are aging typically; it includes skills such as language comprehension, educational qualifications, and life and occupational skills.

D

DASH diet: Dietary Approach to Stop Hypertension diet. See *Mediterranean diet*.

Dehydration: The loss of water and salts essential for normal body function.

Delirium: A serious, rapidly developing state of confusion often associated with surgery or hospitalization. The risk for developing delirium is higher for older adults.

Dementia: Progressive cognitive impairment that eventually interferes with daily functioning. The prevalence of dementia among 60-year-olds is only 1–2%, but it becomes increasingly more common with advancing age.

Demographics of aging: Study of vital statistics of the aging population including size, growth, density, and distribution.

Dental caries: Also known as cavities or tooth decay; a bacterial infection attributed to *Streptococcus mutans.*

Dental plaque (biofilm): A biofilm, usually yellow, that develops on teeth due to bacterial colonization.

Depression: A mood disorder characterized by loss of interest in living. Symptoms that accompany depression can include sadness, hopelessness, loss of energy, tearfulness, loss of appetite, insomnia, and/or excessive sleep.

Diabetes: Any disorder characterized by excessive urine excretion. There are a number of different types of diabetes.

Diabetes mellitus: A condition in which there is insufficient insulin. This can lead to elevated blood glucose levels.

Diaphragm: The dome-shaped skeletal muscle located beneath the lungs. It is the major muscle of ventilation.

Dietary fiber: Non-nutrients that are considered important as a part of a healthy balanced diet because of their crucial role in health maintenance, disease management, and as a component of medical nutrition therapy.

Dietary Guidelines: A federal nutrition policy issued and updated every 5 years by the U.S. government that provides guidelines or qualitative statements for making food choices that will help a person or a population lead a healthy life.

Discrimination: The act of exhibiting prejudicial behavior.

Diverticulosis: The development of small sacs where the large intestinal lining has herniated through the intestinal muscular wall.

Durable power of attorney for health care: Allows an individual to choose a person (agent) to represent that individual and make healthcare decisions on his or her behalf should the individual not be able to.

Dysphagia: Difficulty swallowing.

Dyspraxia: A decreased ability to plan and/or execute purposeful movements.

E

Eden Alternative: A living situation in which the residents have private rooms and are free to do what they like.

Edentulism: The condition of being toothless to at least some degree; it is the result of tooth loss. Loss of some teeth results in partial edentulism, whereas loss of all teeth is complete edentulism.

Elder abuse: Any knowing, intended, or careless act that causes harm or serious risk of harm to an older person—physically, mentally, emotionally, or financially.

Elderly, elders: Older persons.

Embolism: The blockage of an artery by a blood clot or other foreign material such as air or fat.

Emphysema: A loss of functional elastic tissue in the lungs, resulting in the loss of alveolar wall surface area and the premature collapsing of small bronchioles during exhalation.

Empowerment: Related to independence, or perhaps more aptly stated, freedom. It relates not only to people's ability, but also their right to make choices affecting their own lives.

Endurance: The ability to sustain involvement in a physical activity.

Episodic memory: Memory oriented toward the past. This is what most people think of when they think of the global term *memory*. This type of declarative or conscious memory particularly involves remembering episodes or experiences in our lives (e.g., what we ate for lunch, our last birthday party).

Estrogen replacement therapy: Medications including female hormones to increase estrogen in the body, usually prescribed to manage the discomfort associated with menopause.

F

Failure to thrive: A condition in which a person fails to gain weight or in which the person loses weight.

Family caregiver: Unpaid helpers who provide daily care for their family members. Most caregivers in the United States are family members.

Fecal incontinence: The inability to voluntarily control defecation, largely because of the weakening of the external anal sphincter muscle.

Fictive kin: When a niece or a nephew takes on the social role of a child, or a sibling takes on some of the traditional roles of a spouse.

Fluid intelligence: Intelligence that involves the speed and accuracy of information processing, such as discrimination, comparison, and categorization. It has been deemed to be largely evolutionarily and genetically based.

Fluoride gel: Acidic, highly concentrated flouride product that dentists topically apply to a patient's teeth about twice a year. It can help reduce tooth sensitivity, fight cavities, and strengthen tooth enamel.

Fluoride varnish: A highly concentrated form of fluoride that is applied to the tooth's surface by a dentist, dental hygienist, or other healthcare professional.

Free radicals: Molecules that contain at least one unpaired electron in their outer valence shells. Free radicals most notably form in the mitochondria of cells, the site of aerobic respiration.

G

Gastritis: Inflammation of the stomach lining.

Gay: Attracted to others of one's own sex.

Generational Equity: The concept of fairness, in terms of resources and assets, between different age groups (generations) of people.

Geriatrics: A medical term for the study, diagnosis, and treatment of diseases and health problems specific to older adults.

Gerontechnology: An interdisciplinary field that links existing and developing technologies to the aspirations and needs of aging and aged adults.

Gerontology: The scientific study of aging that examines the biological, psychological, and sociological (biopsychosocial) factors associated with old age and aging.

Gerotranscendence: Associated with wisdom and a moving away from early and midlife materialism.

Gluten: A component found in wheat and some other grains.

Gray Panthers: An intergenerational education and advocacy group working on social and economic justice and peace for America.

Guardianship: When a person (usually a family member) is designated to make personal decisions for an incapacitated person, usually in the realm of medical, care, and residential issues.

H

Health literacy: The degree to which a person has the capacity to obtain, process, and understand basic health information and services needed to make appropriate health decisions.

Health Resources and Services Administration: A governmental organization that offers freely accessible online training in multiple areas, including healthcare literacy.

Healthy People 2020: A strategic plan set forth by the U.S. Department of Health and Human Services, the Healthy People Consortium, and other federal agencies to focus on preventable health threats (including disability and death) that affect citizens of all ages.

Heat stroke: A condition caused by excessive exposure to heat in which the body temperature becomes dangerously elevated.

Heterogeneous: Mixed, or consisting of dissimilar elements or parts.

Home health care: Skilled health care provided to patients in the home.

Homelessness: Lack of a consistent or permanent living situation, usually associated with abject poverty.

Homeostasis: The state of equilibrium within the body.

Hospice: Supportive comfort care provided to people at the end of life that focuses on pain relief and quality of life, rather than curative treatments.

Hydrophilicity: Having a strong affinity for water molecules.

Hypertension: High blood pressure.

Hyposmia: A decreased or diminished sense of smell.

Hypothalamus: A small but important structure that controls the activity of the pituitary gland by releasing hormones that stimulate or inhibit its hormonal production and release.

I

Infantilizing: Negative portrayal of older adults that encourages dependency because it devalues the individual and does not foster independence; for example, referring to an unfamiliar older patient as "honey" or "dear."

Insomnia: The inability to fall asleep and/or abnormal wakefulness.

Instrumental activities of daily living (IADLs): A series of life functions necessary for maintaining a person's immediate environment (e.g., shopping, cooking, housecleaning, phone use, medication administration etc.).

Intimacy: Personal closeness between two people usually denoting an affectionate and loving relationship between them. Sexual intimacy is only one form of intimacy.

J

Joint Commission: An organization that establishes standards of quality and performance as well as accreditation for healthcare organizations.

L

Lactose intolerance: An inability to break down milk sugar (lactose), the carbohydrate found in many dairy products.

Learned helplessness: A condition that develops when living beings learn that their responses are independent of desired outcomes. Consequently, they learn to not respond to stimulation from their environments. For example, in experiments when dogs learn they cannot control the onset of electric shocks, they eventually give up and become helpless and apathetic.

Lesbian: A woman who is sexually attracted to another woman.

Lifelong education: A commitment to continuing learning throughout one's life via formal or informal means.

Limited literacy skills: A lack of proficiency in reading documents and prose.

Lipofuscin: Fatty pigments found in aging cells.

Lipophilicity: An affinity for fat.

Literacy: The ability to read and write as needed for daily life.

Living will: A legal document outlining one's wishes regarding medical treatments in the event of a debilitating illness.

Long-distance caregiver: A caregiver who does not live in the vicinity of the care recipient, but still provides care. This may involve living 100 miles or more apart.

Long-term care: An array of long-term services and supports used by people who need assistance to function in their daily lives. It can include personal care, rehabilitation, social services, assistive technology, health care, home modifications, care coordination, assisted transportation, and more.

Long-term care insurance (LTCI): Insurance that provides payment, or supplementary payment, for long-term care.

Long-term memory: Permanent or long-term storage, for example, autobiographic information, early life experiences, or repetitive information.

M

Malabsorption: Difficulty digesting or absorbing nutrients from food. Celiac disease is one of the most common causes of malabsorption.

Malnutrition: A condition in which one suffers from a poorly balanced diet or has a deficiency in the digestive system.

Maximum life span potential (MLP): The oldest age reached by an individual in a population.

Medicaid: A program jointly sponsored by the states and the federal government to provide health care for those who cannot finance their own medical expenses.

Medicaid waivers: Money that can pay for services for people with Medicaid.

Medicare: A federal program that provides health care for those age 65 and older and those with long-term disabilities.

Medication-related problems: Events or circumstances involving a patient's drug treatment that actually, or potentially, interfere with the achievement of an optimal outcome.

Medigap: Private health insurance designed to supplement the coverage provided under governmental programs such as Medicare.

Mediterranean diet: A diet rich in fruits, vegetables, and healthy fats such as olive oil. It is thought to help reduce the risks of heart disease.

Menopause: The time in life when menstruation ceases.

Mild cognitive impairment (MCI): Cognitive losses that may portend the diagnosis of Alzheimer's disease (AD); those with amnestic or memory-related MCI are at higher risk of developing AD.

Motor coordination: Fine and gross motor skills such as writing, self-feeding, and walking/running.

Myocardial infarction: Blockage of the coronary arteries that can cause tissue death to part of the heart (a heart attack).

Myths about aging: Myths or stereotypes about aging often involve the erroneous lack of distinction between pathological and typical aging. For example, one myth is that severe mental deterioration is inevitable with age.

N

Naturally occurring retirement community (NORC): A neighborhood or building in which a large segment of the residents are older adults. In general, they are not purpose-built senior housing or retirement communities and were neither designed nor intended to meet the particular health and social services wants and needs of older adults.

Non-insulin-dependent diabetes mellitus (NIDDM): Also called Type 2 diabetes, it is a mild form of diabetes mellitus that develops gradually in adults. It can be precipitated by obesity, severe stress, or menopause. Usually it can be controlled by diet and lifestyle changes without insulin injections.

Numeracy: The ability to understand and apply day-to-day numerical concepts.

Nutritional supplements: These include multivitamins and individual vitamins and minerals; they are the most commonly used over-the-counter medications.

O

Obstructive sleep apnea (OSA): A cessation of breathing that, when the trachea is either totally or partially obstructed, causes the body's oxygen level to drop.

Old-age dependency ratio: The number of people in the population older than 65 years as compared with those between the ages of 18 and 64 years.

Old-old: Those older than age 75 whose activities are often limited by functional disabilities.

Older adult: People age 65 and older; the preferred term when speaking about aged individuals.

Older Americans Act (OAA): Legislation passed in 1965 to specifically address the needs and rights of older adults. The OAA continues to be reauthorized and is expected to be reauthorized indefinitely. It is one piece of legislation that represents the United States' commitment to promoting the rights and welfare of older adults.

Olfaction: Sense of smell.

Oral and pharyngeal cancers: Cancers that form in the tissues of the oropharynx (the part of the throat at the back of the mouth, including the soft palate, the base of the tongue, and the tonsils).

Oral screening: A quick review of the oral structures to determine if dental disease or oral problems are present.

Orientation: Awareness of self, surroundings, and time.

Osteoarthritis: A degenerative joint disease that is the second most common cause of disability in this country, affecting more than 27 million Americans.

Osteoporosis: A disease in which bones become frail, making them more likely to fracture. It is four times more common in women than in men.

Overnutrition: A condition of excess nutrient and energy (caloric) intake over time. It can be considered a form of malnutrition when it leads to morbid obesity.

P

Peptic ulcer: An ulceration of the stomach, esophagus, or duodenum caused by gastric acid.

Perception: The ability to make sense of incoming sensory information.

Periodontal disease: The inflammatory reaction and dissolution of the bony structures that hold the teeth into the jaws.

Personality: Traits, behaviors, and qualities particular to an individual.

Pharmacodynamics: The biological effects resulting from the interaction between a drug and its receptor site; generally describes the relationship between plasma drug concentrations and an observed effect or response.

Pharmacokinetics: The study of how drugs travel through the body over time. It deals with all aspects of drug disposition in the body, including *absorption* from the administration site, *distribution* into various body compartments, and *clearance* from the body.

Physiatrists: Physicians who specialize in rehabilitation.

Pituitary gland: Under control of the hypothalamus, it releases a battery of tropic hormones that have selective stimulating effects on glands such as the thyroid, adrenal gland, and gonads.

Plain language: Everyday or conversational language.

Plain language standards: Standards of simple language for clients published by organizations such as the National Institute for Aging.

PLISSIT model: A four-level model that defines levels of comfort for practitioners in determining interventions for patients' or clients' sexual problems.

Polypharmacy: The use of multiple medications in one individual.

Postural hypotension: A fall in systemic blood pressure upon rising from a supine to a standing position (usually too quickly).

Power of attorney (POA): A legal document setting out the legal authority of the agent to act for the principal.

Power of attorney for health care (POAHC): Same as a power of attorney, but specific to health care.

Praxis: The ability to carry out purposeful motor actions.

Presbycusis: The most common form of sensorineural hearing loss in adults.

Presbyopia: A condition in which molecular changes render the lens of the eye less elastic and more rigid, which significantly impairs accommodation and thus the ability to focus on near objects.

Primary memory: This type of memory has limited capacity and is used for information that is either used or generally forgotten in a matter of seconds.

Private sector: The segment of the economy that is not controlled by the government, but rather run by individuals or groups of individuals on a for-profit basis.

Procedural memory: Memory that is performance based, for example, remembering how to ride a bicycle or the motoric steps to completing a recipe or self-care task. Because these tasks are often overlearned and have become automatic, this type of memory is often maintained into old age.

Program of All-Inclusive Care for the Elderly (PACE): Designed for people 55 or older needing a nursing-home level of care, this program entails comprehensive services including all medical and supportive services (therapies, day services, meals, counseling, respite, and medication management).

Prospective memory: Relates to remembering to do something in the future (e.g., appointments, medications, meetings, chores).

Protein: One of the three nutrients used as energy sources (calories) by the body. Proteins are essential components of the muscle, skin, and bones.

Public sector: The segment of the economy that includes companies and corporations run by the government.

Q

Quality of Life: Contentment or satisfaction with day-to-day life.

R

Range of motion: The ability of a joint to move through its natural pattern of movement.

Reaction time: The time it takes to respond to a stimulus. For example when driving, stepping on the brake when needed.

Reading levels: The reading level of healthcare literature often exceeds the older adults' ability to comprehend. Several different schemes are used to describe different reading levels. One comprehensive chart is found at: http://steckvaughn.hmhco.com/HA/correlations/pdf/l/LevelingChart.pdf.

Rehabilitation: The process of helping someone regain his or her highest possible level of functioning after an injury or illness.

Residential care facilities: Facilities that can have multiple labels, including adult residential facilities, adult group homes, domiciliary homes, personal care homes, family care, adult foster care, rest homes, board and care homes, and assisted living facilities.

Restless leg syndrome (RLS): A neurological disorder including "creepy crawly feelings" or other unpleasant sensations in the legs, usually while the person is in bed.

Retirement: That period of time after one retires from a work-related occupation.

Reverse mortgage: A program that allows borrowers to use their home as collateral, and the bank sets up either an annuity or a line of credit to be used as needed until the home is sold or the loan repaid. This allows those with inadequate monthly income, but substantial home equity, to continue to reside in their own homes.

Root caries: Dental caries involving the tooth root in the cementum or cervical area of the tooth.

S

Sandwich generation: Adults caught between two caregiving roles, that of caring for older parents and caring for their own children.

Sarcopenia: Loss of muscle mass. This is a common occurrence with aging.

Scotoma: An area of decreased vision (blind spots) surrounded by normal vision.

Self-efficacy: The beliefs that each of us holds about the level of control we have over our future. Those who have strong self-efficacy, or internal locus of control, feel empowered to shape the future of their lives.

Semantic memory: Involves a cumulative knowledge base about the world in general (e.g., language, including the meaning of words and the relationship of words; mathematical facts, symbols, and formulas; vocational information learned during one's career; and recall of current events and worldly facts).

Senescence: Deleterious changes that occur as a result of the aging process.

Senior Service America (SSA): A not-for-profit organization that provides training and employment for disadvantaged older adults throughout the United States.

Senior Volunteer Corps: This group provides opportunities for those 55 and over by connecting older adults who want to volunteer with organizations needing volunteer service providers.

Sensory deficits: Common occurrence with aging that involves a diminishment or defect in one or more senses.

Sexuality: A holistic concept involving intimacy with another person in a mutually satisfying manner.

Shame-free environment: Creating an environment that assures safety and encourages questions.

Shared housing: A household model in which a group of people (usually not part of a family) share a home, as well as household goods and responsibilities.

Short-term memory: Involves remembering information for a short duration. An example of normal short-term memory is being able to recall a seven-digit number (for example, a telephone number) for a few minutes.

Single-room occupancy (SRO) unit: Subsidized housing unit for individuals with very low incomes. SRO units are usually found in cities and offer shared bathroom and kitchen facilities.

Skilled nursing facility (SNF): An establishment that houses chronically ill, usually elderly patients, and provides long-term nursing care, rehabilitation, and other services.

Sleep hygiene: Involves those activities and habits that are conducive to sleeping soundly.

Sleep restriction: Restricting one's time in bed.

Social roles: Roles that define an individual's position in the community and dictate basic behaviors within social groups such as families, workplaces, and communities.

Social Security: A major source of income for older adults in the United States. Ninety percent of older adults collected Social Security in 2004. The Social Security Act was signed into law by President Franklin D. Roosevelt in 1935.

State units on aging: Agencies that administer, manage, design, and advocate for benefits, programs, and services for the elderly and their families and, in many states, for adults with physical disabilities.

Stereognosis: The ability to sense objects by the touch of the tongue, allowing one to perceive problems or alterations in the mouth. Can also refer to sensory perception through touch to identify objects.

Stereotypes: A conventional, oversimplified, and often formulaic conception, option, or image, usually of a person or group.

Stimulus control: Refers to the amount of time spent in bed attempting to get to sleep or back to sleep.

STOPP (Screening Tool of Older Persons' Potentially Inappropriate Prescriptions) Criteria: STOPP comprises 65 common potentially inappropriate prescribing practices including drug–drug and drug–disease interactions, drugs that adversely affect older persons at risk for falls, and duplicate drug class prescriptions.

Streptococcus mutans: Anaerobic bacterium in the oral cavity leading to tooth decay.

Stroke: Infarction in the brain that can occur as a result of occlusion or rupture of a cerebral artery.

Suicide: The deliberate taking of one's life.

Supplemental Security Income (SSI): A program providing resources for lower income individuals including older adults and people with disabilities.

T

Teach-back: Having the client state what he or she just heard and what he or she is supposed to do.

Telehealth: The use of electronic information and telecommunications technologies to support long-distance clinical health care of the patient by a professional.

Third-agers: French method of categorizing elderly persons 65 to 85 years of age.

Thrombus: A stationary blood clot.

U

Universal design: The design of products and environments to be usable by all people, to the greatest extent possible, without the need for adaptation or specialized design.

Urinary incontinence: The loss of voluntary control of micturition.

V

Village to Village Network: An organization that promotes aging in place to foster a person's ability to continue to live in his or her home safely, as independently as possible, and comfortably, regardless of age, income, or ability level. It encourages living in a familiar environment and being able to participate in family and other community activities.

Vision: The ability or act of seeing.

Vitamin B$_{12}$: A vitamin important for the normal formation of red blood cells and the health of nerve tissues.

Vitamin D: Any or all of several fat-soluble vitamins chemically related to steroids, essential for normal bone and tooth structure, and found especially in fish-liver oils, egg yolk, milk, or ultraviolet radiation (sunlight).

Volunteerism: Proactive involvement in helping others without seeking payment or other forms of compensation.

W

Work life: The part of life during which a person is employed.

Working memory: Actively using or manipulating information from a short-term storage base. For example, recalling a telephone number and actually dialing the number to make a call (one must retain the number while dialing).

Weight loss: The involuntary loss of more than just a few pounds of body weight can be a sign of compromised nutrition status.

X

Xerostomia: A condition in which dryness of the mouth occurs as a result of salivary gland dysfunction.

Y

Young-age dependency ratio: The ratio of those younger than age 18 to those between the ages of 18 and 64.

Young-old: Denotes relatively healthy and financially independent older adults of any age, although usually referring to those between 55 and 74 years of age.

INDEX

Note: Page numbers followed by *b*, *f*, and *t* indicate material in boxes, figures, and tables respectively.